# The Practical Guide to
# HIPAA
## Privacy and Security
# COMPLIANCE

# OTHER INFORMATION SECURITY BOOKS FROM AUERBACH

## AUERBACH PUBLICATIONS

www.auerbach-publications.com
To Order Call: 1-800-272-7737 • Fax: 1-800-374-3401
E-mail: orders@crcpress.com

# The Practical Guide to
# HIPAA
## Privacy and Security
# COMPLIANCE

## Kevin Beaver and Rebecca Herold

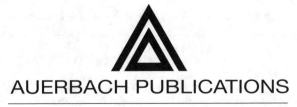

# AUERBACH PUBLICATIONS

A CRC Press Company

Boca Raton   London   New York   Washington, D.C.

## Library of Congress Cataloging-in-Publication Data

Beaver, Kevin.
  The practical guide to HIPAA privacy and security compliance / Kevin
Beaver, Rebecca Herold.
     p. cm.
Includes bibliographical references and index.
  ISBN 0-8493-1953-6 (alk. paper)
  1. Medical records--Law and legislation--United States. 2. Medical
records--United States--Access control. 3. Medical care--Security
measures--United States. 4. Insurance, Health--Continuation
coverage--United States. I. Herold, Rebecca. II. Title.

  KF3827.R4B33 2003
  344.73'041--dc22

2003057900

**Visit the Auerbach Publications Web site at www.auerbach-publications.com**

© 2004 by CRC Press LLC
Auerbach is an imprint of CRC Press LLC

No claim to original U.S. Government works
International Standard Book Number 0-8493-1953-6
Library of Congress Card Number 2003057900
Printed in the United States of America   3 4 5 6 7 8 9 0
Printed on acid-free paper

# Dedication

To my wife Amy

*— Kevin Beaver*

To my two beautiful boys ... Noah Theodore and Heath Xavier.

*— Rebecca Herold*

# Contents

# Limit of Liability and Disclaimer of Warranty

THE AUTHORS HAVE USED THEIR BEST EFFORTS IN THE PREPARATION OF THIS BOOK. THE INFORMATION AND OPINIONS PROVIDED IN THIS BOOK DO NOT CONSTITUTE OR SUBSTITUTE FOR LEGAL OR OTHER PROFESSIONAL ADVICE. THE AUTHORS MAKE NO WARRANTIES OR REPRESENTATIONS REGARDING THE COMPLETENESS OR ACCURACY OF THIS BOOK AND DISCLAIM ANY IMPLIED WARRANTIES OF MERCHANTABILITY OR FITNESS FOR A PARTICULAR PURPOSE. NO WARRANTIES EXIST THAT EXTEND BEYOND THE DESCRIPTIONS IN THIS PARAGRAPH. THE COMPLETENESS AND ACCURACY OF THE INFORMATION AND OPINIONS PROVIDED IN THIS BOOK ARE NOT WARRANTED OR GUARANTEED TO PRODUCE ANY PARTICULAR RESULTS INCLUDING HIPAA COMPLIANCE. READERS SHOULD CONSULT THEIR OWN LEGAL OR OTHER PROFESSIONAL ADVISORS FOR INDIVIDUALIZED GUIDANCE REGARDING THE APPLICATION OF THE HIPAA LAWS TO THEIR PARTICULAR SITUATIONS AND IN CONNECTION WITH OTHER COMPLIANCE-RELATED CONCERNS. THE AUTHORS SHALL NOT BE LIABLE FOR ANY LOSS INCLUDING FINES OR PENALTIES, LOSS OF PROFIT OR ANY OTHER COMMERCIAL DAMAGES, INCLUDING, BUT NOT LIMITED TO SPECIAL, INCIDENTAL, CONSEQUENTIAL, OR OTHER DAMAGES.

# Foreword

This is an important guide. It is important because there is widespread apprehension regarding the privacy and security regulations implementing the Health Insurance Portability and Accountability Act of 1996. This apprehension threatens to block the dissemination of individually identifiable health information in many situations in which the federal government never intended to do so.

There have been widespread media reports of fear in the offices of healthcare providers as to their ability to respond to requests for information from persons other than the patient. Each day those of us who practice in this area receive calls from confused and concerned providers, insurers, and persons seeking to perform services for those sectors. Those calls raise a remarkable array of tough issues.

How can research using health information gleaned across massive data sets continue to be conducted? How can the discovery process in litigation proceed? How can providers determine what disclosures of health information must be "accounted for"? How can insurers provide the information that their employer customers feel they need to answer employee questions and design new benefits across HIPAA covered and noncovered employee welfare benefit plans? How must the electronic data be secured?

Answering these questions is not simple work. First, there are hundreds of pages of regulations to be parsed. The regulations are dense. In the context of privacy, they do not set forth a list of forbidden acts. Instead, they attempt to define the thousands of ways individually identifiable health information could appropriately be used without obtaining the patient or insured's special permission — the so-called "authorization." While the public policy goal may be laudable, in terms of ease of use, it is challenging.

However, the interpretative challenges do not stop there. The regulations are construed in thousands of pages of preamble. The regulations and the preamble are also constantly being interpreted through question and answers published on Web sites by the Office of Civil Rights and the Center for Medicare and Medicaid Services. Distilling this body for relevance is a daunting task. Fortunately, for the reader, Kevin Beaver and Rebecca

Herold have both distilled much of that law and official statements and present it through this guide in a form that makes it understandable to the thousands of persons who must conform their clinical and business practices to its dictates.

Beaver and Herold first give the clinician or businessman an orientation to the purposes of the so-called "Administrative Simplification" provisions of the HIPAA statute and the scope of the privacy, security and transactions, and code set regulations that have emanated from it. The authors then instruct as to the elements of the privacy rule and provide practical guidance as to many issues faced by healthcare providers and plans. Affected parties are given useful checklists for privacy compliance programs and sample forms. The same approach is taken with respect to the security rule — orientation, analysis of areas of challenge, and implementation guidance. Later chapters continue to provide value through in-depth review of issues by industry segment and useful case studies.

The HIPAA regulations are transforming how providers and insurers think about the individually identifiable health information they create and receive every minute of every day. The notices and acknowledgments called for by the regulation are also awakening patients and insureds to the path information about them takes as they are cared for and seek payment for that care.

There is a potential for serious harm to service levels and even to patient health if misunderstandings as to the dictates of these regulations choke off the exchange of patient health information. This guide is a good step toward erasing many of those misunderstandings. I commend the authors for their fine efforts at translating a difficult subject into practical terms.

**Mark Lutes, Esq.**
Washington, D.C.

# Introduction

*The Practical Guide to HIPAA Privacy and Security Compliance* is designed to help you understand what HIPAA is about, what it requires, what you can do to work toward compliance, and how you can maintain compliance on an ongoing basis. We have designed this book as the one-stop, "how-to" reference for real-world HIPAA privacy and security advice that you can immediately apply to your organization's unique and specific situation. This book describes the HIPAA Privacy and Security Rules and compliance tasks in easy-to-understand language. We do not focus on technical and legal theory and jargon but rather lay out what you actually need to do according to the final HIPAA Privacy and Security Rules to become compliant.

HIPAA is very complex. Privacy and security are also very complex. Given that, we do not claim to have coverage in this book on every possible topic or nuance related to these subjects. Our goal, though, is to provide you with guidance on the HIPAA requirements and more commonly discussed topics. We also provide you with a number of checklists and other reference materials that will help you get started down the compliance path and point you in the right direction for references and resources when you need them in the future.

## For Whom this Book Was Written

This book is designed for anyone who needs to prepare their organization, or someone else's organization, for the HIPAA laws. This book is also designed to help you determine how HIPAA may impact you, even if your organization is not a HIPAA Covered Entity. Our target audience includes the following:

- Privacy Officers
- Security Officers
- Physicians
- Nurses
- Clinicians
- Office Managers
- IT Managers
- Network Administrators

- Attorneys
- Consultants
- Compliance Officers
- Chief Information Officers
- Any of the various business associates involved in the healthcare industry

Organizations ranging from rural health clinics to large insurance companies can utilize the material contained in this book. From nontechnical office managers to noncomputer-savvy doctors to highly technical IT specialists, practically anyone who may be touched by HIPAA can benefit from this book.

## How this Book Is Organized

Even if you do not read this book cover to cover, the pertinent information you need should be easy to find by simply referring to the particular section or chapter of interest. This book contains six major sections, as follows:

Section 1: HIPAA Essentials
Section 2: HIPAA Privacy Rule
Section 3: HIPAA Security Rule
Section 4: Covered Entity Issues
Section 5: HIPAA Technology Considerations
Section 6: Managing Ongoing HIPAA Compliance

In addition to these sections, we also provide an abundance of information in the Appendices. You will notice that besides a checklist of highlights at the end of each chapter, we have included a set of quiz questions at the end of each section so you can test your comprehension of some of what we cover in the chapters. You can also utilize these questions as part of your organization's awareness efforts that are required by the HIPAA regulations. The answers to these quiz questions, along with their explanations, are listed in Appendix D of this book. We have also included four different healthcare industry case studies that outline the HIPAA compliance experiences of some representative covered entities. In addition, we have included various sample documents that you can utilize in your HIPAA compliance efforts, along with a listing of various HIPAA-related resources.

Please refer to this book's Web site at www.hipaaprivacyandsecurity.com for critical updates to the issues discussed within this book, along with updates and additions for various HIPAA resources and links. Our goal is to create a living HIPAA resource at our Web site, as well as passing along helpful HIPAA compliance tips, information, and news.

# Acknowledgments

I want to thank Becky Herold for putting up with me during the writing process and for wanting to co-author this book with me in the first place. Her intelligence and drive have really inspired me. She was such a pleasure to work with. I couldn't have had a better person to help write this book. I want to thank the individuals who helped with the HIPAA case studies featured in this book. I also want to thank Rich O'Hanley for giving us the chance to write this book and the staff at CRC Press for all of their behind-the-scenes work to make this book happen. In addition, I want to thank Mark Lutes for the excellent HIPAA insight he expressed in the foreword, and Mike Corby and Micki Krause for their participation in reviewing this book and providing us their feedback. Finally, I want to thank my wife, Amy, for her patience, support, and shoulder massages while I was writing this book – I completely believe that I could not have done this without her!

— *Kevin Beaver*

A huge thanks to my co-author, Kevin Beaver, for having the idea for this book, and for asking me to write it with him. This was a great experience, and I am glad I got to know and work with Kevin and his lovely wife, Amy. Kevin was great to work with, and I really appreciated his professionalism, attention to detail, and depth of knowledge.

Thanks to Rich O'Hanley for publishing our book, and for his continuing support and feedback.

Thanks to Harry Smith and David Ginsberg from PrivaPlan for allowing us to include their fine example Business Associate Agreement in our book.

Thanks to our anonymous contacts for providing information for the case studies. Sharing your experiences helped us immensely.

Thanks to Mark Lutes for contributing so much to our book with his foreword.

A special thanks to Mike Corby for reviewing the raw form of this book early and providing valuable feedback.

Another special thanks to Micki Krause for providing a review of the pre-release of the book and for her constructive comments.

Thanks to all my other postpublishing reviewers: Cherie, Richard, and Robert, and probably others as yet unknown ... you know who you are.

Thanks to all the people who helped with information for this book, and for inspiring me to keep working and writing into the wee hours of the night.

*— Rebecca Herold*

# Section 1
# HIPAA
# Essentials

# Chapter 1
# Introduction to HIPAA

*All that may come to my knowledge in the exercise of my profession or outside of my profession or in daily commerce with men, which ought not to be spread abroad, I will keep secret and will never reveal. If I keep this oath faithfully, may I enjoy my life and practice my art, respected by all men and in all times; but if I swerve from it or violate it, may the reverse be my lot.*

**Hippocrates (460–370 B.C.), the Father of Terran Medicine**
— *Excerpt from the Hippocratic Oath*

## How HIPAA Came to Be

HIPAA is a very well-known acronym in the healthcare industry these days. It consists of old-millennium ideas yet it brings new-millennium realities. A few people love it, a fair amount of people understand the value it brings, and even more people dislike it. So, what is all the fuss about? HIPAA is the Health Insurance Portability and Accountability Act of 1996 and is also known as Public Law 104-191 and the Kennedy–Kassebaum Bill, named after its creators, Senators Edward Kennedy (D-MA) and Nancy Kassebaum (R-KS). This legislation was passed by the Congress, signed into law by Bill Clinton, and became effective on August 21, 1996.

The overall goal of HIPAA is to provide insurance portability, fraud enforcement, and administrative simplification for the healthcare industry. HIPAA was formed out of the growing concerns about keeping healthcare information private, the need to consolidate nonstandard healthcare data and transaction formats, as well as the general consensus to streamline healthcare operations and reduce the cost of providing healthcare services. This legislation has been a long time coming for the healthcare industry — an industry known to be behind the times from a technology perspective. In fact, there have been numerous, well-known stories of privacy and security breaches in the healthcare industry. As listed in the Medical Privacy Stories published by the Health Privacy Project,* here are just a few of the highlights:

* Available at http://www.healthprivacy.org/usr_doc/privacystories.pdf.

---

The information and opinions provided in this book do not constitute or substitute for legal or other professional advice.

- A hacker compromised the medical records, health information, and Social Security numbers of over 5000 medical center patients.
- E-mails, some of them containing sensitive records, were sent out to the wrong people, affecting 858 online members.
- Thousands of medical records en route to be destroyed fell out of a vehicle, causing them to be blown throughout Mesa, AZ.
- A computer disk containing the names of 4000 people who tested positive for HIV was sent to two newspapers.
- A country singer's medical records were sold to tabloid magazines by a hospital employee for $2610.

The Administrative Simplification section (Title II, Subtitle F) of HIPAA — the portion of HIPAA that we will explore in this book — was designed to help decrease the costs of healthcare administration with the goal of spending that money instead on increasing the quality of healthcare. This includes standardizing on electronic transactions, national identifiers, and ensuring the privacy and security of confidential health information.

The Department of Health and Human Services (HHS) is the organization responsible for establishing the HIPAA standards. In February 2003, HHS Secretary Tommy G. Thompson concisely summarized HIPAA Administrative Simplification by stating the following upon final release of the HIPAA Security Rule:

> *Overall, these national standards required under HIPAA will make it easier and less costly for the healthcare industry to process health claims and handle other transactions while assuring patients that their information will remain secure and confidential. The security standards in particular will help safeguard confidential health information as the industry increasingly relies on computers for processing healthcare transactions.*

As published in the final Privacy Rule, HHS states that HIPAA Administrative Simplification has three major purposes:

1. To protect and enhance the rights of consumers by providing them access to their health information and controlling the inappropriate use of that information
2. To improve the quality of healthcare in the United States by restoring trust in the healthcare system among consumers, healthcare professionals, and the multitude of organizations and individuals committed to the delivery of care
3. To improve the efficiency and effectiveness of healthcare delivery by creating a national framework for health privacy protection that builds on efforts by states, health systems, and individual organizations and individuals

There are four administrative simplification sub-sections, or rules, which include mandates for the privacy and security of personal and confidential healthcare information, referred to as the Privacy Rule and the Security Rule; standardized electronic transactions and code sets, referred to as the Electronic Transactions and Code Sets Rule; and national identifiers, referred to as the Unique Identifier Rules. In this book, we provide a brief overview of the Electronic Transactions and Code Sets Rule, which you can find later in this chapter, and in-depth coverage of the Privacy and Security Rules throughout the rest of the book. Moving forward, unless noted otherwise, our references to HIPAA will focus solely on Administrative Simplification and, more specifically, on the Privacy and Security Rules.

## What HIPAA Covers

In addition to the various transactions and code sets standards, HIPAA mandates protection of various forms of confidential health information referred to as protected health information (PHI). PHI is considered any oral or recorded information relating to any past, present, or future physical or mental health of an individual, provision of healthcare to the individual, or the payment for the healthcare of that individual. With very few exceptions, oral or recorded PHI consists of individual health information that is spoken, written, or stored in hard copy or electronically in any way. A similar, more-specific term that relates to this type of information is individually identifiable health information (IIHI). Basically, IIHI identifies or can be used to reasonably identify an individual. There are 18 identifiers defined by HIPAA that can be used to identify an individual, such as name, Social Security number, and medical record number. These 18 identifiers are collectively referred to as PHI when used in activities covered by HIPAA. Information that has been "de-identified " is not covered under HIPAA. We will go into more detail about PHI and IIHI in Chapter 5, where we cover the Privacy Rule in detail.

## Organizations that Must Comply with HIPAA

### Covered Entities

Virtually the entire healthcare industry, as well as a significant number of organizations in other industries, is affected by HIPAA in one way or another. Large insurance companies to hospitals to self-insured employers to small physician practices are required to comply with HIPAA. These organizations are called covered entities (CEs). There are three main categories of CEs:

1. *Healthcare providers:* A healthcare provider can be an individual, a group, or an organization. An individual is a natural person licensed or authorized in some other way to perform or provide medical services, care, equipment, or supplies. A few examples include doctors, nurses, pharmacists, and physical therapists. A group is one that is typically made up of more than one person to provide patient care, including professional services such as billing and payment. For example, two physicians are practicing as a group by billing and

receiving payments as a single entity. An organization is an entity composed of more than one person that is authorized to provide medical services, care, equipment, or supplies as part of their usual business. A few examples include hospitals, laboratories, pharmacies, nursing facilities, and health maintenance organizations (HMOs).

2. *Health plans:* Generally speaking, these are individual or group plans that provide or pay for medical care. Examples include private and governmental health insurance issuers such as HMOs, PPOs, Medicare and Medicaid programs, as well as employer-sponsored health plans with coverage for 50 or more employees. Health plans do not include workers' compensation programs, property and casualty programs, or disability insurance programs, even though they may pay healthcare costs.

3. *Healthcare clearinghouses:* These are public or private entities that process or facilitate the processing of nonstandard data elements of health information into a standard format, or convert from a standard format to one that is nonstandard, for electronic transactions. A few examples include billing services, repricing companies, value-added networks, and even some banks.

So, how do you determine if you are a CE under HIPAA? First, decide if you could possibly be considered a healthcare provider, healthcare clearinghouse, or health plan as described above. Then, acquaint yourself with a few key terms listed below.

### What Does Healthcare Mean?

Healthcare is defined within 45 CFR § 160.103. Beyond care, the services and supplies related to an individual's health are all considered healthcare. A few examples, as discussed in the HIPAA regulations, include:

- A preventive, diagnostic, rehabilitative, maintenance, or palliative care, and counseling service, assessment, or procedure with respect to the physical or mental condition or functional status of an individual or that affects the structure or function of the body
- The sale or dispensing of a drug, device, equipment, or other item in accordance with a prescription

### What Are Covered Transactions?

Covered transactions under HIPAA are those for which the Secretary has adopted standards as described in 45 CFR Part 162. If a healthcare provider uses another covered entity (such as another provider, a health plan, or a clearinghouse) to conduct covered transactions in electronic form on its behalf, the healthcare provider is considered to be conducting the transaction in electronic form. A transaction is a covered transaction if it meets the regulatory definition for a covered transaction. You can find the complete regulatory definitions for each type of covered transaction as indicated in the following list:

- 45 CFR § 162.1101: Healthcare claims or equivalent encounter information transactions
- 45 CFR § 162.1201: The eligibility for a health plan transaction
- 45 CFR § 162.1301: The referral certification and authorization transaction
- 45 CFR § 162.1401: A healthcare claim status transaction
- 45 CFR § 162.1501: The enrollment and disenrollment in a health plan transaction
- 45 CFR § 162.1601: The healthcare payment and remittance advice transaction
- 45 CFR § 162.1701: The health plan premium payment transaction
- 45 CFR § 162.1801: The coordination of benefits transaction

### What Does Electronic Form Mean?

When HIPAA refers to information in "electronic form," it means using electronic media with which to store or transmit information. Such types of electronic media include CDs, disks, magnetic tapes, computer hard drives, dial-up lines, private networks, leased lines, the Internet, extranets that connect businesses with business partners, etc. The term is defined in 45 CFR § 162.103.

### Are You a Covered Healthcare Provider?

Do you furnish, bill, or receive payment for healthcare as part of your business?

- If NO, you are not a covered entity.
- If YES, do you execute covered transactions?
  - If NO, you are not a covered entity.
  - If YES, are the covered transactions transmitted in electronic form?
    - If NO, you are not a covered entity.
    - If YES, you *are* a covered entity healthcare provider. Be sure to read Chapter 16 for information specific to providers.

### Are You a Covered Healthcare Clearinghouse?

Do you facilitate health information processing from a nonstandard format (or content) to a standard format? Or, do you convert standard format (or content) health information into a nonstandard format?

- If NO, you are not a covered entity clearinghouse.
- If YES, do you do these activities for another legal entity?
  - If NO, you are not a covered entity clearinghouse.
  - If YES, you *are* a covered entity clearinghouse. Be sure to read Chapter 17 for information specific to clearinghouses.

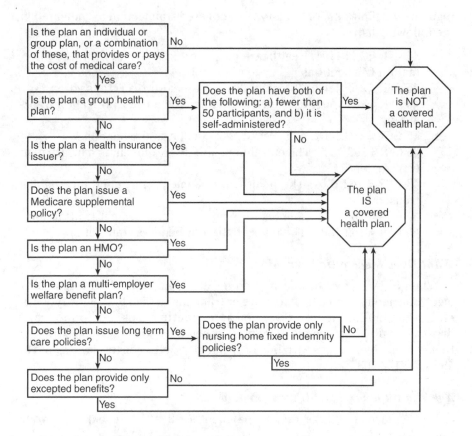

Exhibit 1. **Covered Entity Decision Diagram**

### Are You a Covered Entity Private Benefit Plan?

This is a somewhat detailed analysis best performed by using the decision chart shown in Exhibit 1, based on the one provided by Centers for Medicare and Medicaid Services (CMS). Be sure to read Chapter 18 for information specific to health plans.

### Are You a Covered Government-Funded Health Plan Program?

This is also a detailed analysis and best presented in the decision chart shown in Exhibit 2, also based on a similar one provided by CMS.* Be sure to read Chapter 18 for information specific to covered health plans.

*CMS has a set of covered entity automated decision tools that can help healthcare organizations that are having an identity crisis decide whether or not HIPAA applies to them. These tools can be found at http://www.cms.gov/hipaa/hipaa2/support/tools/decisionsupport/default.asp.

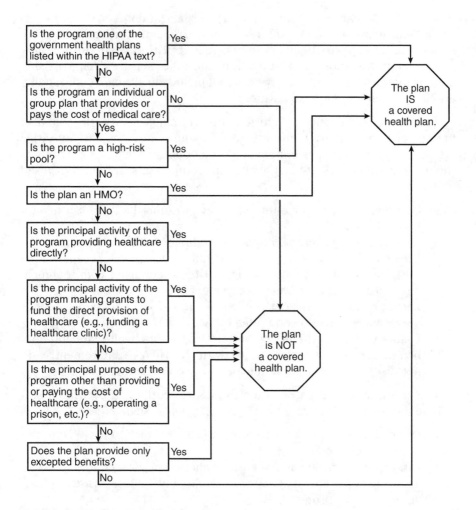

**Exhibit 2. Health Plan Decision Diagram**

## Hybrid Entities

Simply put, a hybrid entity is a covered entity whose covered functions are not its primary functions. An organization that is a single legal entity whose business activities include both covered and noncovered functions can designate itself as a hybrid entity. In that case, only the identified healthcare component is considered as a covered entity.

It is very clear that some entities are covered entities based on their business activities; for instance, networks of hospitals, or a nationwide health plan with millions of members. However, there are many large organizations

9

that have healthcare components, but the organization itself is not primarily a healthcare entity. Consider state governments, for example. State governments support healthcare services, but they also support law enforcement, transportation, education, and other services. Large organizations that provide multiple services that include healthcare components are likely considered hybrid entities.

The Privacy Rule defines a hybrid entity as a single legal entity that also happens to be a covered entity, whose business services and activities include covered as well as noncovered functions, and that has portions of the organization designated as healthcare components. A hybrid covered entity must:

- Designate the components of the organization that perform healthcare-related activities.
- Ensure the healthcare component complies with requirements.
- Create adequate administrative, technical, and physical separations (also commonly called firewalls, not to be confused with technical Internet firewalls) between components.
- Ensure no disclosures between the healthcare component and other parts, except as allowed under HIPAA.
- Ensure workforce members with duties to both healthcare and nonhealthcare components comply with the HIPAA requirements and not disclose PHI to the nonhealthcare component.

The entire organization of which the hybrid entity is a part must still adhere to some of the covered entity requirements, such as:

- Implementing safeguards to protect PHI, and not disclose PHI to the nonhealthcare components
- Establishing privacy and security policies and procedures
- Ensuring applicable language is included in business associate (BA) agreements to protect PHI

There are advantages and disadvantages for an organization to declare itself a hybrid entity. The most apparent advantages are that as a hybrid entity the organization can:

- Limit the scope, and thus expenses and efforts, for HIPAA compliance activities.
- Target the detailed compliance training and administrative procedures to only the identified healthcare component and not the entire organization.
- Designate otherwise noncovered areas of the organization that provide services to the healthcare component (such as legal, accounting, etc.) as part of the healthcare component to facilitate sharing of PHI with these areas, and also eliminate the need for BA agreements and individual authorizations with these components.

Some disadvantages for an organization to declare itself a hybrid entity include:

- Time, effort, and expense must be made to identify the healthcare components.
- Internal systems of administrative, technical, and physical firewalls and safeguards must be established and maintained between the healthcare and nonhealthcare components.
- Information shared outside the healthcare component will likely need to be more limited, and disclosures to the nonhealthcare component must be tracked.
- Workforce members' access to information must be completely evaluated and modified appropriately.
- Clients and business partners may potentially receive or believe they are receiving inconsistent treatment from the different components.
- There will likely be many more forms to administer and maintain.
- Staff confusion and compliance enforcement may be more difficult.
- Challenges may exist with overlapping and shared work areas, computer systems, etc.

Each organization must weigh the advantages and disadvantages of declaring themselves a hybrid entity and make its decision based on its own unique situation.

### Business Associates

Individuals or organizations doing business with CEs, referred to as business associates (BAs), may be affected by HIPAA as well. In order to fall into the business associate category, these individuals or organizations must perform an activity involving the use or disclosure of PHI on behalf of a CE. This does not include performing any activities as an employee of the CE.

CEs may also be BAs to other CEs. For any BA relationship that a CE has, a BA agreement that holds the BAs responsible for certain HIPAA requirements must be in place between the two parties. There are exceptions to this rule as well. These exceptions apply to CEs that disclose PHI to other CEs for purposes of treatment, payment, and operations (TPO) in the course of normal business. We cover business associate issues, including BA agreements, in more detail in Chapter 20.

### Compliance Deadlines

There are several compliance deadlines that must be met for the various HIPAA rules. Each HIPAA rule has both an effective date and a compliance date. Considering there are various extensions, modification dates, and testing dates, it is important to be aware of these dates to ensure your organization is on track and there are no unnecessary surprises that could

**Exhibit 3. Important Dates Associated with HIPAA**

| | Privacy Rule | Security Rule | Electronic Transactions and Code Sets Rule | National Employer Identifier Rule |
|---|---|---|---|---|
| Effective date | April 14, 2001 | April 21, 2003 | October 16, 2000 | July 30, 2002 |
| Compliance deadline[a] | April 14, 2003 | April 21, 2005 | October 16, 2003[b] | July 30, 2004 |

[a] Small health plans (those with annual receipts of $5M or less) have 3 years from the effective date to be compliant. All other CEs must comply within 2 years of the effective date as noted.

[b] The original compliance deadline for the Electronic Transactions and Code Sets Rule was October 16, 2002. This deadline for was extended 1 year to October 16, 2003, for CEs that applied for an extension by October 16, 2002.

catch you off guard. Exhibit 3 outlines the effective and compliance dates associated with the four HIPAA Administrative Simplification rules at the time this book was written (early 2003).

## HIPAA Penalties and Enforcement

Like other laws affecting the healthcare industry such as OSHA, HIPAA must be taken seriously. There are "slap on the hand" civil penalties that start at $100 per incident, as well as severe criminal penalties that include huge fines and possible prison time. If a complaint is lodged against an entity and an investigation or compliance review determines no violation exists, the Secretary of HHS will inform both the entity and the person or organization filing the complaint in writing.

If a complaint is lodged against an entity and the resulting compliance review confirms noncompliance with the HIPAA Rules, the entity will be informed in writing by the Secretary, who will attempt to resolve the situation by informal means if possible. If the situation cannot be resolved in this manner, a formal noncompliance report will be issued to both the complainant and entity. For noncriminal violation of the HIPAA Rules, including disclosures made in error, civil penalties of $100 per violation up to $25,000 per year, per standard, may be issued. Additionally, criminal penalties may be applied for certain violations done knowingly as follows:

- *Wrongful disclosure offense:* $50,000 fine, no more than 1 year in prison, or both
- *Offense under false pretenses:* $100,000 fine, no more than 5 years in prison, or both
- *Offense committed with intent to sell information:* $250,000 fine, no more than 10 years in prison, or both

Additionally, there may be more-stringent state laws that could preempt HIPAA laws and result in different or additional penalties. We will discuss this in more detail in Chapter 8. Regarding the enforcement of HIPAA, the Office of Civil Rights (OCR) of HHS is responsible for enforcing the Privacy Rule. Additionally, CMS will create a new office responsible for enforcing the Electronic Transactions and Code Sets and Security Rules. This office will also provide outreach efforts to ensure that CEs are aware of HIPAA and to provide compliance assistance.

**Insight into the Electronic Transactions and Code Sets Rule**

Although this book focuses on the HIPAA Privacy and Security Rules, it is important for privacy and information security professionals to understand the types and forms of information, as defined within the Electronic Transactions and Code Sets and Unique Identifiers Rules, for which you will need to implement privacy and security safeguards. You will need to include your information technology and services staff, in particular those responsible for implementing the Electronic Transactions and Code Sets and Unique Identifier Rules, when you are planning your HIPAA privacy and security actions.

HHS issued the final electronic transaction standards in August 2000. The intent of these standards was to make the processing of healthcare claims more efficient, reduce the volume of paperwork, and provide better service for providers, insurers, and patients. They established a new standard by which data content, codes, and formats must comply within submitted electronic claims and administrative healthcare transactions. HHS reports that if all healthcare entities follow these standards, the healthcare industry will realize a $29.9 billion net savings over a 10-year period by eliminating inefficient paper forms. While not required, all healthcare providers will be encouraged to use this electronic standard for service billing. Also, all health plans are required to accept claims in this standard electronic form, in addition to accepting referral authorizations and other defined healthcare transactions within this form. The rule is comprised of standards for eight types of electronic transactions and for code sets to be used within these transactions. It also outlines the requirements for using the standards to which health plans, healthcare clearinghouses, and certain healthcare providers must adhere.

Because of the tremendous amount of software implementations and upgrades necessary to establish these electronic transaction standards, Congress adopted legislation in December 2001 that allowed most CEs to obtain a 1-year extension to comply with the standards. If a qualified CE submitted its extension by the deadline, it had until October 16, 2003, to implement the electronic transaction standards. The compliance date for small health plans remained October 16, 2003. For those organizations that filed for an extension, transactions and code sets testing must have begun by April 16, 2003. The official government Web site for information about the HIPAA Electronics Transactions and Code Sets Standards is http://aspe. hhs.gov/admnsimp/bannertx.htm.

Section 1173 of the HIPAA Administrative Simplification requires "a standard unique health identifier for each individual, employer, health plan, and healthcare provider for use in the healthcare system." The wording makes it clear that multiple uses for identifiers would be necessary for multiple classifications of healthcare providers. The proposed unique identifier rules apply to health plans and clearinghouses, as well as any healthcare provider who electronically transmits HIPAA-covered transactions. Collateral impact will be felt by health plan software vendors and also vendors who support the healthcare transactions as they also will need to make changes to incorporate the identifier requirements.

As of early 2003, there have been two rules proposed for identifiers: the National Provider Identifier and the National Employer Identifier. The proposed National Provider Identifier is a new eight-character alphanumeric or ten-digit numeric with a check digit. The National Employer Identifier is the same as the Federal Employer Identification Number (EIN), which is composed of nine digits separated by a hyphen (for example, 00-0000000). The National Health Plan Identifier and the National Health Identifier for Individuals have not yet been proposed as of this writing. The National Health Plan Identifier rules are currently under development. Much controversy accompanied the announcement of the National Health Identifier for Individuals, and HHS has indefinitely postponed this standard. Some view the idea of creating personal identifiers as being a significant privacy threat, and as such, in direct opposition to some of the stated goals of the HIPAA Privacy Rule. The official government Web site for information about the proposed HIPAA Unique Identifiers Standards is http://aspe.hhs. gov/admnsimp/bannerid.htm.

## Summary

In this chapter, we have summarized what HIPAA is about. As you can see, it is quite comprehensive, and compliance will certainly take some time and resources to accomplish. In subsequent chapters on the Privacy and Security Rules we will go into more detail that can provide you some guidance on how to move forward. At the end of each chapter, including this one, you will find practical checklists that will recap some of the major points that we make that can provide a quick reference of key items on which to focus.

## Chapter 1: Practical Checklist

- Does your organization supply, bill, or receive payment for health-care services with payers or with CMS?
- Does your organization provide services that involve PHI on behalf of a covered entity?
- Are you aware that your organization, with the exception of small health plans that have an extra year, was due to be fully compliant with HIPAA Privacy Rule on April 14, 2003?
- Are you aware that your organization, with the exception of small health plans that have an extra year, must be compliant with the HIPAA Security Rule by April 21, 2005?
- Are you aware of the penalties for noncompliance of the HIPAA rules?
- Have you contacted your information systems and software vendors to determine their timetable for releasing HIPAA-compliant software?
- Will your internal and in-house produced systems software be HIPAA compliant?
- Was your HIPAA-compliant software installed and tested prior to the implementation deadline of October 16, 2003?
- If you use a claims clearinghouse, have you checked to ensure it will be compliant with HIPAA, and by what date?
- Are you currently using or have you started implementation of the required coding systems?
- Have you updated your applicable documents to incorporate the required procedures and diagnosis code changes?
- Do you have procedures for obtaining the necessary demographic, charge, and diagnosis information?

### References

Department of Health and Human Services, HIPAA Administrative Simplification Rule links, available at http://aspe.dhhs.gov/admnsimp.

# Chapter 2
# Preparing for the HIPAA Changes

## Background

The magnitude and impact of HIPAA is much greater than most organizations ever anticipated. The resources and business process changes along with the policies, procedures, and technology required to ensure the privacy and security of protected health information (PHI) are overwhelming for most covered entities (CEs), to say the least. There is a common myth that HIPAA compliance is about technology that can simply be bought and put in place, and magically make a CE HIPAA compliant. This is the furthest thing from the truth and any attempts at acquiring "compliance in a box" not only are futile, but likely will leave your organization with huge compliance gaps.

HIPAA compliance is not about technology but rather people. This includes everyone from your receptionist to the highest ranking healthcare executive in your organization. Everyone must be involved in working toward HIPAA compliance. The success of any new and updated policies, procedures, and business processes that are put in place for HIPAA are completely dependent on the awareness and buy-in of everyone involved in daily healthcare operations. Initial HIPAA compliance cannot be achieved without the proper change-management practices in place. Ongoing HIPAA compliance cannot be effectively maintained without the proper culture and mindset.

## Managing Change

Change can be messy. Healthcare organizations are well known for their resistance to change. Quite often things are complicated by multiple changes, differing priorities, and lack of clarity about both short- and long-term goals. In addition, change is often over-managed to the point where people are pushed too hard, too quickly. This can lead to loss of interest, lowered morale, or even severe burn-out. When managing change, there

---

The information and opinions provided in this book do not constitute or substitute for legal or other professional advice.

are quite often many unfavorable decisions and transformations that must be made with which some people will not be happy. HIPAA has been known to strike a few chords in this area. The key to minimizing this is to properly set everyone's expectations in advance. This gets back to instilling the proper mindset and culture. Organizations must also consider the money issue. Change can be costly. A common occurrence is upper management that supports change yet does not want to finance those changes. The changes mandated by HIPAA can be, and must be, managed effectively in order to be rolled out and integrated properly with your business in a cost-effective manner.

Successful HIPAA change management will involve strong leadership, the decision to move forward with compliance efforts, and proactive planning and implementation. The outcome will be the creation of new HIPAA policies, procedures, and organizational structures that foster new ways of thinking and doing business. Remember to monitor and readjust your policies and procedures if your business needs change or if problems arise.

It is human nature to fear change. The new ways of providing healthcare mandated by HIPAA are a lot to take on. One key factor in helping to create a new way of "HIPAA" thinking is persuasion. The best way to persuade others is to motivate them and give them an incentive. Two motivating factors must be considered. The first factor is an individual's desire to gain something and move ahead. You will need to articulate the value of HIPAA and put it in terms of the individual. Answer the question, "What's in it for me?" Then relay that answer to everyone. Think of examples of how HIPAA can make everyone's job easier. For example, standardizing one set of electronic healthcare transactions, having a formal procedure for communicating with patients and other healthcare professionals regarding PHI, and even reducing the number of passwords to keep up with by implementing a unified user log-in system. When people see and hear these types of benefits, they can be motivated to consider and ultimately accept the changes. The second motivating factor is a person's fear of losing something or falling behind. For example, if you can demonstrate to your staff just how easy it is to lose all of their hard work on their computer system when backups are not done properly or, at a higher level, by outlining how serious the HIPAA penalties are, most employees can be motivated to help the organization, and thus their careers. Bottom line: you have got to have an approach that puts it in their terms and shows them what they stand to gain or lose.

### Creating the Mindset

HIPAA requires a new way of thinking and performing daily tasks. Instilling the proper HIPAA-aware mindset begins with creating the proper culture. This culture must be embraced by upper management and HIPAA officers who must lead by example. As difficult as it may initially appear to be, HIPAA must be talked about within your organization in a positive light. HIPAA should be embraced as a standard business practice moving forward, and top-down influence is very important. We are talking about the way people think here — perhaps the most difficult thing to change in the world. There must be buy-in, guidance, and strong leadership from upper managers if HIPAA compliance is going to work properly. Whether you are an office manager, an IT director, or in executive management, you must regularly educate yourself about HIPAA until you understand it. You can attend HIPAA seminars and conferences as well as immerse yourself in the excellent HIPAA resources found on the Internet. See Appendix C for a listing of some of our favorites. You can then take your knowledge and start relating it to your job and your organization's overall mission. This type of activity is contagious. When you start working and behaving with HIPAA in mind, people will notice and, eventually, most will start doing the same.

One of the best ways to get buy-in on HIPAA in your organization is to demonstrate the business value that it brings. Embrace HIPAA with the future in mind and give examples of how HIPAA will pay off long term. No one wants to hear "we've got to become HIPAA compliant because the government is making us." You have got to look beyond that to understand and relay to others why standardized transactions and code sets and the confidentiality of PHI is important. You must be able to relay the overall goal of HIPAA Administrative Simplification to everyone in your organization. Relay to them that HIPAA was designed to help lower costs while increasing the quality of healthcare. More specifically, you can tell them about how, with newer and more formal business policies and procedures, business operations can be streamlined, which can ultimately increase productivity and ultimately make their jobs easier. You can also tell them about the specific risks involved when PHI is not kept secure. For example, the Computer Security Institute (CSI) and the Federal Bureau of Investigation (FBI) publish a "Computer Crime and Security Survey" every year, outlining various statistics related to information threats. It outlines key points such as how the majority of respondents detect computer security breaches, oftentimes by internal employees, year after year. A great resource for medical privacy and security breaches, and interesting reading for almost anyone, is Medical Privacy Stories, published by the Health Privacy Project we mentioned in Chapter 1. It is also a very effective tool to communicate the personal benefits of HIPAA requirements to your staff, and how it will ultimately help protect their own PHI that is processed by their corresponding physicians, insurance companies, etc. When people know they are personally being benefited by regulatory requirements, they are usually more open to making the necessary changes within their work environments.

Most information privacy and security surveys are not comprehensive, or healthcare or HIPAA specific, but certainly provide good cross-section numbers and great insight into what is actually going on regarding the threats and vulnerabilities to healthcare information. Information gleaned from surveys should certainly be considered as part of your organization's information protection program and HIPAA compliance efforts. The key here is to do your research and find specific real-world examples of how the side effects of HIPAA have helped other organizations and apply them to your environment. We outline several Internet resources in Appendix C where you can obtain this type of information.

### It's Up to You

For every healthcare system or business process that is knowingly affected by HIPAA, there may be many more that have not surfaced yet. Do not worry about getting everything right up front — just get started on your compliance efforts. Also, do not worry about having to make yourself a HIPAA expert overnight. Do not let your level of expertise, or lack thereof, in information privacy and security get in your way. Also, do not worry about having to change everyone's mind overnight. It simply will not happen. You can, however, be successful long term if you help influence others a little bit at a time. Remember to start with yourself first. Do not expect others to change their ways of thinking and working. You have got to live and breathe HIPAA every day as well. Be sure to include everyone involved as significant contributors, not simply doers. Keep your eye on the horizon and your mind thinking long term so you can help effect these changes. What we have discussed in this chapter is only the tip of the iceberg regarding the importance of a HIPAA-aware culture. In Chapter 24, we go further into detail on creating ongoing training, education, and awareness programs that will help maintain a HIPAA mindset and ways of providing and improving healthcare in the future.

### Chapter 2: Practical Checklist

- Establish a strong leadership role to drive the HIPAA changes.
- Has a shared "change" vision been created and communicated to everyone in the organization?
- Create a plan to monitor ongoing changes and readjust if necessary.
- Have you researched and studied HIPAA to the point where you feel that you really understand it?
- Is upper management leading by example?
- Are you leading by example?
- Be prepared to articulate the value that HIPAA brings.
- Focus on what motivates people — the desire to gain and the fear of loss.
- Consider tying employees' HIPAA change efforts and attitudes into performance evaluations.

## References

1. CSI/FBI Computer Crime and Security Survey, available at http://www.gocsi.com.
2. Health Privacy Project Medical Privacy Stories, available at http://www.healthprivacy.org/usr_doc/privacystories.pdf.

# Chapter 3
# HIPAA Cost Considerations

## Background

Actual costs for HIPAA compliance will vary among covered entities (CEs) because of various factors such as size, type of business, organizational culture, geographic locations, and number of business associates. In addition, costs will depend on how "compliant" that CE can be and the amount of risk it can feasibly accept. Obviously, costs will vary depending on whether the organization chooses to implement completely new systems and business processes, only the bare minimum requirements, or something in between. Unfortunately, there is no one good answer to how much HIPAA will cost. However, we believe it is safe to say that initial HIPAA compliance will most likely range from a few thousand dollars for small CEs to a few hundred thousand dollars or more for larger CEs.

Research firm Gartner Group has estimated that HIPAA is expected to cost the healthcare industry at least $3.8 billion between 2003 and 2008, and potentially even 10 times that. The American Hospital Association (AHA) reported* early in 2001 that doctors and healthcare providers are spending vast amounts of money and time to comply with state and federal privacy laws. According to AHA-funded research, hospitals nationwide are planning to spend as much as $22 billion during the first 5 years to comply with applicable HIPAA laws. For example, they project that implementing minimum necessary requirements will cost a minimum $1.3 billion over 5 years for hospitals and up to $19.8 billion if hospitals must invest in new or upgraded computer systems.

The AHA has compiled several other compelling statistics** with regard to estimated HIPAA Privacy Rule implementation costs. A sampling includes:

* Available at http://www.healthdatamanagement.com.
**Available at http://www.hospitalconnect.com.

---

The information and opinions provided in this book do not constitute or substitute for legal or other professional advice.

- Baylor University Medical Center in Dallas has budgeted $7.5 million over 5 years to pay for implementation of HIPAA.
- Texas Health Resources trained 22,000 workers before the April 14, 2003 deadline, and it expects to spend more than $10 million to comply with the law.

The Department of Health and Human Services (HHS), on the other hand, estimated that implementation of the Privacy Rule will cost CEs $17.6 billion over the first 10 years. At the same time, HHS performed a regulatory impact analysis on the Administrative Simplification standards and expects them to save the industry $29.9 billion over 10 years. These estimates were made prior to the Privacy Rule NPRM changes that were released in August 2002, which, with eased requirements, will likely lower the cost estimates and possibly even raise the savings estimates.

In December 2000, Clinton administration officials did some number crunching to determine what costs may be involved. Peter Swire, the Chief Privacy Counsel for the administration at that time, projected the Privacy Rule cost would equate to $6.25 per year for every insured American. According to the administration numbers, the electronic transactions and code sets requirements will save the industry $29.9 billion over 10 years, leaving a net savings of $12.3 billion after paying for privacy implementation costs. These numbers do not incorporate the Security Rule implementation costs.

Studies are showing that HIPAA compliance will cost as much or more than Y2K preparations did for CEs. The positive side of this is that HIPAA costs can be spread out over a longer period of time, perhaps making them a little easier to deal with. Regardless of who turns out to be closest in their estimates of savings or costs related to implementing the HIPAA requirements, the fact remains that CEs will need to spend at least a fair amount of money up front to implement the requirements. Time, probably over a decade or so, will tell if and when the savings occur for HIPAA implementation activities.

**Privacy Implementation Costs**

Exhibit 1 contains the Privacy Rule implementation activities that will likely involve costs. Use this table to estimate and keep track of your organization's Privacy Rule implementation costs. The estimated costs will vary greatly among organizations, depending on the type of CE, the size, the amount of computer systems used, the number of business associates involved, and other aspects unique to each organization. There may be no cost involved with some of these activities if your organization already has the personnel or resources indicated.

**Exhibit 1. Estimated Privacy Rule Implementation Costs**

| Privacy Rule Implementation Activity | Estimated Cost |
|---|---|
| Performing a privacy gap analysis to establish your baseline compliance state | |
| Performing a privacy risk assessment to identify risks to PHI | |
| Creating and distributing a notice of privacy practices | |
| Creating required policies | |
| Creating required supporting procedures | |
| Assigning personnel to be responsible for privacy | |
| Assigning personnel to be the point of contact for individuals with questions about their privacy rights, and to report complaints | |
| Providing initial personnel privacy training | |
| Implementing electronic technologies to provide safeguards | |
| Printing, paper, and other notice- and procedures-related costs | |
| Updating the provider facility directory | |
| Establishing PHI disclosure accounting mechanisms | |
| Establishing resources to archive and maintain necessary documentation for at least 6 years per document | |
| Establishing business continuity plans, including backup and recovery facilities and resources | |
| Establishing sanctions and the related resources | |
| Implementing physical safeguards where necessary | |
| Reviewing and updating marketing and fundraising plans | |
| Reviewing and updating research procedures and associated forms and documents | |
| Establishing identity verification mechanisms and practices | |
| Establishing mitigation mechanisms and practices | |
| Creating alternative communications methods to give individuals copies of their PHI | |
| Establishing mechanisms to update and correct PHI in response to individual requests | |
| Establishing mechanisms to review authorizations and ensure their currency | |
| Establishing mechanisms to obtain and document acknowledgment of receipt of notices | |
| Reviewing and updating business associate agreements as necessary | |
| Establishing mechanisms to de-identify PHI | |
| **Other Expenses** | |
| **Total Estimated Costs** | |

## Privacy Ongoing Maintenance Costs

Once you have implemented the Privacy Rule requirements, you will not be finished with your compliance obligations. There are ongoing responsibilities that are necessary to maintain compliance. Exhibit 2 below will help you estimate these costs.

## Costs Related to Providing Access to PHI

One of the most hotly debated cost recoup issues is whether or not the Privacy Rule allows CEs to charge individuals who request copies of their records. The rule is pretty clear about this. CEs are permitted to charge a cost that is based on the actual expenses involved with sending the copy of PHI to the requester. These costs include, but are not necessarily limited to, the following:

- Copy supplies (paper, toner cartridges, etc.)
- Postage
- Labor involved with the actual copying

If the individual wants a summary or explanation of PHI, the CE may also charge a fee for the actual clerical preparation of this summary or explanation. The CE must communicate this to the individual and get agreement for the cost before preparing this summary or explanation. This cost may not include the costs related to searching for and retrieving the information, however. Some states have established a cap on the fees that can be charged for the clerical time used. For example, California has set a limit of $6 per hour for the clerical charges incurred in the course of copying and providing access to the PHI. HIPAA does not allow a CE to charge for the time someone supervises an individual within facilities while the individual reviews the PHI. Even though some state laws may allow for such a charge, HIPAA preempts this allowance.

## Privacy Officer Costs

A requirement of HIPAA is to appoint a person or position the responsibility of ensuring compliance with the Privacy Rule. A Medical Records Briefing (MRB) survey* reveals that most hospitals are not spending money to create new positions to meet this requirement, but rather the responsibility is being assigned to existing health information management (HIM) directors or someone else within the information technology department. The 329 MRB survey respondents indicate 64 percent of hospitals have appointed a privacy official to address HIPAA requirements, but in only 5.5 percent of these situations acting as the privacy officer is the person's only job. It is likely that smaller organizations will need to assign the privacy responsibilities to existing staff because of their limited budgets.

*Available at http://www.hin.com.

**Exhibit 2. Estimated Ongoing HIPAA Privacy Costs**

| Privacy Rule Maintenance Activity | Estimated Cost |
|---|---|
| Doing regularly scheduled follow-up privacy gap analysis (recommend every 1 to 2 years) to see where you may now be out of compliance | |
| Doing follow-up privacy risk assessments to identify new risks and ensure previous risks have not reoccurred | |
| Creating and distributing a notice of privacy practices | |
| Personnel to be responsible for privacy | |
| Personnel answering individuals' questions about their privacy rights, and to report complaints | |
| Providing ongoing personnel privacy training | |
| Maintenance of technologies to provide safeguards | |
| Printing, paper, and other notice-related costs | |
| Health plans establishing mechanisms to distribute notices on an ongoing basis (at least every 3 years and when significant changes occur within the notice) | |
| Performing PHI disclosure accounting activities | |
| Archiving and maintaining necessary documentation for at least 6 years | |
| Maintaining, testing, and updating business continuity plans, including backup and recovery facilities and resources | |
| Applying sanctions | |
| Maintaining and upgrading physical safeguards where necessary | |
| Maintaining identity verification mechanisms and practices | |
| Performing mitigation activities | |
| Utilizing alternative communications methods to give individuals copies of their PHI | |
| Updating and correcting PHI in response to individual requests | |
| Reviewing authorizations to ensure their currency | |
| Obtaining and documenting acknowledgment of receipt of notices | |
| Reviewing and updating business associate agreements | |
| Maintaining mechanisms to de-identify PHI | |
| **Other Expenses** | |
| **Total Estimated Costs** | |

However, in larger organizations it will probably be necessary to assign a person to dedicate his entire time to addressing the privacy requirements. AHIMA indicates* the salary range for a privacy officer will be in the $80,000 to $140,000 range.

Use Exhibit 2 to help you plan for and estimate all the various costs related to ongoing Privacy Rule compliance.

## Security Implementation Costs

If you do not have thousands of dollars to completely harden your information systems, fear not. There are plenty of things you can do to secure your PHI that will not break the bank or your budget. Remember, there is no such thing as 100-percent information security and there will always be residual risks. You can, however, implement certain measures to reduce your exposure. The risks identified during your security risk analysis combined with security measures that are already in place will help you determine how much money will be spent on Security Rule compliance. Sure, HIPAA is a set of laws that must be adhered to, but the costs associated with protecting information (i.e., time, effort, and money) cannot exceed the value of the information or the consequences if the information is compromised. Your goal should be to align what is needed to reasonably protect PHI with your overall business objectives.

Do not worry about return on investment (ROI) on technology infrastructure and security spending. You have got to spend money on HIPAA compliance anyway, right? True; just make sure you are spending it wisely. Besides, it is difficult changing the lens through which executives see IT and security investments. They need to see money spent on information security as a business expense or investment — not just another IT expenditure. Why? Because it is a business expense — it is the cost of federal compliance, the cost of reasonably protecting confidential health information, the cost of demonstrating due diligence, and the cost of embracing IT to streamline operations and provider higher-quality healthcare.

As discussed in the final Security Rule, HHS utilized Gartner Group to study the impact changes in the healthcare industry might have on the expected impact of the final Security Rule. Gartner estimated that the cost of implementing the Security Rule standards in 2002 is less than 10 percent higher than it would have been in 1998. They go on to say that the preparation for the Security Rule that many CEs have begun offsets this cost difference, making it essentially the same now as it was in 1998. Gartner also determined that compliance with the Privacy Rule may even slightly reduce the overall cost impact of the Security Rule.

*Available at http://www.healthcare-informatics.com.

A really positive aspect of the Security Rule is its flexibility regarding costs. There are many security standards that are "addressable," meaning that CEs have some flexibility, depending on their specific situation. In addition, there are several information security best practices that can be put in place with relatively little or no cost at all, such as:

- Sending out periodic security reminders
- Applying critical patches
- Using stronger passwords
- Turning on logging functions that are built into existing applications and operating systems

There is specific verbiage in the final Security Rule backing HHS' stance on the flexibility of this final rule:

> *While cost is one factor a covered identity may consider in determining whether to implement a particular implementation specification, there is nonetheless a clear requirement that adequate security measures be implemented...*

> *Our decision to classify many implementation specifications as addressable, rather than mandatory, provides even more flexibility to covered entities to develop cost effective solutions.*

> *...the implementation of these security requirements will reduce the potential overall cost of risk to a greater extent than additional security controls will increase costs.*

> *With respect to security, covered entities will be able to blend security processes now in place with new processes. This should significantly reduce compliance costs.*

You should keep these things in mind when the time comes to budget for and spend money on Security Rule compliance.

If you end up outsourcing some HIPAA initiatives to consultants, systems integrators, or large accounting firms, you can expect to be presented with a wide range of hourly rates. The following estimates will vary, depending on your location and the current state of the economy, but should give you a good idea of what some of the going rates are:

- $50 to $100 per hour for basic computer and network work
- $150 to $225 per hour for highly skilled information security experts
- $275 to $350+ per hour for larger accounting/consulting firms that can provide brand recognition

Exhibit 3 contains the Security Rule implementation activities that will likely involve costs. Use this table to estimate and keep track of your organization's Security Rule implementation costs. Like the privacy costs outlined previously, these estimated costs will vary greatly or in some cases not even apply, depending on your needs.

**Exhibit 3. Estimated Security Rule Implementation Costs**

| Security Rule Implementation Activity | Estimated Cost |
|---|---|
| **Administrative Security Costs** | |
| Performing a security gap analysis to establish your baseline state of Security Rule compliance | |
| Performing a security risk assessment to identify risks to PHI — this may include hiring outside experts to help with penetration testing and vulnerability assessments | |
| Hiring internal information security experts to build up your compliance team | |
| Establishing security incident plans, including specific technologies and external resources/expertise to assist in these efforts | |
| Establishing contingency plans, including backup and recovery systems and facilities and resources such as Uninterruptible Power Supplies (UPS), generators, failover sites, backup devices, and backup media storage and retrieval services | |
| Implementing security awareness reminders such as screen savers, posters, and mouse pads, along with the necessary training programs and materials | |
| Establishing employee sanctions along with the associated HR and legal resources | |
| Reviewing and updating current business associate agreements as necessary | |
| Creating required security policies and their supporting procedures | |
| Establishing resources to archive and maintain necessary documentation relating to Security Rule implementation for at least 6 years | |
| **Physical Security Costs** | |
| Implementing physical safeguards where necessary, including facility access controls such as card readers, biometrics, cameras, and alarm systems | |
| Implementing shredders or other physical media destruction mechanisms | |
| **Technical Security Costs** | |
| Implementing network infrastructure technologies to facilitate confidential data transmission such as VPNs, firewalls, secure e-mail servers, and intrusion-detection systems | |
| Implementing computer and network strong authentication mechanisms, including tokens and biometrics | |

**Exhibit 3. Estimated Security Rule Implementation Costs (Continued)**

| | |
|---|---|
| Implementing encryption systems to ensure confidential data transmission | |
| Implementing secure fax servers and fax machines | |
| Establishing computer and network access control mechanisms such as new operating system upgrades, policy servers, and possibly even routers and firewalls | |
| Establishing computer and network auditing mechanisms, including log monitoring and analysis software | |
| **Other Expenses** | |
| **Total Estimated Costs** | |

## Security Ongoing Maintenance Costs

Once you have implemented the Security Rule requirements, you will also have ongoing maintenance costs to consider. These ongoing costs of delivering secure information services that adhere to the Security Rule and meet your customers' needs must be low enough so that it is not cost-prohibitive to continue with them. Rather than using theoretical models of total cost of ownership (TCO) and ROI that do not always apply in the real world, look at the overall value that these security investments are bringing to your organization. Look at how it not only enables you to be compliant but also makes your business better by enabling newer technologies that can streamline operations and ultimately lower your overall IT costs.

## Security Officer Costs

As with the mandated Privacy Officer position, HIPAA mandates that an individual be assigned as your HIPAA Security Officer for ensuring compliance with the Security Rule. Salaries for this position will vary greatly, depending on the size of the CE and specific needs. Most of the smaller CEs cannot afford to hire a dedicated Security Officer. These CEs will most likely make an existing position, typically the Office Manager, responsible for both privacy and security compliance. This is reasonable in a small environment, especially if most information security services are outsourced. Medium-sized CEs of 50 employees or more might consider hiring a dedicated HIPAA Officer that is responsible for both privacy and security and possibly other areas of IT or operations. Large CEs such as hospitals and health plans will most likely want to have a dedicated Security Officer that focuses solely on security compliance efforts.

Based on various general surveys and job postings, the annual salary ranges for a Security Officer position could vary widely — anywhere from

31

$30,000 to $300,000 and up. This position is new to a lot of healthcare organizations so there are no specific criteria to determine exactly how much the Security Officer should make. As the healthcare industry sees just how important this position is, more-specific salaries and job descriptions will evolve. For comparative purposes, according to study done by Giga Information Group, Security Officers in the financial services industry can expect to make between $125,000 and $400,000 plus bonuses, depending on who they report to within the organization. This will very likely be lower for the healthcare industry, but shows you how important the position is within larger organizations.

Exhibit 4 lists potential activities that will cost money for ongoing maintenance of your Security Rule compliance.

Moving ahead, you should always assess information security purchases in terms of what is the best fit for your organization — you might not be able to afford the best or need the solution with all the whistles and bells. The "best" for others might be the worst for your particular situation. So do not always assume that the highest priced, or even highest rated, security products or services are the best ones for you. Shop around, try stuff out, and always make sure there is some sort of contingency in case the product or service ends up being a bad match. By all means never, ever, make security purchasing decisions based on price alone.

**Chapter 3: Practical Checklist**

- Decide how to staff your Privacy Officer and privacy contact responsibilities.
- Decide how to staff your Security Officer responsibilities.
- Do not position technology expenses required by HIPAA as IT expenses but rather as business expenses.
- Budget for your Privacy Rule implementation activities.
- Budget for your Security Rule implementation activities.
- Budget for your Privacy Rule ongoing and maintenance activities.
- Budget for your Security Rule ongoing and maintenance activities.
- Obtain budget approval.
- Keep track of your Privacy Security Rule related spending.

**Exhibit 4.  Estimated Ongoing HIPAA Security Costs**

| Security Rule Maintenance Activity | Estimated Cost |
|---|---|
| **Administrative Security Costs** | |
| Performing ongoing security gap analyses (recommended every 1 to 2 years) to ensure ongoing compliance with HIPAA | |
| Performing follow-up security risk assessments (recommended at least every year) to identify new risks and ensure previous risks have not reoccurred | |
| Performing risk mitigation activities | |
| Testing and maintaining your security incident plans to ensure they are still viable for new information systems and business changes | |
| Testing and maintaining your contingency plans to ensure they are still viable for new information systems and business changes | |
| Ongoing training costs for personnel, including class and conference registrations, publication subscriptions, and association dues | |
| Reviewing and updating business associate agreements as necessary | |
| Maintaining security policies and their supporting procedures | |
| Establishing resources to archive and maintain necessary documentation relating to Security Rule implementation for at least 6 years | |
| Applying sanctions | |
| Ongoing maintenance of the risk management function | |
| **Physical Security Costs** | |
| Ongoing maintenance of physical safeguards and systems | |
| Management of facility maintenance records | |
| **Technical Security Costs** | |
| Administering and maintaining network infrastructure technologies | |
| Administering and maintaining computer and network authentication mechanisms | |
| Administering and maintaining encryption systems | |
| Administering and maintaining secure fax servers and fax machines | |
| Administering and maintaining computer and network access control mechanisms | |
| Administering and maintaining computer and network auditing mechanisms | |
| **Other Expenses** | |
| **Total Estimated Costs** | |

# Chapter 4
# The Relationship between Security and Privacy

## Background

In many organizations the people responsible for privacy are completely separated from and in entirely different departments from the people responsible for security. Often these departments do not communicate, or even acknowledge or understand the compelling relationship that essentially exists between the two. Too often privacy is considered a purely legal issue, the responsibility for which is often handed to organizational legal counsel. Or, it is ignored altogether as a separate issue, and management assumes it will be addressed by all the various business units during the course of doing business. Security is too often viewed as a purely technical issue, and the responsibility for security is more often than not placed within the information technology or networking support area — often buried beneath several layers of management. And the twain never meets. Security personnel must be actively involved in privacy issues and crafting privacy policies, and privacy personnel must be actively involved in security issues and crafting security policies.

Likewise, with regard to HIPAA, many organizations believe they can treat the HIPAA Privacy Rule and Security Rule as completely separate, independent regulations. Many organizations have created a HIPAA Privacy Rule compliance team and a HIPAA Security Rule compliance team, and unfortunately the two teams do not share any members, nor do they even communicate. It is mistakenly assumed that because the Security Rule only applies to electronic PHI that there will be no overlap with the Privacy Rule, which applies to PHI in electronic form and all other forms. Some organizations are focusing solely on the Privacy Rule and do not plan to start addressing the Security Rule requirements until they are completely finished with the Privacy Rule implementation.

So, to the crux of this topic: how is security different than privacy? It is really pretty simple; you must implement security to ensure privacy. You must use security to obtain privacy. Security is a process, privacy is a consequence. Security is action, privacy is a result of successful action. Security is a condition, privacy is the prognosis. Security is the strategy, privacy is the outcome. Privacy is a state of existence, security is the constitution supporting the existence. Security is a tactical strategy, privacy is a contextual strategic objective. Security is the sealed envelope, privacy is the successful delivery of the message inside the envelope. Rather than digress any further, we will stop the metaphors and assume you understand what we are trying to get across. The bottom line: enterprise privacy management strategies and security management architecture must be effectively and actively integrated.

What is a common mistake an organization can make that can lead to potentially devastating public press, irreversible damage to personal lives, and huge fines and lawsuits? Often when the privacy responsibility lies in a different part of the organization from the security responsibility, or the two areas do not communicate, privacy policy notices are issued, then no security policies, procedures, or mechanisms are implemented to ensure the now-published privacy policies are enforced. These published privacy policies are in effect a contract with your patients, customers, and consumers. The privacy policies are often the first and main point of contact between the public and your organization. If you are telling customers that your organization is performing certain activities to ensure their privacy, you had better well make sure your organizational personnel know what they have committed to, whether or not they were involved with the privacy choices.

Privacy with respect to many of the current legislated regulations, such as HIPAA, means people are able to make informed choices when seeking care and reimbursement for healthcare based on how protected health information (PHI) may be used, or are able to make choices about how their personally identifiable financial information is used and shared by the organizations with which they do business. Privacy enables patients to find out how their information may be used and what disclosures of their information have been made. Privacy enables consumers to find out how financial information is going to be protected and know that the people handling their information have been properly trained to protect their privacy. Privacy limits release of information to the minimum reasonably needed for the purpose of the disclosure. Privacy gives people the right to examine and obtain a copy of their own personal records and request corrections.

Security with respect to these same regulations constitutes those reasonable and prudent policies, processes, steps, and tools that are used to maintain confidentiality and privacy. It involves all methods, processes, and technology used to ensure the confidentiality and safety of the once-private information that has been entrusted to a third party by the customer or patient.

Closely reviewing the HIPAA Privacy Rule and the HIPAA Security Rule reveals many overlaps in requirements. To achieve compliance with all the Privacy Rule requirements you will need to understand and implement many of the Security Rule requirements. If you try to implement the safeguards required within the Privacy Rule without considering the Security Rule, you may end up making more work for yourself in the long run; if you implement a security procedure or mechanism to satisfy a Privacy Rule requirement, but that solution is in contradiction to a Security Rule requirement, you will need to redo the establishment and implementation of that security safeguard — spending precious money, time, personnel resources, etc. — in essence, reinventing the wheel. You should plan to implement the security safeguards required in the Privacy Rule as they are required within the Security Rule.

### Privacy Rule and Security Rule Overlaps

To most effectively achieve HIPAA compliance, you need to understand where the Privacy Rule and Security Rule overlap. The Privacy Rule requires CEs to safeguard all PHI it has, regardless of the form the PHI is in, such as on paper, electronic, or spoken. The Security Rule applies to PHI in electronic form only, a subset of the PHI that the Privacy Rule covers. The Privacy Rule often directs covered entities (CEs) to restrict access to PHI; to implement these multiple directives you must implement security controls. The Privacy Rule also explicitly requires security safeguards. Exhibit 1 lists the significant Privacy Rule statements that specifically require security safeguards.

It should be clear that the Privacy Rule regulations require security to be implemented to achieve compliance; whenever you see the terms "protection" or "safeguards" within the text, think "security." From a topical view, how do security and privacy relate?

### *Appropriate and Reasonable Safeguards*

Both the Privacy Rule and the Security Rule require CEs to evaluate their organizational requirements and needs, and to identify security and privacy protections that are appropriate for their unique environment. In both rules CEs are directed to do a risk analysis to ensure the risk is balanced with the costs of the solutions.

### *Protecting Appropriate Information*

The Privacy Rule requires all individually identifiable information, in any medium, collected and directly used in or documenting healthcare or health status, to be adequately safeguarded. This covers a significant amount of information, many different types of PHI, and can be achieved

### Exhibit 1.  Privacy Rule Statements Requiring Security Safeguards

§ 164.504 Uses and disclosures: organizational requirements

(c)  (2)  Implementation specification: application of other provisions

*Safeguard requirements.* The covered entity that is a hybrid entity must ensure that a healthcare component of the entity complies with the applicable requirements of this subpart. In particular, and without limiting this requirement, such covered entity must ensure that:

(i)  Its healthcare component does not disclose PHI to another component of the covered entity in circumstances in which this subpart would prohibit such disclosure if the healthcare component and the other component were separate and distinct legal entities.

(ii)  A component that is described by paragraph (c)(3)(iii)(B) of this section does not use or disclose PHI that it creates or receives from or on behalf of the healthcare component in a way prohibited by this subpart.

(iii)  If a person performs duties for both the healthcare component in the capacity of a member of the workforce of such component and for another component of the entity in the same capacity with respect to that component, such workforce member must not use or disclose PHI created or received in the course of or incident to the member's work for the healthcare component in a way prohibited by this subpart.

(d)  Standard: affiliated CEs safeguards

(3)  *Implementation specifications:* Safeguard requirements. An affiliated covered entity must ensure that:

(i)  The affiliated covered entity's use and disclosure of PHI comply with the applicable requirements of this subpart.

(ii)  If the affiliated covered entity combines the functions of a health plan, healthcare provider, or healthcare clearinghouse, the affiliated covered entity complies with paragraph (g) of this section.

(e)  (2)  *Implementation specifications:* Business associate contracts. A contract between the covered entity and a business associate must:

(ii)  Provide that the business associate will:

(A)  Not use or further disclose the information other than as permitted or required by the contract or as required by law.

(B)  Use appropriate safeguards to prevent use or disclosure of the information other than as provided for by its contract.

(C)  Report to the covered entity any use or disclosure of the information not provided for by its contract of which it becomes aware.

(D)  Ensure that any agents, including a subcontractor, to whom it provides PHI received from, or created or received by the business associate on behalf of the covered entity agrees to the same restrictions and conditions that apply to the business associate with respect to such information

**Exhibit 1.  Privacy Rule Statements Requiring Security Safeguards (Continued)**

§ 164.514 Other requirements relating to uses and disclosures of PHI

(c) (2) *Security.* The covered entity does not use or disclose the code or other means of record identification for any other purpose, and does not disclose the mechanism for reidentification to another covered entity.

§ 164.530 Administrative requirements

(c) (1) *Standard: Safeguards.* A covered entity must have in place appropriate administrative, technical, and physical safeguards to protect the privacy of PHI.

(2) Implementation specification: Safeguards.

(i) A covered entity must reasonably safeguard PHI from any intentional or unintentional use or disclosure that is in violation of the standards, implementation specifications, or other requirements of this subpart.

(ii) A covered entity must reasonably safeguard PHI to limit incidental uses or disclosures made pursuant to an otherwise permitted or required use or disclosure.

only by incorporating appropriate security procedures and mechanisms in addition to the other tasks involved, such as using the correct forms, using correct wording, notifying appropriate people, etc.

### Mapping PHI Data Flows

Both the Privacy Rule and the Security Rule require CEs to identify their PHI, and to know and understand the flow of PHI through their organizations. Related to this is identifying where PHI comes into their organization, and where it leaves their organization. This encompasses the identification of business associates (BAs) who have access to or process their PHI. In order to identify and implement appropriate security safeguards and procedures, you must know the flow of PHI.

### Access Control and Information Integrity

The Privacy Rule contains many access control requirements, and access controls are fundamentally security mechanisms. For instance, the Privacy Rule requires:

- Role-based access controls to ensure that only appropriate people have access to the minimum necessary PHI to perform their job responsibilities. So, policies and procedures must be created to specify the groups and positions that need access to PHI to perform their job responsibilities, as well as the types of PHI to which they need access. Technological, procedural, and physical security controls will be required to implement and enforce these policies and procedures.

- Safeguards (security) to ensure that the PHI does not get altered or destroyed in an unauthorized manner.
- A formal process for ending a person's employment or a user's access so that inappropriate access to PHI does not occur. This will involve implementing security access controls and mechanisms.
- Consistent, secured control of media (such as papers, diskettes, tapes, laptops, personal digital assistants, CDs, etc.) containing PHI to ensure that unauthorized use or disclosure does not occur.
- Allowing only properly authorized persons to have physical access into your facilities where PHI is stored and resides.
- Definition of the appropriate functions for and locations of workstations to ensure PHI is not inappropriately stored or viewed on a workstation.
- A well-defined change control process to ensure information system changes do not result in the inappropriate use or disclosure of PHI.
- Regular audits of information system activity to ensure that PHI is being used or disclosed only by properly authenticated and authorized persons.
- PHI sent across open systems, such as the Internet, is protected from unauthorized access.

### Assigned Security and Privacy Accountability

The Privacy Rule and the Security Rule both require a specific position or group to be assigned responsibility to appropriately safeguard PHI. Referenced as "Designating a Privacy Official" in the Privacy Rule and as "Assigned Security Responsibility" in the Security Rule, assigning responsibility creates accountability and helps to ensure that a specific position or group is accountable for PHI use and disclosure.

### Policies and Procedures

Both rules require CEs to implement reasonable and appropriate policies and procedures to comply with the standards, specifications, and other requirements. Additionally, both the privacy and security policies and procedures must be documented, maintained, and updated as appropriate, and retained for at least 6 years. The policies and procedures for security and privacy include the following similar issues:

- Identity Verification
- Mitigation of Security Incident Effects
- Risk Analysis
- Background and Security Checks

### Business Associate Agreements

Both rules require CEs to establish agreements between themselves and all other entities with whom PHI is shared to protect the information they exchange. This is to ensure that PHI is safeguarded at all times, even when it is no longer under the CE's direct control. CEs are also expected to periodically verify that the other entities are complying with the agreements. This principle is defined as a Business Associate Contract in both the Privacy Rule and Security Rule.

### Training and Awareness

The Privacy Rule and the Security Rule both require ongoing training for protecting PHI to ensure all personnel understand why they must protect PHI, as well as how they must protect PHI. This is one of the most important aspects of safeguarding PHI.

### Contingency Plans

The Privacy Rule and the Security Rule require contingency plans to ensure that you can effectively respond to incidents and disasters as soon as possible, and ensure the appropriate access and availability of PHI. Develop and implement security incident response procedures so that you can effectively detect, report, and respond to inappropriate use or disclosure of PHI. This includes procedures for handling security incidents at organizations with which your organization has exchanged PHI.

### Compliance Monitoring and Audit

The Privacy Rule and Security Rule require monitoring PHI access, audit activities, and audit logs to verify the appropriate use and disclosure of PHI. Related to this, both rules also require you to maintain an accounting of PHI disclosures and other applicable HIPAA-related documentation for at least 6 years. PHI will continue to be stored increasingly in electronic form. To keep comprehensive track of accounting, you need to develop and implement security policies, procedures, and mechanisms that will track, log, and maintain the use and disclosure of PHI.

### Sanctions

Sanctions, meaning disciplinary actions, are required by both rules. You must document the sanctions in formal policies as well as document evidence that you support and follow the sanctions.

### Individual Rights

**Access and Amendment.** Individuals have rights to access, view, request amendments to, and request restrictions over how their PHI is used. Both rules require that you document these disclosures and any subsequent changes, and maintain the documentation for such access to PHI. Both require, indirectly or specifically, for such access to PHI to be made using secure methods.

**Uses and Disclosures.** The Privacy Rule requires minimum necessary access to PHI. The Security Rule requires administrative, physical, and technical safeguards, all involving access based on minimum requirements as they relate to job responsibilities. Key concepts overlapping between the Privacy Rule and the Security Rule related to this issue include:

- Accounting for Disclosures
- Minimum Necessary
- Restrict Access
- Emergencies

## Conclusion

The Privacy Rule and the Security Rule do not contradict each other, nor are they mutually exclusive of each other. The Security Rule requirements should be used to implement the safeguard requirements of the Privacy Rule. You should not wait until 2005 to start implementing the Security Rule requirements; many of them need to be implemented as soon as possible to contribute to Privacy Rule compliance. Additionally, by starting your Security Rule implementation now, you will have a head start on Security Rule compliance and help to avoid the potential civil suits that could be brought based on the Security Rule and associated noncompliance.

### Chapter 4: Practical Checklist

- You must have security to have privacy.
- The Privacy Rule and the Security Rule are not mutually exclusive. Each rule must be implemented by taking into account the requirements of the other rule.
- Safeguard requirements are basically security requirements.
- Some of the Security Rule requirements must be implemented now to support the Privacy Rule safeguard requirements.
- Do not implement the Privacy Rule without reviewing and understanding the Security Rule.

# Section 1: HIPAA Essentials Quiz

1. What section of HIPAA was designed to help decrease the costs of healthcare administration with the goal of spending that money instead on increasing the quality of healthcare?
   A. Accounting and Budget
   B. Administrative Simplification
   C. Costs and Analysis
   D. Low Price Healthcare

2. What organization is responsible for establishing the HIPAA standards?
   A. CIA
   B. CMS
   C. HHS
   D. FCC

3. HHS reports that if all healthcare entities follow the electronic transaction standards, the healthcare industry will realize what amount of savings over a 10-year period?
   A. $1.2 million
   B. $29.9 billion net
   C. Over $500,000
   D. 42 cents

4. What are the two rules proposed for identifiers?
   A. National Provider Identifier and the National Employer Identifier
   B. Certified Physician Identifier and the Patient Privacy Set
   C. Federated Healthcare Identifier and the Home Health Identifier
   D. National Safety and Privacy Codes and the Employer Regulations Identifier

5. Successful HIPAA change management will involve which of the following?
   A. A large budget
   B. A strong leadership role
   C. A 10-person technical team
   D. Outside consultants

6. Which of the following is one key factor in helping to create a new way of "HIPAA" thinking?
   A. Bribery
   B. Signed contracts
   C. The right software
   D. Persuasion

7. Instilling the proper HIPAA-aware mindset begins with which of the following?
   A. Creating the proper culture
   B. Convincing the patients
   C. Handing out flyers
   D. Online research

8. What is one of the best ways to get buy-in for HIPAA in your organization?
   A. Enforcement of rules
   B. A three-day seminar
   C. Demonstrate the business value
   D. Long-term planning

9. How much are hospitals nationwide planning to spend during the first 5 years to comply with applicable HIPAA laws?
   A. As much as $22 billion
   B. An estimated $400,000
   C. Close to 1 million
   D. Under $50,000

10. Peter Swire, the Chief Privacy Counsel for the administration in the year 2000, projected compliance with which of the following would equate to $6.25 per year for every insured American?
    A. EDI
    B. Privacy Rule
    C. Administrative Simplification Act
    D. Disability Insurance

11. AHIMA indicates the salary range for a privacy officer will be in what range?
    A. $20,000 to $30,000
    B. $8.00 to $12.00 hourly
    C. $80,000 to $140,000
    D. Will vary widely

12. What is a really positive aspect of the Security Rule?
    A. The enforcement deadlines
    B. The lack of technical requirements
    C. The control given to the patients
    D. The flexibility regarding costs and implementation requirements

13. Which of the following best describes security (as opposed to privacy)?
    A. Enables consumers to find out how financial information is going to be protected
    B. Limits release of information to the minimum reasonably needed for the purpose of the disclosure
    C. Is the implementation of reasonable and prudent policies, processes, steps, and tools that are used to maintain confidentiality
    D. Enables patients to find out how their information may be used and what disclosures of their information have been made

14. The Privacy Rule generally does not refer directly to security requirements, but instead uses another term that basically means the same thing as security. Which of the following terms is used to represent all types of security in this way within the Privacy Rule?
    A. Administrative Requirements
    B. Safeguard Requirements
    C. Technical Requirements
    D. Physical Requirements

15. Which of the following is the most apparent difference between the Privacy Rule and the Security Rule?
    A. The Security Rule will cost more to implement
    B. The Privacy Rule applies to international locations
    C. The Security Rule applies only to electronic PHI, and the Privacy Rule applies to PHI in any form
    D. The Security Rule contains very specific technology requirements and vendor specifications, and the Privacy Rule contains only broad requirement specifications

# Section 2
# HIPAA
# Privacy Rule

# Chapter 5
# HIPAA Privacy Rule Requirements Overview

## Background

In today's high-tech and increasingly network-connected world, depending on locking file cabinets alone to protect the privacy of health information is not feasible. In addition to technology challenges, the laws in force to protect patient information have historically been very patchwork and greatly diverse under the large collection of state and federal laws. In the past, patient and health information could be distributed without notice for almost any reason, including those not even related to healthcare or medical treatments. For example, such health information could be passed from an insurer to a lender, who subsequently could deny the person's application for a mortgage or a loan. The health information could even be sent to the person's employer, who could then consider it for making personnel decisions.

By enacting HIPAA, Congress has mandated that organizations must take specific actions to protect personally identifiable health information. HIPAA contains an important section called "Administrative Simplification." Provisions of this section are intended to reduce the costs and administrative burdens of healthcare by standardizing many administrative and financial forms and transactions. Administrative Simplification includes sub-sections on the privacy and security of patient information that mandate standards for safeguarding for physical storage and maintenance, transmission, and access of health information. The privacy requirements are collectively referred to as the Privacy Rule.

The Privacy Rule was passed on April 14, 2001, and updated on August 14, 2002, with compliance required by most health plans and healthcare providers by April 14, 2003. Those entities that do not comply with these regulations will be subject to severe civil and criminal penalties.

---

The information and opinions provided in this book do not constitute or substitute for legal or other professional advice.

The Privacy Rule intends to safeguard protected health information (PHI) by:

- Giving patients more control over their health information
- Setting limitations on the use and release of health records
- Establishing safeguards covered entities (CEs) must implement to protect the privacy of health information
- Holding those in noncompliance responsible through civil and criminal penalties for privacy violations
- Attempting to create a balance between public responsibility for disclosure of some forms of information and the personal information of individual patients
- Giving patients the opportunity to make informed choices when seeking care and reimbursement for care based on considering how personal health information can be used
- Enabling patients to learn how their information can be used along with the disclosures of their information
- Limiting release to only the minimal amount of information needed for required disclosures
- Giving patients the right to examine and correct any mistakes in their personal health records

### Uses and Disclosures

#### *General Rules for PHI Uses and Disclosures*

"Use" means the sharing, employment, application, utilization, examination, or analysis of individually identifiable health information within a CE. "Disclosure" means the release, transfer, provision of access to, or divulging of information outside the entity holding the information.

CEs may use or disclose PHI for living and deceased individuals only under certain conditions, including:

- To the individual about whom the PHI applies
- With individual authorization or other legal agreement
- Generally without individual authorization for treatment, payment, and operations (TPO), with a few exceptions

The Privacy Rule allows disclosure of medical information to parents if state law allows such disclosures. So, even if a minor has a legal right to certain types of medical care without parental consent, the Privacy Rule does not grant the child the right to withhold this information from parents or guardians.

When using, disclosing, or requesting PHI from another CE, reasonable precautions must be implemented to limit PHI access to only those people who need the access to accomplish their valid job responsibilities related to TPO. A CE may create and use aggregate information without authorization if the PHI cannot be connected to a specific individual, in other words ensuring "de-identification" of the individual PHI. De-identification is discussed later in this chapter.

With exceptions related to HMOs and government programs, a CE generally may disclose PHI to a business associate (BA) and allow a BA to create or receive PHI on its behalf if the CE can ensure the BA will provide adequate security over the PHI. The CE must have written documentation showing the evidence of adequate security within agreements or other types of contracts. When communicating PHI in any form, the CE must take measures to ensure the confidentiality of the PHI is maintained. PHI may not be used or disclosed in any way that conflicts with the entity's notice.

### Uses and Disclosures: Organizational Requirements

There will be situations where a CE performs one or more other functions that are not related or covered by the Privacy Rule. Such an organization is referred to within the regulation as a "hybrid entity." (Chapter 1 discusses hybrid entities at more length.) Legally separate CEs can be considered as a single affiliated CE if all of the CEs designated are under common ownership or control. A hybrid entity must ensure that the healthcare component of the organization complies with the Privacy Rule. For example, such a CE must ensure that the healthcare component does not disclose PHI to the other component of the entity in the same manner, as if the other component were distinctly and legally separate.

If a person within a hybrid organization has job responsibilities for both the healthcare component and another aspect of the organization, the person must not disclose PHI within the nonrelated role. To help ensure protection of PHI in this and similar types of situations, CEs must implement policies and procedures to ensure compliance and awareness of the Privacy Rule by all persons working with PHI.

Affiliates and BAs of a CE must also ensure that their use and disclosure of the entity's PHI complies with the Privacy Rule. The Privacy Rule includes model BA contract provisions. With the exception of small health plans, the Privacy Rule gives CEs up to an additional year to change existing contracts, so it is more realistic to renegotiate contracts one or a few at a time instead of all at once.

If a CE knows one of its affiliates or BAs is in violation of the Privacy Rule, then the CE will be considered in noncompliance if it does not take reasonable steps to end the violation. To help ensure such compliance, CEs must ensure that BA contracts clearly establish the permitted and required uses and disclosures of the entity's PHI by the BA. The regulations list specific activities that can and cannot be included within BA contracts. See Chapter 20 for more information.

The following are organizational tasks you need to address for your privacy provisions:

- Amend employee sanctions and disciplinary policies
- Communicate the employee HIPAA obligations
- Apply disciplinary actions for improper use and disclosure of PHI
- Confirm employee awareness and understanding of HIPAA policy
- Appoint a privacy official
- Develop complaint processes and sanctions
- Implement personnel training and awareness programs
- Establish a plan to comply with the minimum necessary requirement
- Implement physical, administrative, and technical safeguards for PHI
- Establish a minimum 6-year records retention policy
- Implement procedures to ensure beneficiary rights
- Ensure the covered plan participants receive the Notice of Privacy Practices (NPP)
- Obtain authorizations as applicable to HIPAA requirements
- If you are going to declare your organization as a hybrid entity, designate in writing the operations that perform covered functions as one or more healthcare components; if you do not do this, your entire organization is subject to the Privacy Rule
- If your organization is affiliated by common ownership or control to another CE, you may designate in writing (including the healthcare components) as a single covered entity for Privacy Rule compliance; you must operate the different covered functions in compliance with the Privacy Rule provisions applicable to those covered functions
- If you are in an organized healthcare arrangement, you can share PHI with others within the organized healthcare arrangements (OHCA) for joint healthcare operations
- If you are a CE with multiple covered functions, you must operate the different covered functions in compliance with the Privacy Rule provisions applicable to those covered functions

### Uses and Disclosures: Consent for TPO

As stated within the original Privacy Rule, a consent agreement was intended to give healthcare providers who have a direct relationship with a patient permission to use and disclose all PHI for performing TPO. The consent purpose was to give permission to that specific provider and not to any other person.

The Privacy Rule as updated on August 14, 2002, no longer requires healthcare providers to obtain a patient's written consent before using or disclosing the patient's PHI to carry out TPO. Prior to passage of the Privacy Rule many healthcare providers routinely obtained a patient's consent for disclosure of information to insurance companies or for other purposes. The Privacy Rule originally mandated such practices by establishing a consistent standard for covered healthcare providers to obtain patient consent for uses and disclosures of PHI to carry out TPO. However, the requirement to obtain a signed consent for uses and disclosures of PHI to carry out TPO was removed in the Privacy NPRM (Notice of Proposed Rulemaking). Patient authorizations are still required to use and disclose information for non-TPO purposes. It is important to note, however, that CEs may still choose to use consents if they believe the use of consents is beneficial to their business organization and environment, if required by their applicable state laws, or if they want to continue their existing consent agreement practices.

If a CE chooses to use consents for use or disclosure of PHI, the consents can be combined with other types of legal documents from the patient if the PHI consent is clearly separated from the other legal permissions, and if it is signed and dated by the individual.

Additional disclosures were allowed within the 2002 Privacy NPRM for certain types of payments and healthcare operations by a second CE. The 2002 Privacy NPRM removed the original restrictions and allows the general sharing of TPO information between healthcare providers concerning a common patient.

### *Uses and Disclosures: Authorization*

As stated earlier, the Privacy Rule allows but does not require a CE to voluntarily obtain patient consent for uses and disclosures of PHI for TPO and to create associated processes that best serve their situation. In contrast, an authorization is more customized, detailed, and specific than a consent agreement. An authorization gives CEs permission to use specified PHI for specified purposes, generally other than TPO, or to disclose PHI to a specified third party. An authorization is required by the Privacy Rule for uses and disclosures of PHI not otherwise allowed by the Privacy Rule. It is critical for CEs to understand that voluntary consent is not sufficient to permit a use or disclosure of PHI unless it also satisfies the Privacy Rules requirements for an authorization.

An authorization is detailed and gives CEs permission to use PHI for the specific purposes listed within the document. These purposes are typically other than for TPO or for disclosing PHI to a third party. An authorization must include a description of the PHI to be used and disclosed, the name of the person authorized to make the use or disclosure, the name of the person to whom the CE may disclose the PHI, an expiration date, and, depending on the situation, the purpose(s) for which the PHI may be used or disclosed. CEs may generally not make authorization a condition for treatment or coverage for an individual, with a few specific exceptions.

Generally, an authorization is required for all purposes that are not part of TPO and are not described as acceptable uses and disclosures that do not require authorization. All CEs must obtain an authorization to use or disclose PHI for these purposes. A provider may have to obtain multiple authorizations from the same patient for different uses or disclosures. For example, an obstetrician may obtain an authorization from a patient for marketing, and need another authorization from the patient to have her participate in a research project.

A few examples of disclosures that require authorization include disclosures to:

- A life insurer for coverage purposes
- An employer of the results of a preemployment physical or lab test
- A pharmaceutical firm for their own marketing purposes

The 2002 Privacy NPRM changes allowed the use of a single type of authorization form to get a patient's permission for a specific use or disclosure that otherwise would not have been permitted under the original Privacy Rule. Patients still need to grant permission in advance for each type of use or disclosure, but the updated rule eliminates the requirement for CEs to use different types of forms to obtain advance permission. The Privacy Rule requires providers to obtain authorization to use or disclose PHI maintained in psychotherapy notes for treatment by persons other than the originator of the notes, for payment, or for healthcare operations purposes.

Generally, an authorization for use or disclosure of PHI cannot be combined with another document to create a compound authorization unless the use or disclosure is for research purposes, related to psychotherapy notes, or if the provider has conditioned treatment, payment enrollment in a health plan, or benefits eligibility according to the specific allowances within the Privacy Rule.

Individuals can revoke, in writing, authorizations at any time, except to the extent that the CE has taken action as a result of the authorization, or if the authorization was a condition of getting insurance coverage.

Here are some points to remember about authorizations:

- A CE must obtain an individual's written authorization for any use or disclosure of PHI that is not for TPO or otherwise permitted or required by the Privacy Rule.
- A CE may not condition TPO or benefits eligibility upon receiving an individual's authorization, except in limited circumstances.

- An authorization must be written in specific terms. It may allow use and disclosure of PHI by the CE seeking the authorization or by a third party.
- Authorizations must be written in plain language, and must contain specific information regarding the information to be disclosed or used, the person(s) disclosing and receiving the information, expiration, right to revoke in writing, as well as other information, depending on the situation.
- The Privacy Rule contains transition provisions applicable to authorizations and other express legal permissions obtained prior to April 14, 2003.
- A CE must obtain an individual's authorization to use or disclose psychotherapy notes, with a few exceptions (discussed later).
- A CE must obtain an authorization to use or disclose PHI for marketing, except for face-to-face marketing communications between a CE and an individual, and for a CE's provision of promotional gifts of nominal value. (No authorization is needed to make a communication that falls within one of the exceptions to the marketing definition, as discussed later.)
- An authorization for marketing must state that the CE is receiving direct or indirect remunerations from a third party, if applicable.

CEs may use and disclose PHI without individual authorization for certain activities. This is a long and detailed list; be sure you discuss these situations and how they apply to your organization with your legal counsel. A general listing of such purposes is shown in Exhibit 1.

### *Uses and Disclosures Requiring Opportunity for the Individual to Agree or Object*

HIPAA allows a CE to use or disclose PHI without the written authorization of the individual in certain situations if the individual is informed in advance of the use or disclosure. Informal permission may be obtained by asking the individual outright, or by circumstances that clearly give the individual the opportunity to agree or object. Where the individual is incapacitated, in an emergency situation, or not available, covered entities generally may make such uses and disclosures, if in the exercise of their professional judgment, the use or disclosure is determined to be in the best interests of the individual.

In general, individuals must be given the opportunity in advance to agree or object to uses and disclosures of PHI in the situations listed in Exhibit 2. The CE may orally inform the individual and obtain oral agreement or objection to use or disclosure.

Individuals may ask a CE to restrict further use and disclosure of PHI (with the exception of uses or disclosures required by law). The CE does

## Exhibit 1.  General Listing of Purposes

PHI may be used and disclosed by CEs without an authorization in the following situations:

- For its own TPO activities.
- For the treatment activities of any healthcare provider.
- For the payment activities of another CE and of any healthcare provider.
- For the healthcare operations of another CE involving either quality or competency assurance activities or fraud and abuse detection and compliance activities, if both CEs have or had a relationship with the individual and the PHI pertains to the relationship.
- For another CE that has, or had, a relationship with the individual.
- For another CE that participates in an organized healthcare arrangement.
- Use and disclosure for health oversight activities.
- Disclosure to coroners and medical examiners.
- Use and disclosure for governmental health data systems.
- Disclosure for facility directory information.
- Disclosure for banking and payment processes.
- Use and disclosure for research as described in the research section of this chapter.
- In emergency circumstances.
- For next-of-kin information.
- As required by other laws.
- For treatment by a CE that originated psychotherapy notes to use them for treatment.
- A CE may use or disclose psychotherapy notes for its own training, and to defend itself in legal proceedings brought by the individual, for HHS to investigate or determine the covered entity's compliance with the Privacy Rules, to avert a serious and imminent threat to public health or safety, to a health oversight agency for lawful oversight of the originator of the psychotherapy notes, for the lawful activities of a coroner or medical examiner, or as required by law.
- Communications to describe health-related products or services, or payment for them provided by or included in a benefit plan of the CE making the communication.
- Communications about participating providers in a provider or health plan network, replacement of or enhancements to a health plan, and health-related products or services available only to a health plan's enrollees that add value to, but are not part of, the benefits plan.
- Communications for treatment of the individual.
- Communications for case management or care coordination for the individual, or to direct or recommend alternative treatments, therapies, healthcare providers, or care settings to the individual.
- To the individual (unless required for access or accounting of disclosures).
- When the opportunity to agree or object provisions (discussed later in this chapter) apply.
- Incidental to an otherwise permitted use and disclosure.
- When disclosure or use of the PHI is for public interest and benefit activities.
- When creating and using a limited data set (discussed later in this chapter) for the purposes of research, public health, or healthcare operations.
- To funeral directors as needed, and to coroners or medical examiners to identify a deceased person, determine the cause of death, and perform other functions authorized by law.

## Exhibit 1.  General Listing of Purposes (Continued)

- To facilitate the donation and transplantation of cadaver organs, eyes, and tissue.
- CEs may disclose PHI that they believe is necessary to prevent or lessen a serious and imminent threat to a person or the public, when such disclosure is made to someone they believe can prevent or lessen the threat (including the target of the threat).
- To law enforcement if the information is needed to identify or apprehend an escapee or violent criminal.
- For certain essential government functions, including assuring proper execution of a military mission, conducting intelligence and national security activities that are authorized by law, providing protective services to the President, making medical suitability determinations for State Department employees, protecting the health and safety of inmates or employees in a correctional institution, and determining eligibility for or conducting enrollment in certain government benefit programs.
- As authorized by, and to comply with, workers' compensation laws and other similar programs providing benefits for work-related injuries or illnesses.
- For quality assurance reviews by authorized authorities.
- For emergencies or concerns affecting public health or safety.
- For suspected abuse of the individual.
- For research with documented authorization waiver approval from the Institutional Review Board (IRB) or Privacy Board.
- For reviews preparatory to research.
- For research on decedent information.
- For government health data and specialized functions.
- For financial institution payment processing for healthcare.
- For utilization review.
- For credentialing.
- When mandated by other laws.
- For other activities that are part of ensuring appropriate TPO.
- To public health authorities authorized by law to collect or receive such information for preventing or controlling disease, injury, or disability and to public health or other government authorities authorized to receive reports of child abuse and neglect.
- To entities subject to FDA regulation regarding FDA-regulated products or activities for purposes such as adverse event reporting, tracking of products, product recalls, and postmarketing surveillance.
- To individuals who may have contracted or been exposed to a communicable disease when notification is authorized by law.
- To employers, regarding employees, when requested by employers, for information concerning a work-related illness or injury or workplace related medical surveillance, because such information is needed by the employer to comply with the Occupational Safety and Health Administration (OSHA), the Mine Safety and Health Administration (MHSA), or similar state law.
- In certain circumstances, to appropriate government authorities regarding victims of abuse, neglect, or domestic violence.
- To health oversight agencies (as defined in the Privacy Rule) for purposes of legally authorized health oversight activities, such as audits and investigations necessary for oversight of the healthcare system and government benefit programs.

## Exhibit 1. General Listing of Purposes (Continued)

- In a judicial or administrative proceeding if the request for the information is through an order from a court or administrative tribunal. Such information may also be disclosed in response to a subpoena or other lawful process if certain assurances regarding notice to the individual or a protective order are provided.
- To law enforcement officials for law enforcement purposes under the following six circumstances, and subject to specified conditions:
  1. As required by law (including court orders, court-ordered warrants, subpoenas) and administrative requests.
  2. To identify or locate a suspect, fugitive, material witness, or missing person.
  3. In response to a law enforcement official's request for information about a victim or suspected victim of a crime.
  4. To alert law enforcement of a person's death, if the covered entity suspects that criminal activity caused the death.
  5. When a covered entity believes that protected health information is evidence of a crime that occurred on its premises.
  6. By a covered healthcare provider in a medical emergency not occurring on its premises, when necessary to inform law enforcement about the commission and nature of a crime, the location of the crime or crime victims, and the perpetrator of the crime.

## Exhibit 2. Uses and Disclosures Requiring Opportunity to Agree or Object

- Disclosure of name, location, general condition, and religion within the entity's facility directory or to clergy or persons asking for the individual by name. The provider may then disclose the individual's condition and location in the facility to anyone asking for the individual by name, and also may disclose religious affiliation to any clergy inquiring about patients with certain religious affiliations.
- Disclosure of medical condition and location to a family member, other relative, or a close personal friend of the individual, or any other person identified by the individual.
- To an individual's family, relatives, friends, or other persons identified by the individual, for notification and other purposes directly relevant to that person's involvement in the individual's care or payment for care. For example, this allows a pharmacist to dispense filled prescriptions to a person acting on behalf of the patient.
- Notifying (including identifying or locating) family members, personal representatives, or others responsible for the individual's care of the individual's location, general condition, or death.
- For notification purposes to public or private entities authorized by law or charter to assist in disaster relief efforts.

not have to agree to such a request. But, if the CE and the individual agree to such a restriction, the CE is then bound by the agreement, even when the agreement is given orally.

It is also important to note that although HIPAA allows CEs to use or disclose PHI in these specific situations, it does not mean the CE must do so. Each entity must decide what is best and what is in compliance with the applicable state laws for each situation and act accordingly.

### Other Requirements Relating to Uses and Disclosures of PHI

The Privacy Rule makes many other requirements for a vast array of situations relating to virtually every conceivable type of PHI use and disclosure. Again, it is important for CEs and their legal counsel to thoroughly review and understand the Privacy Rule and these many sundry requirements. These issues are explored in detail later in this chapter. Following is an overview of the other requirements:

- PHI must be handled in specific ways for de-identification requirements.
- Covered entities must ensure minimum necessary requirements are implemented related to PHI use and disclosure.
- PHI may not be used for marketing purposes without the specified authorizations described within the Privacy Rule.
- A CE may use or disclose demographic information relating to an individual and dates of healthcare provided to an individual for its own fundraising purposes without authorization to a BA or to a related foundation.
- PHI used by a heath plan for underwriting, premium rating, or other activities relating to the creation, renewal, or replacement of a contract of health insurance or health benefits, may not be used or disclosed for any other purpose, except as may be required by law, if such the PHI is not placed with the health plan.
- Before CEs disclose PHI, they must verify the identity and authority of the person requesting the PHI.

### Limited Data Set

A limited data set is PHI that excludes the specific direct identifiers of the individual and the relatives, employers, or household members of the individual as outlined within the Privacy Rule. A CE may use or disclose a limited data set if the recipient of the data set signs a data-use agreement promising specified safeguards for the PHI within the limited data set. A limited data set may only be used for the purposes of research, public health, or healthcare operations. A CE must ensure that anyone using the limited data set agrees to all the same restrictions and conditions specified within the data-use agreement, and the entity must not identify the information or contact the individuals.

If a CE discloses only a limited data set to a BA to carry out a healthcare operations function, the CE satisfies the Privacy Rule requirement to obtain satisfactory assurances from the BA with the data-use agreement. A separate BA agreement is not also necessary. A good example provided by the Department of Health and Human Services (HHS) Office of Civil Rights (OCR) is if a state hospital association receives only limited data sets of PHI from member hospitals for the purposes of conducting and sharing comparative quality analyses with these hospitals, the member hospitals need only have data-use agreements in place with the state hospital association.

- A CE may contract with a BA to create a limited data set the same way it can use a business associate to create de-identified data. The OCR provides another great example: if a researcher needs county data, but the CE's information contains only the postal address of the individual, a BA may be used to convert the CE's geographical information into the form needed by the researcher. Additionally, the CE may hire the intended recipient of the limited data set as the BA for this purpose in accordance with the BA requirements.
- A CE can combine the data-use agreement and BA contract in order to hire the intended recipient of a limited data set to also create the limited data set as a BA. Because the CE is providing the recipient with PHI that includes direct identifiers, a BA agreement is required in addition to the data-use agreement to protect the information. The agreement must require the recipient to return or destroy the information that includes the direct identifiers once it has completed the conversion for the CE.

### Fundraising

When a CE does fundraising for its own benefit, it is defined as part of the CE's healthcare operations. A CE may use or disclose the demographic information and date of healthcare for an individual to a BA or an institutionally related foundation for the purpose of it own fundraising efforts for mailings and similar communications. An authorization is not necessary in these types of situations. However, the individual must be given the opportunity to opt out of receiving any further types of communications.

The Department of Health and Human Services (HHS) does not define demographic information within the Privacy Rule but indicates that for the purpose of fundraising it generally includes name, address and other contact information, age, gender, and insurance status. HHS further clarifies the meaning of demographic information and the use of non-demographic information in fundraising as follows:

- In the final rule, HHS limits the information that can be used or disclosed for fundraising, and excludes information about diagnosis, nature of services, or treatment.
  a. *Permissible Information.* [Note: There is no regulatory source for this advice, other than the Preamble to the 2000 Final Rule.]

Protected health information that can be utilized for fundraising purposes without obtaining a patient's authorization includes:
- Date of Service [45 CFR § 164.514(f)(1)]
- Demographic Information [45 CFR § 164.514(f)(1) (all of the above are discussed as "demographic information" in the Preamble) to the 2000 Final Rule]
- Name
- Address
- Other contact information (phone numbers, e-mail, etc.)
- Age
- Gender
- Insurance status

b. *Impermissible Use and Disclosure.* PHI that cannot be used without a patient first signing an authorization includes:
- Diagnosis
- Nature of services
- Treatment
- Place within healthcare provider where patient receives treatment that identifies the treatment, such as:
  - Department of Psychiatry
  - Department of Obstetrics
  - Department of Radiation Oncology

c. *Questionable Use and Disclosure.* Although not discussed in the regulations or any of the Preambles to the proposed or adopted regulations, a covered entity may be able to use information about the department in which the patient was treated to filter patient names for fundraising purposes if the department name does not identify the type or nature of treatment. For example, when a patient is treated by the medical/surgery or another type of general department, using or disclosing this information for fundraising filtration purposes would not appear to reveal the diagnosis or nature of the services or treatment received by the affected individuals, and would appear to fit within the minimum necessary information to accomplish the goal: fundraising.

- Implement policies to ensure that fundraisers receive only limited PHI, while allowing them to request some other department of the healthcare provider to review patient PHI to ensure that data received fits within the limitation. Using procedures to ensure that individuals with access to PHI limit the information given to fundraisers to only that which is appropriate should be consistent with the responsibility of the healthcare provider to use reasonable efforts to limit use of PHI to the minimum necessary to accomplish the task.
- Always keep in mind that the Privacy Rule does not preempt state laws that are more restrictive than HIPAA, or other federal laws. So, while HIPAA permits limited disclosure of healthcare provider directory

information, other federal laws may prohibit a healthcare provider from even responding to an inquiry about a patient receiving treatment for substance abuse, and applicable state laws on the privacy of medical records must be considered by the fundraising entity. However, in most cases the most common information used for fundraising (name, age, gender, date of treatment, and address) can be used safely for fundraising efforts. See Chapter 8 for full discussion of state preemption issues.

## Underwriting Purposes

When a health plan receives PHI for the purpose of underwriting, premium rating, or other activities relating to the creation, renewal, or replacement of a health insurance contract or health benefits, and if such health insurance or health benefits are not placed with the health plan, the health plan may not use or disclose the PHI for any other purpose, except as may be required by law. Prior to any disclosure of PHI, a CE must verify the identity of a person requesting PHI and validate their authority to access the PHI. The CE must also obtain any documentation, statements, or representations, whether oral or written, from the person requesting the PHI when it is a condition of the disclosure.

## Public Health

The Privacy Rule allows but does not require CEs to share PHI with public health authorities that are authorized by law to collect the information when necessary to protect the health of the public. A CE may disclose PHI for public health activities and purposes to:

- A public health authority authorized by law to collect or receive PHI for the purpose of preventing or controlling disease, injury, or disability. Such activities include, but are not limited to, reporting disease, injury, vital events such as birth or death, and the conduct of public health surveillance, public health investigations, and public health interventions. The activities may also be directed by a public health authority to a foreign government agency official acting in collaboration with a public health authority.

- A public health authority authorized by law to receive reports of child abuse or neglect.

- A person who may have been exposed to a communicable disease or may otherwise be at risk of contracting or spreading a disease or condition, if the CE or public health authority is authorized by law to notify such a person as necessary in the conduct of a public health intervention or investigation.

## Research

Research is not considered TPO under the Privacy Rule. Therefore, unless an exception applies, as listed earlier, authorizations are generally required for use or disclosure of PHI for research purposes. These authorizations may be combined with any other type of written permission for the same research study, including other authorizations for the use or disclosure of PHI or consents to participate in such research. Healthcare providers may also condition the provision of research-related treatment on receipt of a prior authorization for the use or disclosure of PHI.

While this seems very restrictive, there are many ways PHI may be obtained for research purposes. For instance, CEs may use or disclose PHI for research regardless of funding, when they obtain documentation that a waiver of the individual authorization required for use or an institutional review board (IRB) or a privacy board has approved disclosure of PHI. CEs may also use or disclose PHI if a researcher demonstrates that the PHI is necessary to prepare a research protocol, or if the researcher demonstrates the PHI is needed exclusively for research on decedents.

Limited data sets are applicable to PHI for research. Limited data sets are similar to de-identified data sets except they have 15 identifiers removed instead of 18. Limited data sets may include the following identifiers: date of birth; dates of hospital admissions and discharges; and an individual's residence by city, county, state, and five-digit zip codes. Researchers using PHI via limited data sets must enter into data-use agreements with CEs. These researchers may serve as BAs to CEs, however, and create limited data sets from fully identifiable health information.

Accounting is not required when PHI is disclosed to researchers pursuant to an authorization or as part of a limited data set. Research performed under IRB or privacy board waivers, reviews in preparation for research, or research on decedents are subject to accounting requirements for disclosures. Research disclosures prior to the regulatory compliance date of April 14, 2003, are not subject to the accounting requirement.

A CE needs to accomplish one of the following to use PHI for research purposes:

- Obtain documentation that an alteration or waiver of the authorization for the use or disclosure of PHI about an individual for research purposes has been approved by an Institutional Review Board or Privacy Board.
- Obtain documented representations from the researcher that the use or disclosure of the protected health information is solely to prepare a research protocol or for similar purpose preparatory to research, that the researcher will not remove any protected health information from the covered entity, and that protected health information for which access is sought is necessary for the research.

- Obtain documented representations from the researcher that the use or disclosure sought is solely for research on the protected health information of decedents, that the protected health information sought is necessary for the research, and, at the request of the covered entity, documentation of the death of the individuals about whom information is sought.
- A CE may use or disclose a limited data set of PHI or de-identified information for research purposes without authorization. See the section on limited data sets in this chapter for more information.

What should you consider if you do research with PHI?

- Obtain an authorization whenever possible to use or disclose PHI for research protocols.
- Authorizations should be combined with informed consent documents if you use them.
- Consider using de-identified PHI and limited data sets. They do not need IRB/privacy board approval and have no accounting requirement. Limited data sets require data-use agreements between researchers and CEs.

### *Workers' Compensation*

Unless they are also CEs, the Privacy Rule does not apply to workers' compensation insurers, workers' compensation administrative agencies, or employers. Regardless, these entities need access to individuals' health information to process workers' compensation claims and to coordinate care under workers' compensation systems. This information is typically obtained from the healthcare providers treating the individuals. The Privacy Rule likely covers these providers. The Privacy Rule recognizes the need of insurers and other entities involved in the workers' compensation systems to have access to individuals' health information as authorized by state or other applicable laws. Because of the vast differences between these other laws, the Privacy Rules allow disclosures of health information for workers' compensation purposes in a number of different ways that tend to vary depending upon the type of organization. These issues are explored in more detail in Section 4, Covered Entity Issues.

### Incidental Uses and Disclosures

The nature of many customary healthcare communications and practices and the various environments in which individuals receive healthcare create the potential for health information to be disclosed incidentally. However, these types of communications are often necessary to ensure prompt healthcare treatment. For example, someone visiting in a hospital may overhear the physician's confidential discussion with a patient in the same room. The Privacy Rule was written so it would not prevent these customary communications. The Privacy Rule does not require that 100 percent of all risks of incidental use or disclosure be eliminated; this would be impractical. The Privacy Rule allows certain incidental uses and disclosures of PHI if there are reasonable safeguards and minimum necessary policies and procedures in place to protect an individual's privacy to the greatest possible practical extent.

The Privacy Rule permits certain incidental uses and disclosures that occur as a result of other acceptable uses or disclosures if reasonable safeguards have been implemented according to the minimum necessary standard. Safeguards cannot guarantee the privacy of PHI from all potential risks. Reasonable safeguards depend on many factors, such as size, location, nature of the business, etc. What are considered reasonable safeguards will vary from organization to organization. An incidental use or disclosure is a secondary use or disclosure that cannot reasonably be prevented as a result of an acceptable use or disclosure, and is limited in nature. An incidental use or disclosure is not permitted if it results from a violation of the Privacy Rule.

Here are some examples of reasonable safeguards CEs should consider implementing:

- Speak quietly when discussing a patient's condition with family members in a public area such as a waiting room.
- Avoid using patients' full names in public locations, such as elevators and public hallways.
- Post signs reminding employees to protect patient privacy.
- Physically isolate or lock file cabinets or records rooms.
- Secure workstations and computers containing personal information by requiring passwords and the other security mechanisms as detailed in this book.

## Minimum Necessary

The minimum necessary requirement is based on the premise that PHI should not be used or disclosed when it is not necessary to perform job responsibilities or healthcare-related activities. Covered entities need to examine and evaluate their health information handling practices to meet the minimum necessary requirements to ensure safeguards exist to limit unnecessary or inappropriate access to PHI.

Covered entities must take reasonable actions to limit the use and disclosure of PHI to the minimum necessary to accomplish a necessary task. The minimum necessary requirement does not apply to the following situations:

- Disclosures to or requests by a healthcare provider for treatment purposes
- Disclosures to the individual who is the subject of the information

- Uses or disclosures made with an individual's authorization
- Uses or disclosures required for compliance with HIPAA
- Disclosures to HHS for Privacy Rule enforcement purposes
- Uses or disclosures required by other law

The Privacy Rule requirements necessitate the development and implementation of policies and procedures appropriate for each CE's own unique organization, business practices, and personnel. Use the following guidance to help develop the policies and procedures necessary for your organization. Chapter 7 describes two important policies you must create, and Appendix B provides a few sample policies.

- Develop and implement policies and procedures that identify the persons, positions, groups, or departments who need access to PHI to perform job responsibilities, and the conditions appropriate for the access. For example, hospitals may implement policies that permit doctors, nurses, or others involved in treatment to have access to the entire medical record, as needed. Where the entire medical record is necessary, the CE's policies and procedures must state so explicitly and include a justification.
- Develop criteria for determining and limiting the disclosure of PHI necessary for nonroutine disclosures and requests to only the minimum amount to accomplish the purpose. Nonroutine disclosures and requests must be reviewed on an individual basis in accordance with these criteria and limited accordingly.
- Standard protocols for routine or recurring requests and disclosures must limit the PHI disclosed or requested to the minimum necessary for that particular type of disclosure or request. Individual review of each disclosure or request is not required.
- The Privacy Rule permits a CE to rely on the judgment of the requester to be asking for the minimum amount of information necessary in the following circumstances:
  - A public official or agency who states that the information requested is the minimum necessary for a purpose permitted, such as for public health purposes
  - Another CE
  - A workforce member or BA of the CE holding the information and who indicates the information requested is the minimum necessary for the stated purpose
  - A researcher with appropriate documentation from an Institutional Review Board (IRB) or Privacy Board [Note: The Privacy Rule does not require disclosure or use under these circumstances. It is still at the determination of the CE to make the minimum necessary determination for disclosures it makes and to which the standard applies]

- Implement policies and procedures that limit how much PHI is used, disclosed, and requested for certain purposes. These must limit who within the entity has access to PHI, and under what conditions, based on job responsibilities and the nature of the business.
- Uses and disclosures that are authorized by the individual are exempt from the minimum necessary requirements.
- The Privacy Rule does not prohibit the use, disclosure, or request of an entire medical record; and a CE may use, disclose, or request an entire medical record without a case-by-case justification, if the CE has documented in its policies and procedures that the entire medical record is the amount reasonably necessary for certain identified purposes. For uses, the policies and procedures would identify those persons or classes of person in the workforce that need to see the entire medical record and any conditions that are appropriate for such access. Policies and procedures for routine disclosures and requests and the criteria used for nonroutine disclosures and requests would identify the circumstances under which disclosing or requesting the entire medical record is reasonably necessary for particular purposes.

The minimum necessary standard does not apply to the following situations:

- Disclosures to or requests by a healthcare provider for treatment purposes
- Disclosures to the subject of the information
- Uses or disclosures made pursuant to an individual's authorization
- Uses or disclosures required for compliance with the HIPAA Rules
- Disclosures to HHS when disclosure of information is required under the Privacy Rule for enforcement purposes
- Uses or disclosures that are required by other laws

### Reasonable Reliance

There are certain circumstances where the Privacy Rule permits a CE to rely on the judgment of the requester as to the minimum amount of information that is needed. These circumstances are called reasonable reliance, and must be reasonable under the particular circumstances of the request. Reasonable reliance is allowed for requests made by:

- A public official or agency that indicates that the information requested is the minimum necessary for a purpose permitted under the Privacy Rule, such as for public health purposes
- Another covered entity
- A professional who is a workforce member BA of the CE holding the information and who states that the information requested is the

minimum necessary for the stated purpose of providing services to or for the CE

- A researcher with appropriate documentation from an Institutional Review Board (IRB) or Privacy Board

The Privacy Rule does not require reasonable reliance allowances. A CE may make its own minimum necessary determination for disclosures to which the standard applies.

## De-Identification

Covered entities can generally use de-identified information for any of their healthcare purposes without seeking authorization or other agreements. De-identified information is health information that does not identify a specific individual, so there is no reasonable basis to believe that the information can be used to identify an individual. De-identified information is not necessarily anonymous information. The purpose of de-identification is to ensure there is a reasonable and feasible balance between the risks of identifying individuals using the information and the usefulness of the information.

Covered entities must remove the following pieces of information from a designated record set to de-identify the PHI:

- Name
- Geographic subdivisions smaller than a state
- Dates (excluding year) of:
  - Birth
  - Admission
  - Discharge
  - Death
- Telephone number
- Fax number
- E-mail address
- Social Security number
- Medical records numbers
- Health plan beneficiary numbers
- Account numbers
- License and certificate numbers
- Vehicle identifiers (such as license plate number)
- Device identifiers (such as serial numbers)
- URLs (Internet Universal Resource Locators)
- Internet Protocol (IP) address
- Biometric identifiers (such as finger and voice prints)
- Full face photographic images (and any comparable images)
- Other unique identifiers that can be attributed to a specific individual

A CE may need to modify the data set even more if the CE believes the information could still be used to identify the individual after the eighteen items are removed.

Removing the 18 items and any further information as previously indicated is commonly referenced as the "Safe Harbor" method of de-identification. Age is allowed in de-identified information; however, all dates that might be directly related to the individual must be removed or aggregated to the level of year to prevent the determination of birth date because this could be used to help identify an individual. The Safe Harbor method does not allow a month or day of any date, so does not allow for judgment calls about what to include in a data set based on what may or may not be deduced from the data.

## Business Associates

A BA is a person or business that performs a function or activity for a CE involving the use or disclosure of PHI. This includes claims processing and administration; data analysis, processing or administration; utilization reviews, quality assurance; billing; benefits management; practice management; repricing; or any other activity HIPAA covers. A BA is also a person, not a member of the CE's workforce, who provides legal, actuarial, accounting, consulting, data aggregation, management, administrative, accreditation, or financial services for a CE or for an organized healthcare arrangement in which the CE participates, and where the service involves the disclosure of PHI. A CE may be a BA of another CE. Chapter 20 discusses BA issues at length.

## Marketing

Covered entities generally cannot conduct marketing of health-related products and services without authorization from the patient. Covered entities need to scrutinize and thoroughly assess their marketing plans to determine whether their current marketing activities or plans are in compliance with the HIPAA Privacy Rule.

The Privacy Rule distinguishes marketing communications from communications about goods and services that are necessary for quality healthcare. The Privacy Rule defines marketing as "a communication about a product or service that encourages recipients of the communication to purchase or use the product or service." This definition of marketing has certain exceptions. A communication is not marketing if it is made:

- To describe a health-related product or service (or payment for such product or service) that is provided by, or included in a plan of benefits of, the CE making the communication
- For treatment of the individual

**Exhibit 3. HHS Marketing Advice**

The following are examples of marketing communications that require authorization:
- A communication from a health insurer plan to subscribers informing them about a clinic that can provide a physical for $39.
- A communication from a health insurer promoting a mortgage product offered by the same parent company.
- A health plan selling a list of its members to a company that plans to send the members brochures advertising the benefits of purchasing and using their blood pressure monitors.
- A health plan receiving remuneration from a drug manufacturer for sending it a list of plan members who have made claims for antidepressant medication, then the drug manufacturer sends coupons for their drugs directly to the listed plan members.

- For case management or care coordination for the individual, or to direct or recommend alternative treatments, therapies, healthcare providers, or settings of care to the individual

The Privacy Rule defines marketing as "a communication about a product or service that encourages recipients of the communication to purchase or use the product or service." A CE can only make a marketing communication if the CE first obtains an individual's authorization. There are some exceptions to this rule. The HHS Web site (Appendix C) has some very good information providing guidance for marketing compliance with HIPAA. Exhibit 3 highlights some of HHS' marketing advice.

Marketing also means "an arrangement between a CE and any other entity whereby the CE discloses PHI to the other entity, in exchange for direct or indirect remuneration, for the other entity or its affiliate to make a communication about its own product or service that encourages recipients of the communication to purchase or use that product or service." There are no exceptions to this part of the marketing definition. Basically, a CE may not sell PHI to a BA or any other third party for its own purposes. Additionally, health plans may not sell lists of enrollees to third parties without obtaining authorization from each person on the list.

There are three categories of exceptions to the Privacy Rule marketing definition:

1. A communication is not marketing if it is made to describe a health-related product or service, or payment for the product or service, which is provided by, or included in the plan of benefits of, the CE making the communication. These include communications about:
   - CEs participating in a health plan network
   - Replacement of, or enhancements to, a health plan
   - Health-related products or services available only to a health plan member that add value to, but are not part of, the plan benefits

This exception allows a CE to make communications about its own healthcare related products or services. A few examples of when communications are not marketing include:

- When a health plan uses its subscriber list to announce the addition of new physicians within the approved preferred providers

- When a health plan sends a mailing to subscribers nearing Medicare-eligible age with information about its Medicare supplemental plan and an application form

2. A communication is not marketing when it is made for treatment of the individual. For example, it is not marketing when:

- A pharmacy or other healthcare provider mails prescription refill reminders to patients, or contracts with a mailing service to do so

- A primary care physician refers an individual to a specialist for a follow-up test or provides free samples of a prescription drug to a patient

3. A communication is not marketing when it is made for case management or care coordination for the individual, or to tell or recommend alternative treatments, therapies, healthcare providers, or care facilities to the individual. For example, it is not marketing when:

- An endocrinologist shares a patient's medical record with several behavior management programs to determine which program best suits the ongoing needs of the individual patient

- A hospital social worker shares medical record information with various nursing homes in the course of recommending that the patient be transferred from a hospital bed to a nursing home

For each of these three categories of exceptions, the activity being considered must also be permissible under the Privacy Rule, and a CE can use a BA to make the communication. The CE must obtain the BA's agreement to use the PHI only for the communication activities of the CE, which follows the other BA requirements.

A communication does not require an authorization, even if it is marketing, if it occurs during a face-to-face communication between the CE and an individual, or if it is a promotional gift of nominal value provided by the CE. For example, no prior authorization is necessary when:

- A hospital provides a free sample of formula or other baby products to new mothers leaving the maternity ward

- An insurance agent sells a health insurance policy in person to a customer and also discusses (markets) a casualty and life insurance policy

## Notice of Privacy Practices for PHI

Health plans and healthcare providers must provide individuals a notice document specifying their information use and disclosure practices. The notice must include information describing how the information is protected, stored, used, and the conditions under which is it shared. More specifically, the notice must:

- Contain the following statement, prominently displayed:
  THIS NOTICE DESCRIBES HOW MEDICAL INFORMATION ABOUT YOU MAY BE USED AND DISCLOSED AND HOW YOU CAN GET ACCESS TO THIS INFORMATION. PLEASE REVIEW IT CAREFULLY
- Contain a description, including at least one example, of the types of uses and disclosures that the CE is permitted to make for TPO
- Contain separate statements if the entity will use PHI for appointment reminders, information about treatment alternatives, to raise funds for the entity, in information sent to the HMO or health insurance insurers
- Contain a statement that the individual may revoke or restrict authorization for the CE to use PHI
- Describe the patient's right to inspect and copy PHI
- Describe the patient's right to amend PHI
- Describe the patient's right to receive an accounting of PHI disclosures and make formal complaints
- Contain a statement that the CE is required by law to maintain the privacy of PHI
- Contain the name, or title, and telephone number of a person or office to contact for further information regarding the handling of PHI
- Be made available at enrollment, within 60 days of a material revision to the notice, and not less than every 3 years

A CE must revise and distribute its notice without delay whenever there is a material change to the uses or disclosures, the individual's rights, the CE's legal duties, or other privacy practices stated in the notice. Except when required by law, a material change to any part of the notice cannot be implemented prior to the effective date of the notice in which such material change is reflected.

If a CE provides information about its customer services or benefits on a Web site, it must prominently post the notice on the Web site in addition to allowing requests for the notice from the Web site. The requested notice can be sent by e-mail if the requestor agrees to this type of response. If the CE knows that an e-mail transmission failed, a paper copy of the notice must be sent to the individual. Covered entities must document compliance with the notice requirements by retaining all copies of the issued notices.

Keep the following points in mind with regard to your NPP:

- Each health plan and healthcare provider that is a CE must have an NPP.
- The NPP must contain the elements previously listed.
- A covered healthcare provider with a direct treatment relationship with individuals must deliver the NPP to patients starting April 14, 2003, as described in Chapter 16.
- All CEs must give an NPP to anyone on request.
- A CE must post the NPP on any Web site it maintains for customer service or benefits information.
- CEs in an OHCA may use a joint NPP, as long as each agrees to abide by the NPP content with respect to the PHI created or received in connection with participation in the OHCA.
- Distribution of a joint NPP by any CE participating in an OHCA arrangement at the first point that an OHCA member has an obligation to provide notice satisfies the distribution obligation of the other participants in the OHCA.
- A health plan must distribute its NPP to each enrollee by the Privacy Rule compliance date. Following this, the health plan must give the NPP to each new enrollee at enrollment, and send a reminder to every enrollee at least once every 3 years that the NPP is available upon request. A health plan satisfies the distribution obligation by giving the NPP to the "named insured," or subscriber, for coverage that also applies to spouses and dependents. See Chapter 18 for further discussion.
- A covered healthcare provider with a direct treatment relationship with individuals must make a good-faith effort to obtain written acknowledgment from patients of receipt of the NPP. The Privacy Rule does not describe particular content for the acknowledgment. However, the provider must document the reason for any failure to obtain the patient's written acknowledgment in such situations. Providers do not need to request acknowledgment in emergency treatment situations.

See Chapter 7, Writing Effective Privacy Policies, for further discussion of the NPP.

## Individual Rights to Request Privacy Protection for PHI

Covered entities must permit an individual to request restrictions for uses or disclosures of PHI about the individual to carry out TPO and other disclosures. A CE is not required to agree to a restriction request. However, if the entity agrees to a restriction, then the entity is then bound to comply with the restriction for that individual except for emergency situations and as required by other laws. A CE may terminate its agreement to a restriction if:

- The individual agrees to or requests the termination in writing
- The individual orally agrees to the termination and the oral agreement is documented
- The CE informs the individual that it is terminating its agreement to a restriction. The termination is only effective with respect to PHI created or received after it has informed the individual.
- Covered healthcare providers must permit individuals to request and must accommodate reasonable requests by individuals to receive communications of PHI from the covered healthcare provider by alternative means or at alternative locations if the individual indicates that disclosure of all or part of the PHI could endanger the individual. For example, an individual may request that a CE communicate using a method other than through the use of the telephone or a specific telephone number; perhaps through a specific mailing address or alternate phone number. An individual may also request CEs to send printed communications in sealed envelopes instead of on a postcard. Health plans must also accommodate reasonable requests from individuals indicating that disclosure of all or part of the PHI could put them in danger. A health plan may not question the individual's statement of endangerment. All CEs may condition compliance with a confidential communication request on the individual specifying an alternative address or method of contact and explaining how any payment will be handled.

### Individual Access to PHI

An individual generally has a right to access, inspect, and obtain a copy of his or her own PHI in a CE's designated record set for as long as the PHI is maintained. The designated record set is the group of records maintained by or for a CE that is used, in whole or part, to make decisions about individuals, or that is a provider's medical and billing records about individuals or a health plan's enrollment, payment, claims adjudication, and case or medical management record systems. There are a few exceptions, including:

- Psychotherapy notes
- Information that is, or could be used for, a civil, criminal, or administrative action or legal proceeding
- PHI that is subject to access prohibitions described in the Clinical Laboratory Improvements Amendments (CLIA) of 1988
- PHI held by certain research laboratories

A CE can deny an individual access to PHI without providing an opportunity for review under certain circumstances. For instance, providers for correctional institutions can deny an inmate's request to access PHI if it could jeopardize the health, safety, security, custody, or rehabilitation of the individual or of other inmates, or the safety of any officer, employee, or other person at the correctional institution or responsible for the transporting of the inmate. Access can also be denied if the healthcare professional believes the access could cause harm to the individual or some other person. The individual can also be denied access if the PHI was used for research that does not allow such access, if the access is subject to the denial of access requirements within the Privacy Act, or if the PHI was obtained from another provider with the condition the PHI cannot be given to anyone else.

Individuals have the right to have such denials reviewed by a licensed healthcare professional designated by the CE to act as a reviewing official. The reviewer must be someone who did not participate in the original decision to deny. Such circumstances include:

- Access is likely to endanger the life or physical safety of the individual or another person
- The PHI references another person and the access would likely cause substantial harm to the other person
- The request for access is made by the individual's personal representative and access to the individual's PHI is likely to cause substantial harm to the individual or another person

A CE must provide or deny an access request in writing generally no later than 30 days after receipt of the request for PHI it maintains on-site, and generally no later than 60 days for PHI maintained offsite. If a denial, it must explain, in plain language, the basis for the denial, and if applicable, the individual's review and complaint rights. The CE must provide the individual with access to the protected health information in the form requested by the individual if it already exists in the form, or, if it does not, in another form agreed to by the CE and the individual. When providing an individual a copy of PHI, the CE may impose a reasonable, cost-based fee, provided that the fee includes only the costs of copying, postage, and preparing an explanation or summary.

If a CE does not maintain the PHI requested but knows where it is maintained, it must inform the individual where to direct the request for access. A CE must document the PHI files that are subject to access by individuals, in addition to the titles of the persons or offices responsible for receiving and processing individual requests for access.

### Amendment of PHI

The CE must permit an individual to request amendment to PHI maintained in a designated record set. The CE may require the requests to be in writing and require a reason to support a requested amendment. A CE must accept requests to amend PHI for individuals for as long as it maintains PHI records. A CE can deny an individual's amendment request if the PHI was not created by the CE (unless the originator of PHI is no longer available), if the PHI is not part of the designated record set, or if the PHI is determined to be accurate and complete.

A CE must make the requested amendment, or deny the amendment, no later than 60 days after receipt of the amendment request. If the CE denies in part or in whole the requested amendment, the entity must give the individual a written denial. If the CE is unable to act on the amendment within 60 days, the CE can extend the time to take action by no more than 30 days, provided the entity gives the individual a written statement of the reasons for the delay and the date by which action will be completed on the request. The CE can have only one extension of time for action on a request for an amendment.

If the CE accepts the requested amendment, in whole or in part, the entity must make the appropriate amendment to the PHI by, at a minimum, identifying the records that are affected by the amendment, and appending or otherwise providing a link to the location of the amendment. Then the CE must inform the individual that the amendment is accepted and obtain the individual's identification of and agreement to have the entity notify the relevant persons with which the amendment needs to be shared. Notice of the amendment must be made to persons identified by the individual as having received PHI about the individual and needing the amendment, and all persons that the CE knows have the PHI that is the subject of the amendment.

If the CE denies the requested amendment, it must provide the individual with a written denial. The denial must describe the basis for the denial in plain language and describe the individual's right to submit a written statement disagreeing with the denial. The denial must also state that if the individual does not submit a statement of disagreement, the individual may request the CE provide the individual's request for amendment and the denial with any future disclosures of the PHI, and a description of how the individual can submit formal complaints. The description must include the name, or title, and telephone number of the designated contact person or office.

A CE must permit the individual to submit a written statement disagreeing with a denial of a requested amendment describing the basis of the disagreement, and the entity can prepare a written rebuttal to the individual, but this is not a required action. Whenever a rebuttal is prepared, the CE must provide a copy to the individual who submitted the statement of disagreement. The CE must also identify the PHI that is the subject of the disputed amendment and amend it with information regarding the individual's request for amendment, related denial, and any resulting statement of disagreement and rebuttal. These amendments must then be included with any subsequent PHI disclosures related to the disagreement.

A CE that is informed by another CE of an amendment to an individual's PHI must amend the PHI in designated record sets. A CE must document and retain the titles of the persons or offices responsible for receiving and processing requests for amendments.

## Accounting Disclosures of PHI

An individual generally has a right to receive an accounting of disclosures of PHI made by a CE and the CE's BAs in the 6 years prior to the date on which the accounting is requested. The exceptions to this include accounting of disclosures:

- To carry out TPO
- To individuals of PHI about them
- To the personal representatives of individuals
- For notification of or to persons involved in an individual's healthcare or payment for healthcare
- For disaster relief
- For the facility's directory or to persons involved in the individual's care or other notification purposes
- For national security or intelligence purposes
- To correctional institutions or law enforcement officials for certain purposes regarding inmates or individuals in lawful custody
- That occurred prior to the compliance date for the CE
- For incidental disclosures
- For disclosures made pursuant to an authorization
- For limited data sets

The CE must temporarily suspend an individual's right to receive an accounting of disclosures to a health oversight agency or law enforcement official if the agency or official indicates in writing that such an accounting to the individual would impede the agency's activities.

If, during the period covered by the accounting, the CE has made multiple disclosures of PHI to the same person or entity for a single purpose, the accounting may include the number of the disclosures made during the accounting period and the date of the last disclosure during the accounting period.

A CE must act on the individual's request for an accounting no later than 60 days after receipt of the request. The action must either be providing the individual with the accounting requested, or a written statement explaining the reason for delay. If there is a delay, the time can be extended no more than 30 days, and the CE must provide the individual a written statement explaining the reasons for the delay and the date by which the CE will provide the accounting.

The CE must provide the first accounting to an individual in any 12-month period without charge. However, the CE may impose a reasonable, cost-based fee for each subsequent request for an accounting by the same individual within the 12-month period, provided that the CE informs the individual in advance of the fee and provides the individual with an opportunity to withdraw or modify the request for a subsequent accounting in order to avoid or reduce the fee. In addition, a CE must document the information that will be included in an accounting, including the specific pieces of information and the titles of the persons or offices responsible for receiving and processing requests for an accounting by individuals.

The original Privacy Rule required that all CEs keep a log of all authorized disclosures for disclosure-accounting purposes, except disclosures made to the individual, for TPO, "verbal agreement" disclosures, or national security or law enforcement disclosures. The 2002 Privacy NPRM added disclosures that the subject individual has authorized to this exception list. So, a patient who has signed an authorization to disclose the results of a pre-employment physical to a prospective employer would not see this event in a disclosure-accounting report.

## PHI Restrictions Requests

The Privacy Rule gives individuals the right to request CEs to restrict use or disclosure of PHI for TPO, disclosure to persons involved in the individual's healthcare or payment for healthcare, or disclosure to notify family members or others about the individual's general condition, location, or death. A CE is not obligated to agree to these restriction requests. If a CE agrees to a restriction request, though, it must comply with the specified and agreed-upon restrictions, except for purposes of medical emergency treatment for the individual.

## Administrative Requirements

CEs are required to implement basic administrative procedures to protect PHI. Some high-level descriptions of administrative requirements include obligations to:

- Designate a privacy official responsible for the development and implementation of the entity's policies and procedures.
- Designate a contact person or office responsible for receiving complaints and answering questions related to the notice.
- Document the associated personnel designations (for example, Privacy Officer, contact person, etc.).

- Train all personnel and workforce members on the privacy policies and procedures with respect to PHI as necessary and appropriate to carry out their job responsibilities. Workforce members include employees, volunteers, trainees, and may also include other persons whose conduct falls under the CE's direct control, whether or not they are paid by the entity.
- Document training that has occurred.
- Implement appropriate administrative, technical, and physical safeguards to protect the privacy of PHI.
- Safeguard PHI from any intentional or unintentional unauthorized use or disclosure.
- Maintain reasonable and appropriate administrative, technical, and physical safeguards to prevent intentional or unintentional use or disclosure of PHI in violation of the Privacy Rule and to limit incidental use and disclosure resulting from otherwise permitted or required use or disclosure. A safeguard example is shredding documents containing PHI before having a trash service haul it away, locking access to physical print-out of medical records, requiring access to electronic PHI only with passwords and user IDs, etc.
- Provide a process for individuals to make complaints concerning the policies and procedures CEs must explain these procedures in the NPP.
- Document all complaints received and their resolution.
- Consistently apply and document sanctions against personnel who fail to comply with the privacy policies and procedures, and document applied sanctions.
- Mitigate as much as possible any harmful effect that is known to the CE of a use or disclosure of PHI in violation of its policies and procedures by the CE or a BA.
- Maintain, until at least 6 years after the later of the date of the creation or last effective date, the CE's privacy policies and procedures, NPP(s), documentation of complaints, and other actions, activities, and designations that the Privacy Rule requires to be documented.

CEs may not intimidate or take any type of retaliatory action against any individual for exercising the right to submit a complaint, request a review, request an amendment for their PHI, or any other type of action described previously as being a right of the individual under the Privacy Rule. Additionally, CEs may not require individuals to waive their rights as a condition of medical treatment, payment, enrollment in a health plan, or eligibility for benefits.

Covered entities must implement PHI privacy policies and procedures designed to comply with the Privacy Rule. The policies and procedures must be designed to take into account the size of and the type of activities that relate to the CE's PHI. When developing policies and procedures to meet Privacy Rule compliance, a CE needs to:

- Review and change its existing policies and procedures as necessary and appropriate.
- Promptly document and implement a revised policy and procedure whenever there is a change in the law that necessitates a change. If the change affects the content of the notice, the CE must promptly make the appropriate revisions to the notice.
- Maintain the policies, procedures, and related communications in written or electronic form for at least 6 years from the date of creation or the date when it last was in effect, whichever is later.

A group health plan is not subject to most of the above requirements if it provides health benefits solely through an insurance contract with a health insurance issuer or an HMO, and does not create or receive PHI other than summary health information or information indicating whether the individual is participating in the group health plan, or is enrolled in or has disenrolled from a health insurance issuer or HMO offered by the plan.

The only administrative obligations with which a fully-insured group health plan that has no more than enrollment data and summary health information is required to comply are:

- Ban on retaliatory acts and waiver of individual rights
- Documentation requirements with respect to plan documents if such documents are amended to provide for the disclosure of PHI to the plan sponsor by a health insurance issuer or HMO that services the group health plan

### Privacy Officer

A CE must designate a privacy officer to be responsible for developing and implementing the CE's privacy policies and procedures. A contact person or office must also be designated to be responsible for receiving complaints and answering questions about the entity's privacy practices, notice, and HIPAA compliance. See Appendix B for a job description of a privacy officer.

### Training

All personnel must receive initial and ongoing training that covers the privacy policies and procedures to ensure they perform their job responsibilities in compliance with the requirements. While not specifically required within the HIPAA text, you should consider including the following actions items within your training project plan:

- Establish a timeline for mandatory initial HIPAA privacy training.
- Establish procedures to train new personnel as soon as feasible following their employment.

- Provide training that helps personnel relate the policy to their working environment.

- Provide training on how to report a privacy problem.

- Consider competency tests or quizzes to evaluate and ascertain the training effectiveness.

- Require regular follow-up training, and training following significant changes in policies and procedures. Train the personnel who are most impacted as soon as possible either immediately before or immediately following these changes.

Document the training in written or electronic form and retain the records for at least 6 years.

See Chapter 24 for a detailed discussion of awareness and training.

### Safeguards

A CE must establish appropriate and reasonable administrative, technical, and physical safeguards to protect PHI. These safeguards must protect PHI from any intentional or unintentional use or disclosure that is in violation of the standards, implementation specifications or other requirements of the Privacy Rule. Perform a risk analysis and, based on the results, create and implement a risk management plan for both electronic and non-electronic information assets. Request the privacy officer to work closely with the security officer, and other personnel as appropriate, to determine the most feasible safeguards for your organization.

### Complaints

A CE must establish policies and processes for adequately taking and responding to complaints from individuals concerning the CE's privacy policies and procedures, or concerns with its compliance with the policies and procedures. All complaints received must be documented, along with the associated actions that were taken to address the complaints. Documentation must be retained for at least 6 years.

### Sanctions

Sanction policies and procedures must be established and applied when appropriate. The procedures must ensure disciplinary actions are taken against personnel who do not comply with the CE's privacy policies and procedures or the requirements of the Privacy Rule. Assign an individual or group to review policy and procedural violations and specify corrective and disciplinary action. Apply disciplinary action as necessary and appropriate. Each sanction that is applied must be documented.

Some suggestions to consider for sanctions:

- Make sanctions progressive and appropriate for the severity, frequency, and intent of violations.
- Apply sanctions equitably without regard to the person's role or position within the CE.
- Include termination of employment or contract relationship and criminal prosecution as possible sanctions.
- Include provisions for sanctions within contract and labor agreements.
- Coordinate sanctions with your Human Resources department.
- Consider establishing progressive sanctions, such as verbal warning, written warning, up to termination, and determine when progressive sanctions are appropriate.
- Make sure workforce members are aware of the sanction procedures.

### *Mitigation*

A CE must mitigate as much as possible any harm that occurs as a result of a use or disclosure of PHI that occurred in violation of its policies and procedures or the requirements of the Privacy Rule by the CE or any BA.

Here are just a few of the methods you can consider using for mitigating (and containing) the damage from inappropriate disclosure of PHI. Keep in mind that mitigation procedures also include those that help to mitigate (prevent) a PHI disclosure from occurring:

- Use a fax cover sheet for all PHI transmittals and include a notice asking people who have received the fax in error to contact you immediately and to destroy the information.
- Inform the area responsible for the policy or procedural breach to determine if it needs to be updated to prevent future actions that would have harmful effects.
- Meet with your legal counsel to determine if inappropriate use or disclosure may in itself constitute a harmful effect with regard to HIPAA and other applicable legal requirements.
- Discuss with your legal counsel how and when your organization should notify individuals if misuse or inappropriate disclosure of PHI will likely lead to a harmful effect.
- Consult with your legal counsel to determine appropriate contract language to use to transfer the potential financial burden of harm to BAs.
- Notify the individual immediately when an improper disclosure has occurred. Determine if there is anything you can do to prevent the further unauthorized spread of the PHI.

### Refraining from Intimidating or Retaliatory Acts

Establish policies and procedures to make sure members of your workforce do not intimidate, threaten, coerce, discriminate against, or take other retaliatory action against any individual who exercises any of the rights established by the Privacy Rule, such as filing a complaint with regard to privacy practice compliance.

### Waiver of Rights

Individuals cannot be required to waive their rights provided by the Privacy Rule as a condition for providing treatment, payment, enrollment in a health plan, or to be eligible for benefits.

### Policies and Procedures

A CE must create and implement privacy policies and procedures designed to ensure the entity's compliance with the standards, implementation specifications, or other Privacy Rule requirements.

### Documentation

Documented privacy policies and procedures must be maintained in written and electronic form, and kept available for at least 6 years from the date of its creation or the date when it was last in effect, whichever is later.

### Personal Representatives

A CE must treat a personal representative of an individual the same as the individual with respect to uses and disclosures of the individual's PHI, as well as the individual's rights under the Privacy Rule. A personal representative is a person legally authorized to make healthcare decisions on an individual's behalf or to act for a deceased individual or the individual's estate. The Privacy Rule permits an exception when a CE believes the personal representative may be abusing or neglecting the individual, or that treating the person as the personal representative could otherwise endanger the individual.

### Minors

In most cases, parents are personal representatives for their minor children. And, in most cases, parents can exercise individual rights, such as access to the medical record, on behalf of their minor children. However, in certain exceptional cases, the parent is not considered the personal representative. In these situations, state and other applicable laws determine the rights of parents to access and control the PHI of their minor children. If state and other laws do not address parental access to a minor's PHI, a licensed healthcare professional on behalf of the CE has discretion to provide or deny a parent access to the minor's PHI.

## *Some Points from HHS Regarding Personal Representatives and Minors*

- An individual given a healthcare power of attorney has the right to access PHI of the individual related to this representation to the extent permitted by the Privacy Rule. However, when a CE believes that an individual, including an unemancipated minor, has been or may be subjected to domestic violence, abuse, or neglect by the personal representative, or that treating a person as an individual's personal representative could endanger the individual, the CE may choose not to treat that person as the individual's personal representative.

- With the exception of decedents, a CE must treat a personal representative as the individual only when that person has authority under other law to act on the individual's behalf on matters related to healthcare. A power of attorney that does not include decisions related to healthcare in its scope would not, therefore, authorize the holder to exercise the individual's rights under the Privacy Rule. Additionally, a CE does not have to treat a personal representative as the individual if it believes doing so would not be in the best interest of the individual because of a reasonable belief that the individual has been or may be subject to domestic violence, abuse, or neglect by the personal representative, or that doing so would otherwise endanger the individual.

- With respect to personal representatives of deceased individuals, the Privacy Rule requires a CE to treat the personal representative as the individual as long as the person has the authority under law to act for the decedent or the estate. The power of attorney needs to be valid after the individual's death to qualify the holder as the personal representative of the decedent.

- An individual who is the subject of PHI can exercise all rights granted by the Privacy Rule with respect to all corresponding PHI, including information obtained while the individual was an unemancipated minor consistent with state or other applicable law. Generally, the parent would no longer be the personal representative of his or her child once the child reaches the age of majority or becomes emancipated, and therefore, would no longer control the PHI about the child. Any individual can have a personal representative, including a parent, who can exercise rights on his or her behalf.

- A deceased individual's PHI may be relevant to a family member's healthcare. The Privacy Rule provides two ways for a surviving family member to obtain the PHI of a deceased relative:
  - Disclosures of PHI for treatment purposes, including the treatment of another individual, do not require an authorization. So,

a CE may disclose a decedent's PHI without authorization to the healthcare provider who is treating the surviving relative.

- A CE must treat a deceased individual's legally authorized executor or administrator, or a person who is otherwise legally authorized to act on the behalf of the deceased individual or his estate, as a personal representative with respect to PHI relevant to the representation. If it is within the scope of the personal representative's authority under other law, the Privacy Rule permits the personal representative to obtain the information or provide the appropriate authorization for its disclosure.

## Transition Provisions

A CE may continue to use or disclose PHI under a consent, an authorization, or other type of legal permission that was obtained from an individual before the April 14, 2003, compliance date, as long as the entity complies with all limitations placed by the permission. For example, a provider that obtained consent for use or disclosure for billing purposes would be able to continue to use PHI obtained prior to the compliance date and covered by the consent form for all TPO activities to the extent not expressly excluded by the terms of the consent.

If a permission obtained prior to April 14, 2003, is a general consent to participate in a research project, and a CE is conducting or participating in the research, the entity may continue to make use or disclosure of PHI for purposes of that project. If a CE agrees to a restriction requested by an individual, subsequent use or disclosure of PHI is subject to that restriction.

## Compliance Dates and Penalties

The following are the compliance dates for initial implementation of the HIPAA Privacy Rule standards:

- *Healthcare providers:* No later than April 14, 2003
- *Health plans:* No later than the following date, as applicable:
  - *Health plans other than small health plans:* April 14, 2003
  - *Small health plans:* April 14, 2004
- *Healthcare clearinghouses:* No later than April 14, 2003

If a complaint is lodged against an entity and an investigation or compliance review determines no violation exists, the Secretary of HHS will inform both the entity and complainant in writing.

If a complaint is lodged against an entity, and the resulting compliance review confirms noncompliance with the Privacy Rule, the CE will be informed by the Secretary in writing, who will attempt to resolve the situation by informal means if possible. If the situation cannot be resolved in this manner, a formal noncompliance report will be issued to both the person filing the complaint and the CE.

- For noncriminal violation of the Privacy Rule, including disclosures made in error, civil penalties of $100 per violation up to $25,000 per year, per standard may be issued. Additionally, criminal penalties may be applied for certain violations done knowingly as follows:
- Up to $50,000 and 1 year in prison for obtaining or disclosing PHI
- Up to $100,000 and up to 5 years in prison for obtaining or disclosing PHI under false pretenses
- Up to $250,000 and up to 10 years in prison for obtaining PHI with the intent to sell, transfer, or use it for commercial advantage, personal gain, or malicious harm

**Looking Forward**

How long will it be until HHS makes more changes to the HIPAA Privacy Rule? HIPAA gives HHS the authority to modify the Privacy Rule as the Secretary determines is appropriate. Nonetheless, a standard such as the Privacy Rule can, by law, only be modified once in a 12-month period. Additionally, future modifications to the Privacy Rule must be made in accordance with the Administrative Procedure Act (APA). Any changes HHS proposes must be published in the Federal Register through an NPRM, and comments must be accepted from the public. After HHS has reviewed and addressed the comments, and the 12-month period has passed, then a modified rule can be issued.

**Chapter 5 Practical Checklist**

- Assign, document, and communicate about your privacy official.
- CEs include healthcare providers, health plans, and healthcare clearinghouses.
- Creating an NPP is the action that will be the most obvious to the public.
- You may want to create more than one NPP based on your locations and jurisdictions.
- HIPAA gives individuals many explicit rights to their corresponding PHI; create procedures to support these rights.
- Know the circumstances under which you must obtain signed authorizations, as well as those requiring you to give an individual the opportunity to agree or object to a use or disclosure.
- Document! Document!! Document!!!

# Chapter 6
# Performing a Privacy Rule Gap Analysis and Risk Analysis

Considering the potential costs and effort associated with HIPAA compliance, it is a mistake to install a HIPAA "solution" without first understanding your current organizational HIPAA compliance situation. Your organization may already have in place policies, procedures, systems, and technology that adequately address at least some of the HIPAA requirements. To determine where HIPAA compliance requirements must be addressed, or your HIPAA gaps, you must perform a HIPAA Privacy Rule gap analysis and risk analysis. Using the results of these analyses, along with any existing business and financial plans, your organization will be ready to develop a HIPAA compliance plan, including a listing of compliance priorities.

Use the following checklist to help you perform your own Privacy Rule gap analysis and identify privacy risks.

**Gap Analysis and Risk Analysis**

1. *Is someone within your organization responsible for addressing privacy issues and compliance?* This should be someone who has been assigned privacy official responsibilities, often designated as the Privacy Officer. (See Appendix B for a sample job description.) The Privacy Officer should be someone who knows not only your business well, but also is very familiar with the healthcare industry, is experienced with security and privacy activities, and is knowledgeable in the HIPAA regulations. Typically this person has filled one or more of the following positions:
   - Information Security Officer
   - Chief Privacy Officer
   - Director of Information Technology
   - Director of Medical Records
   - Director of Patient Accounting
   - Director of Patient Registration/Admitting

---

The information and opinions provided in this book do not constitute or substitute for legal or other professional advice.

2. **Do you have an inventory of all your organizational policies, procedures, training, and technical controls?** Besides collecting all these documents from within your organization, also collect HIPAA plans from your business associates (BAs), including vendors, clearinghouses, payers, etc. Obtain copies of all forms related to release of protected health information (PHI) or authorizations to release or disclose PHI to third parties. Document and inventory everything you collect.

3. **Have you reviewed all your documents and identified the directives and practices that apply to PHI?** Determine and document the following:
   - What rules, if any, exist for protecting health information?
   - Identify all current non-IT-specific policies and procedures related to information access, disclosure, and integrity.
   - What are the procedures for allowing access to PHI and medical records?
   - What are the procedures for responding to complaints?
   - How is your Notice of Privacy Practices (NPP) worded?
   - What PHI-related security and privacy training do you provide and require?
   - If written policies and procedures for the privacy of PHI meeting the HIPAA Privacy Rule exist, have they been completely implemented?
   - Are any existing privacy policies and procedures monitored, incidents documented, and corrective action taken?
   - Identify the policies, procedures. and forms that need to be revised to comply with HIPAA requirements.
   - Identify which policies, procedures. or forms do not currently exist and need to be created to comply with HIPAA.
   - Identify all reports containing PHI that are distributed on paper, electronically, faxed, e-mailed, or using some other method (technical or nontechnical).
   - Identify all organized healthcare arrangements (OHCA).
   - Interview key staff to confirm or expand upon findings. What reports need to be changed to comply with HIPAA requirements?
   Do not forget to review your Web sites to see if you have any forms or databases with health information. It is typical in many organizations for the Web administrators to place forms or databases onto Internet Web sites at the request of almost any manager within the organization. Marketing areas in particular have a tendency to want to collect as much information from Web site visitors as possible, very possibly including PHI. Review carefully the information collected from and stored on your Internet Web servers to determine if any is PHI. Be sure to check *all* Web pages — some sites have thousands of Web pages.

4. ***Have you determined the security and privacy practices of your BAs?*** Carefully review your BA contracts. How does your organization ensure privacy protection by BAs? Do you have a standard BA agreement that has been executed by all BAs? Have the noncompliant BAs been replaced? Determine HIPAA compliance and the adequacy of BA privacy practices; ask each of your BAs to provide the following information:
   - Identify all electronic data interchange (EDI) transactions and their associated purposes and types.
   - Identify all EDI standards used by your BAs.
   - Identify and document BA systems that process your organization's PHI.
   - Obtain and review copies of BA and third-party agreements involving the transmission of PHI in any form.
   - Identify code sets used.
   - Document how identifiers are used.
   - Identify third parties and BAs receiving or sending PHI. This includes information received or sent via export, file transfer, e-mail, paper, disk, tape, Web, or transactional interface.
   - Meet with third parties and BAs receiving or sending PHI. Are they aware of HIPAA requirements? What are their plans for meeting HIPAA compliance?
   - Identify contracts that need to be revised to comply with HIPAA. Include BA agreements as appropriate to meet HIPAA requirements for third-party data processing vendors.
   - Meet with vendors to determine their HIPAA compliance plans. Will they offer system upgrades? At a cost? Will new products be offered? In what timeframe?
   - If applicable, meet with your healthcare clearinghouse to determine their plans. Review your contract with the clearinghouse to ensure appropriate language exists for exchange of data.
   - Identify legal counsel with HIPAA expertise within your organization. You will need their help to make business and third-party contract revisions.
   - Determine and document HIPAA compliance for your BAs and third-party partners based on all your previous research.

   Implement a methodology to identify all your organization's BA and third-party contracts. Include the following in your methodology:
   - Develop standard contract terminology to ensure consistency for BA provisions to help ensure HIPAA compliance.
   - While you are reviewing your BA contracts, identify terminology and HIPAA requirements that must be included.
   - Update your contract renewal process to incorporate HIPAA BA terminology and requirements into existing contracts.

5. *Have you conducted a security review to determine what security technology and practices exist to help ensure health information privacy?* Have you reviewed the security of PHI during transmission and in storage of all forms to ensure privacy and security? For example, if you send PHI over the Internet, carefully consider implementing encryption to prevent unauthorized interception. Most of the privacy requirements for a security review will be met when you perform your security risk analysis. At a high level you must determine:
   - What administrative security exists for PHI?
   - What physical security exists for PHI?
   - What technical security exists for PHI?

However, there are a few additional security review actions you should perform that fall under these categories.
   - Identify all information systems (including Web servers) containing PHI.
   - Identify all PHI code sets and determine those that are not in compliance with HIPAA requirements.
   - Determine the systems and related software applications that must be upgraded or changed to comply with HIPAA EDI requirements.
   - Assess the functionality, changes, and upgrades that must be made. For example, will you need to add security breach and incident tracking and reporting capabilities? Do you have a way to track and report new code releases? Do you have capabilities for tracking data access and changes?
   - Identify all current policies and procedures related to system security and information sharing.
   - Identify contingency and disaster planning practices.
   - Determine how your organization's Web sites need to be modified based on code-set and reporting changes.
   - Document your overall architecture, including internal and external networks, and identify potential security risks and issues.
   - Verify the use of virus detection software, firewalls, and other security and intrusion detection mechanisms.
   - Identify, document, and evaluate the effectiveness of the applications and operating system security features.
   - Identify how information communications are secured. For instance, how does your organization secure e-mail, fax transmissions, Internet connections, etc.? Are encryption, digital signatures, and other such privacy-enhancing technologies used?
   - Identify and document access points to your networks and systems, both internal and external.
   - Map the PHI data flows through your systems and applications.
   - Identify and review backup systems and procedures.

- Identify and determine the purposes for your Internet and intranet Web sites.
- Identify user security policies and practices such as log on/log off, passwords, etc.
- Determine where workstations that can access PHI are located, and the policies and practices that govern their use.
- Identify the physical security mechanisms that help to protect access to PHI; for example, locks, badges, pass codes, guards at entrances, etc.
- Identify your organization's incident-reporting and follow-up procedures.

6. ***Have you documented your organization's uses and disclosures of PHI?*** When you do your gap analysis and risk analysis correctly you will discover all the ways that PHI is used and disclosed. To determine risks that exist during use and disclosure, and then determine how to address those risks, you must know what use and disclosure means. Use means the sharing, employment, application, utilization, examination, or analysis of individually identifiable information within an entity. Disclosure means the release, transfer, provision of access to, or divulging of information outside the entity holding the information.

   Use and disclosure typically occur during face-to-face communications, mail, fax, e-mails, phone calls, or access to your computer systems. To effectively mitigate unauthorized use and disclosure you must implement good policies and procedures and train your workforce well.

   - Understand current uses and disclosures
   - List all privacy measures in place
     - Forms of notice in use
     - Authorization forms in use
     - Disclosure request forms in use
     - Copies of all agreements in use
     - Copies of all consent in use
   - Obtain operational procedure documentation
   - Examine security and privacy policies in place

7. ***Have you identified uses and disclosures that require authorizations? Does your organization follow the promises made within the authorizations?*** Authorizations give CEs permission to use or disclose indicated PHI for indicated purposes that are typically other than treatment, payment, and operations (TPO). Except as otherwise permitted or required by the HIPAA Privacy Rule (see Chapter 5), your organization may not use or disclose PHI without a valid authorization as indicated by the HIPAA regulations. When you obtain or receive a valid authorization for the use or disclosure of PHI, the use or disclosure must be consistent with the authorization.

8. ***Have you identified your organization's uses and disclosures of health information that do not require authorizations, but allow for opportunity to object?*** Your organization may use or disclose PHI without the written authorization of the individual, or the opportunity for the individual to agree or object, in several situations as detailed within the HIPAA Privacy Rule. When your organization is required by the HIPAA Privacy Rule to inform the individual of a use or disclosure permitted by the HIPAA Privacy Rule, or when the individual may agree to such, the individual's agreement may be given orally. The situations for which authorization are not required, but opportunity to agree or object must be presented to the individual, for use or disclosure of PHI, include the following:
   - Name, location, condition, and religion within the entity's facility directory or to clergy or persons asking for the individual by name.
   - Medical condition to a family member, other relative, or a close personal friend of the individual, or any other person identified by the individual.
   - See Chapter 5 for detailed information on this subject.

9. ***Have you determined which PHI needs to be de-identified?*** Identify PHI that must be de-identified per HIPAA Privacy Rule requirements (see Chapter 5) so that it does not identify an individual and with respect to which there is no reasonable basis to believe that the information can be used to identify an individual is not individually identifiable health information. Eighteen specific types of information must be removed from a data set for it to be de-identified.

10. ***Have you established procedures for using PHI for marketing purposes to meet HIPAA requirements?*** Your organization may not use or disclose PHI for marketing without an authorization that meets the applicable HIPAA Privacy Rule requirements. (See Chapter 5.) Generally, a CE may use or disclose PHI for marketing communication in the following three situations:
    1. The communication occurs in a face-to-face encounter with the individual.
    2. The products or services have a "nominal" value; for example, when giving calendars, pens, etc.
    3. To direct or recommend alternative treatments, therapies, healthcare providers, care settings, or similar topics within a case management or care coordination situation.

11. ***Have you identified all the uses and disclosures of PHI for fundraising purposes?*** Your organization must provide an opt-out method for individuals to deny your use of their PHI for fundraising purposes. You must take reasonable steps to ensure that opt-outs are honored throughout all areas of your organization. Additionally,

you must maintain a record of disclosures made for fundraising purposes. Review your organization's privacy practices notice to determine whether it permits the use of other PHI for fundraising.

12. *If you are a health plan organization, do you have policies and procedures governing the use of health information received for policy processing purposes?* Health plans that receive PHI for the purposes of underwriting, premium rating, or other activities relating to the creation, renewal, or replacement of a contract of health insurance or health benefits may not use or disclose the PHI for any other purpose, except as may be required by law, if health insurance or health benefits are not placed with the health plan.

13. *Have you identified all your organization's uses of PHI for which authorization and opportunity to object are not needed?* These special situations include:
    - Uses and disclosures required by law
    - Uses and disclosures for public health activities
    - Disclosures about victims of abuse, neglect, or domestic violence
    - Uses and disclosures for health oversight activities
    - Disclosures for judicial and administrative proceedings
    - Disclosures for law enforcement purposes
    - Uses and disclosures about decedents
    - Uses and disclosures for cadaveric organ, eye, or tissue donation purposes
    - Uses and disclosures to avert a serious threat to health or safety
    - Uses and disclosures for specialized government functions
    - Disclosures for workers' compensation

14. *Has your organization established and implemented identity verification policies and procedures to use when it receives requests for PHI?* Your organization must develop policies and procedures to verify the identity and authority of people requesting PHI. We recommend you consider using the following activities as appropriate for your situation and organization:
    - Require requesters to provide documentation detailing the purpose for requesting the PHI.
    - Verify the identity of persons requesting PHI before giving them access.
    - Confirm that persons acting on behalf of a public official have appropriate statements on official letterhead or credentials before giving them the PHI.
    - Establish a policy that legal authority is presumed when a request is made in relation to a legal proceeding, warrant, subpoena, or order.
    - Develop a formal procedure to authorize disclosure of PHI using other verification items in the absence of a written verification.

- Establish procedures requiring your personnel to make every effort to identify and document the people requesting disclosure and the circumstances of disclosure as detailed within the HIPAA Privacy Rule.
- Develop policies that clearly define the sources of identification and documents of authority that are acceptable to verify permission for disclosure.
- Provide your personnel with comprehensive guidelines and back-up resources to help them obtain answers to their verification questions.
- When PHI is released to a legal authority, send a cover letter with the information to remind the recipients that the information is PHI and must be handled in a confidential manner. Retain a copy of the letter for your records.
- Inform frequent requestors of PHI of the procedural changes required by the HIPAA Privacy Rule.

15. ***Does your organization provide individuals with an NPP that meets HIPAA requirements?*** Except as provided by the HIPAA Privacy Rule, individuals have a right to adequate notice of the uses and disclosures of their PHI that may be made by your organization, in addition to a right to know their rights and your organization's legal duties with respect to PHI. Your organization must document compliance with the notice requirements by retaining copies of the notices issued.

- Include a brief, easy-to-read explanation of the primary points within the notice along with the detailed version. This will help to reinforce individuals' understanding of their privacy rights.
- Incorporate the privacy practice notice into your organization's "patient rights" literature and procedures to minimize the expense and inconvenience, and maximize the informational impact.
- Develop a procedure to account for the delivery of the privacy practices notice as your organization delivers it.

16. ***Have you identified your organization's confidential communications requirements and established procedures to fulfill requests for alternative communications methods?*** Review your organization's facilities to verify that all areas of your organization enable privacy when communicating patient information. A covered healthcare provider must permit individuals to request and must accommodate reasonable requests by individuals to receive communications of PHI from the covered healthcare provider by alternative means or at alternative locations. A health plan must permit individuals to request and must accommodate reasonable requests by individuals to receive communications of PHI from the health plan by alternative means or at alternative locations, if the individual

clearly states that the disclosure of all or part of that information could endanger the individual. Consider the following as appropriate for your organization:

- Establish procedures for patients or plan members to request alternative means of communication for PHI, and accommodate the requests when feasible.
- Establish procedures and training for all personnel who receive and fulfill requests from patients for PHI so they are aware of the need for and use of alternate means of communication as appropriate.
- Document the most common causes for requests for special restrictions, and determine a set of restriction methods to accommodate these situations; for example, for celebrities, government officials, social stigma, physical danger, etc.
- Establish a way to communicate the restrictions quickly and effectively to workforce members. Remember, some workforce members may not yet have received training on this issue when they receive the restriction request.
- Keep the possible communications restrictions as simple as possible.
- When an individual asks for restrictions you cannot make, refer them to a facility that can honor their request, if appropriate.
- Identify how to provide aliases for patients when using them to comply with this provision.

17. ***Does your organization have procedures in place to archive your PHI and allow authorized individuals access to their corresponding information?*** With the few exceptions detailed within the HIPAA Privacy Rule, individuals have a right to inspect and obtain a copy of their corresponding PHI for as long as the PHI is maintained in the designated record set. Your organization must develop and document policies and procedures to receive and act upon an individual's request to access, inspect, and receive a copy of PHI, including the denial of such requests. Be sure you:

- Respond to access requests within the timeframe specified within the HIPAA Privacy Rule as is appropriate to the situation, typically 30 or 60 days.
- Develop procedures to release required PHI to verified requestors.
- Develop documented and legally defensible grounds for denials of information requests.
- Develop procedures to review denial of information access requests.
- Develop procedures to allow for the appeal of access denial decisions.

- Identify a person within your organization with the authority to release PHI, and a person authorized to process denials and appeals.
- We recommend you include a temporary suspension of the patient's right of access to research records within your research authorization and consent forms if applicable.

18. ***Do you have procedures in place to allow individuals to amend their PHI?*** An individual has the right to ask your organization to amend PHI or a record about the individual in a designated record set for as long as the PHI is maintained in the designated record set. A designated record set is a group of records you maintain that consists of:

- Medical records and billing records about individuals maintained by or for a covered healthcare provider; enrollment, payment, claims adjudication, and case or medical management record systems maintained by or for a health plan; or being used, in whole or in part, by or for your organization to make decisions about individuals.
- You need to develop and document policies and procedures to receive and act upon these requests, as well as policies and procedures providing guidance and directives on when to deny such requests.
- Respond to amendment requests within the timeframe specified for the specific situation within the HIPAA Privacy Rule.
- Consider providing resources from your organization to assist patients with their record reviews.
- Establish procedures for retrieving PHI about individuals following a request to amend information.
- Establish procedures for evaluating and accepting or rejecting requests for correction and implementing corrections.
- Establish procedures to amend paper and electronic records (including accepted requests for removal of a record).
- We recommend you date-stamp PHI amendment requests.

19. ***Do you have procedures and mechanisms implemented to record the disclosures of PHI and maintain them for at least 6 years as required by HIPAA?*** Individuals have a right to receive an accounting of disclosures of their PHI made by your organization in the 6 years prior to the date on which they request the accounting. You need to establish policies and procedures to ensure these disclosure records are retained.

- Maintain a record of all individuals requesting reports of disclosure as required by the HIPAA Privacy Rule, as well as the nature of those requests.

- Identify a person or group to determine on a case-by-case basis whether disclosures must, may optionally, or must not be reported in accordance with the HIPAA Privacy Rule.
- Establish a procedure to ensure all covered disclosures are reported as quickly as possible in accordance with HIPAA Privacy Rule requirements.
- If an extension of the time limit for providing an accounting is needed, notify the requestor of the delay as required by the HIPAA Privacy Rule, and ensure the extension does not exceed permissible limits.

20. ***Does your organization have someone to handle HIPAA- and privacy-related complaints and questions?*** Your organization must designate a contact person or department to be responsible for receiving and addressing HIPAA-related complaints, in addition to being able to provide further information in response to HIPAA- and privacy-related issues and questions.
    - Designate an individual or department to receive complaints and provide information about issues covered in your Notice of Privacy Practices, as well as questions or complaints regarding your organization's compliance with HIPAA policies and procedures.
    - Document the contact information within your Notice of Privacy Practices.
    - Document and maintain this personnel designation.
    - Establish a reporting structure and procedures to involve persons with appropriate authority to investigate and track complaints.
    - Ensure the procedures for responding to complaints are consistent with good public relations practices as well as good privacy policy.
    - Maintain a record of complaints and brief explanations of how they were resolved.
    - Establish procedures governing how the person or department that receives complaints will handle them, and under what circumstances they will triage them to be handled by others.
    - Establish timeframes and procedures for handling and reporting complaints.
    - Use complaints to evaluate your HIPAA compliance procedures to improve upon them where warranted.
    - Identify the person or position responsible for reviewing and accessing complaint information and for what purposes.
    - Establish a method to track complaints.
    - Create reports to periodically communicate to appropriate management complaint resolutions.
    - Ensure your complaint procedures are synchronized with your NPP and your organization's Patient Rights policy, if applicable.

21. **Do you require all personnel to participate in ongoing privacy training?** A CE must train all members of its workforce on the policies and procedures with respect to PHI required by the HIPAA Privacy Rule as necessary to allow personnel to perform their job responsibilities. See Chapter 24 for additional training and awareness guidance.
    - Establish a timeline for mandatory initial HIPAA privacy training.
    - Establish procedures to train new personnel as soon as feasible following their employment.
    - Require regular follow-up training, and training following significant changes in policies and procedures. Train the personnel who are most impacted as soon as possible either immediately before or immediately following these changes.
    - Document the training in written or electronic form and retain the records for at least 6 years.
    - Give copies of the NPP to each workforce member.
    - Require each member to sign an acknowledgment that they have received, read, and understand their responsibilities with regard to the privacy practices.
    - Provide training that relates the privacy practices to how personnel are expected to perform their job responsibilities.
    - Train personnel on how to report a privacy problem.
    - Provide ongoing refresher training and periodic reminders for workforce members about privacy practices.
    - Consider competency tests or quizzes to evaluate training effectiveness. (*Hint:* Use the quizzes in this book!)

22. **Have you implemented administrative, technical, and physical safeguards to help ensure the privacy of PHI?** Your organization must establish administrative, technical, and physical safeguards to protect the privacy of PHI from unauthorized use or disclosure. These safeguards must be appropriate and reasonable.
    - Perform a risk analysis and, based on the results, create and implement a risk management plan for both electronic and non-electronic PHI.
    - Request the privacy officer to work closely with the security officer and other personnel as appropriate to determine the safeguard appropriate and feasible for your organization.
    - Establish the privacy and security positions at a high enough level within your organization to ensure they have the authority to implement effective safeguards.
    - Document reasonably anticipated threats and hazards to the privacy of PHI and unauthorized uses or disclosures.
    - Meet with the appropriate areas of your organization to gather details about how they address specific aspects of the safeguard requirements (for example, training, sanctions, complaints, etc.).

- Be sure to dispose of PHI appropriately (for example, shred papers or reformat hard drives of PCs you are no longer going to use).

23. ***Does your organization have enforced sanctions for policy non-compliance?*** Develop sanctions to apply for workforce members who do not comply with your organization's privacy policy and privacy practices.
   - Identify an individual or group to review policy and procedural violations and to determine the appropriate disciplinary action.
   - Document corrective and disciplinary action taken.
   - Make the sanctions appropriate to the violation.
   - Discuss the sanctions with your legal counsel and obtain their approval for the wording.
   - Apply sanctions equitably without regard to an offender's role or position within the organization.
   - Termination of employment or contract relationship or criminal prosecution or both should be included as possible sanctions.
   - Include provision for sanctions in contract and labor agreements.
   - Coordinate sanctions with your Human Resources department.
   - Communicate the sanctions policy and possible disciplinary actions to your personnel.

24. ***Does your organization have mitigation procedures to address unauthorized use or disclosure of PHI?*** Consider using the following methods for containing or minimizing the damage, or potential for damage, and stopping further compromise:
   - Inform the area responsible for the policy or procedural breach to determine if the policy needs to be updated to prevent future actions that would have harmful effects.
   - Meet with your legal counsel to determine if inappropriate use or disclosure may in itself constitute a harmful effect with regard to HIPAA and other applicable legal requirements.
   - Discuss with your legal counsel how and when your organization should notify individuals if misuse or inappropriate disclosure of PHI will likely lead to a harmful effect.
   - Consult with your legal counsel to determine appropriate contract language to use to transfer the potential financial burden of harm to BAs as appropriate to situations where the unauthorized use or disclosure occurred at a BA.

25. ***Has your organization implemented procedures to prohibit intimidation following patient requests allowed by HIPAA?*** Establish policies and procedures that prohibit intimidation, threats, coercion, discrimination, or retaliatory action against individuals who exercise their rights under this provision.

26. ***Has your organization established policies prohibiting your personnel from requiring individuals to waive their rights if they file complaints?*** Your organization cannot require individuals

to waive their rights to file a complaint or their other rights under the privacy standards as a condition of treatment, payment, and enrollment in a health plan or eligibility for benefits. Do not put waivers of rights on consent forms if you use them. Covered entities cannot ask patients to waive their privacy rights.

27. ***Has your organization developed and implemented policies and procedures to address all the HIPAA Privacy Rule requirements?*** A CE must implement policies and procedures with respect to PHI that are designed to comply with the standards, implementation specifications, or other requirements of this sub-part. The policies and procedures must be reasonably designed, and take into account the size and the type of activities that relate to PHI within your organization. You cannot create policies and procedures that would violate any of the HIPAA requirements, or any other applicable privacy regulations.

28. ***Has your organization established and implemented procedures to update your policies whenever changes in the law occur, or when your organization makes changes in your practices or your NPP?*** A CE must change its policies and procedures as necessary and appropriate to comply with changes in the law, including the standards, requirements, and implementation specifications of the Privacy Regulations. When you change your NPP, you must update your policies and procedures appropriately, and make the changes effective for PHI that was created or received before the effective date of the notice revision if you included in the notice a statement reserving the right to make such a change in the privacy practices. You can make changes to your other policies and procedures at any time if you document them and meet the HIPAA requirements.

   – Consider reserving the right to change your privacy policy within your NPP.

   – When creating your privacy policies, procedures, and notices, take into consideration how you will need to communicate any necessary updates.

   – Consider your organization's size and complexity when creating and updating your policies and procedures.

29. ***Does your organization maintain your policies and procedures in written or electronic form, and keep copies for at least 6 years from the effective date?*** You must maintain your privacy policies, notices, and related procedures for at least 6 years. You must also retain related communication for this period as well.

   – Document required communications, designations, actions, and activities.

   – Record the creation date and last effective date of documents.

- Maintain the documentation for at least 6 years from date of creation or the date when the policy or procedure was last in effect, whichever is later.
- Assign responsibility for policies and procedures documentation.
- Indicate the expiration and review dates for documentation.
- Centralize retention of policy and procedure documentation so that it is easily accessible.
- Communicate to appropriate personnel the importance of documentation, and that lack of documentation is considered a HIPAA noncompliance action.
- Organize documentation in such a way that it can be identified when necessary.

30. ***Have you identified existing consents, authorizations, and other legal permissions that are not in compliance with the HIPAA Privacy Rule requirements?*** You may continue to use or disclose PHI under a consent, authorization, or other type of legal permission obtained from an individual permitting the use or disclosure of PHI that does not comply with HIPAA, depending on when it was created.
   - Decide whether or not to treat PHI created or received before the HIPAA compliance date with a different set of privacy consents and authorizations from PHI created or received after the HIPAA compliance date.
   - If PHI will be handled in different ways depending on the date it was created or received, clearly identify the PHI that existed before the HIPAA compliance date.
   - Handle PHI in accordance with the consent, authorization, or other documented wishes of the individual that were effective at the time the PHI was created or received.

31. ***Have you identified all PHI, and developed and implemented procedures to limit access to the PHI to only that which is minimally necessary to perform job responsibilities?*** Is PHI accessed, used, and disclosed based on the minimum amount of information necessary to accomplish the required purpose? Are patient information access, use, and disclosure by personnel based only on a need-to-know basis, to accomplish the required business purpose?
   - Document all PHI access allowed and the relationship to job functions.
   - Identify PHI that can be de-identified without interfering with needed functions.
   - Calculate personnel and technology costs for limiting information disclosure and de-identifying PHI.
   - Identify appropriate persons to determine what PHI should be used, disclosed, and requested consistent with the minimum necessary standard.

- Create methods to determine minimum access allowances on an individual basis.
- Define and implement policies and procedures that are reasonable and appropriate for your organization.

32. *Analyze your responses to the previous questions to identify the gaps between your organization's current state and the HIPAA Privacy Rule requirements. Do you have gaps?* Use your inventory to assess and document compliance levels, gaps, and vulnerabilities.

- Rank the gaps according to their immediacy. It is usually most efficient and effective to use a "high, medium, and low" ranking system.
- Include your applicable state regulatory requirements within the gap analysis.
- Identify situations requiring de-identification of PHI.

33. *Have you created a summary risk analysis report and created an action plan to close gaps and address the risks?* This will establish your current baseline compliance status. Prepare the final report, with details on specific areas of observed and potential risk.

- Include dates.
- Label as your baseline.
- Set a target date to perform next gap analysis.
- Clearly identify the noncompliance items.
- Document the observed and potential risks.
- Identify disparities between procedure, practice, and culture, and HIPAA requirements.
- Determine the availability of archived PHI.
- Determine the impact of potential HIPAA-related changes on secondary uses of PHI; for instance, in clinical systems, medical devices, support applications, etc.
- Indicate opportunities for operational streamlining and cost savings.
- Use any existing analysis of security risk management priorities strategies.
- Consider applicability of HIPAA provisions for hybrid and affiliated CEs.
- Indicate alternative HIPAA solutions, including beneficial EDI advances and their costs.
- Note available resources for performing remediation activities.
- Identify opportunities for HIPAA-related changes that will facilitate your business goals.
- Make recommended HIPAA-related remediation and strategic actions.

## Chapter 6: Practical Checklist

- Perform a Privacy Rule gap analysis and risk analysis now to determine your current and baseline compliance status.
- Perform another gap analysis after you have completed all your compliance activities.
- Continue performing gap and risk analyses following Privacy Rule changes, major organizational changes, and major technology changes.
- Always communicate results to organization leaders, appropriate compliance officers, and legal counsel.

# Chapter 7
# Writing Effective Privacy Policies

HIPAA requires two kinds of privacy policies. People sometimes consider the required Notice of Privacy Practices (NPP) the only necessary privacy policy. HIPAA also requires covered entities (CEs) to document their organizational privacy policies and procedures that will support the multiple requirements of the HIPAA Privacy Rule. First we will address the NPP, and then address writing organizational privacy policies.

**Notice of Privacy Practices**

The NPP is covered within 45 CFR 164.520 parts (a), (b), (c), and (d). The notice requires CEs to inform individuals of their rights for accessing and modifying their protected health information (PHI), in addition to describing the security the CE has established to protect individuals' privacy. CEs must make the NPP available to generally any individual who asks, and CEs must take the initiative to make their NPP available and known to individuals for whom they process or handle PHI. We will look at the specific distribution and communication issues related to the notices in the chapters specific to each type of covered entity in Section 4. Here we will examine specifically how to write an NPP.

**Example NPP**

*Header*

The HIPAA Privacy Rule requirements are very specific and straightforward when it comes to specifying the wording for the heading of the privacy notice (45 CFR 164.520(b)(1)(i)). The header, or a prominently displayed message, must be written exactly as follows:

*THIS NOTICE DESCRIBES HOW MEDICAL INFORMATION ABOUT YOU MAY BE USED AND DISCLOSED AND HOW YOU CAN GET ACCESS TO THIS INFORMATION. PLEASE REVIEW IT CAREFULLY.*

---

The information and opinions provided in this book do not constitute or substitute for legal or other professional advice.

### Content of the Notice

There are three requirements related to the content of an NPP.

1. Your NPP must be written clearly, in plain language, describing:
   - How your organization may use and disclose PHI. Include an example of each use and disclosure.
   - All the individual's rights with regard to the corresponding PHI, and how an individual may execute his rights; this includes the right to submit formal complaints to your organization. This section may be quite lengthy, depending on other state laws that have more stringent requirements related to health information privacy.
   - Your organization's legal duties for handling PHI, including a statement clearly stating your organization is required by law to maintain the privacy of PHI.
   - The name of the person to contact when an individual wants more information about your organization's privacy policies.
2. Your organization's notice must include an effective date.
3. Your organization must revise and distribute its notice promptly following material changes to its privacy practices.

### Layered Notices

CEs are allowed to use "layered" notices to implement the HIPAA Privacy Rule notice requirements. When a layered notice is used, all the elements listed above must still be present within the notice. For example, your organization can choose to create a short notice that briefly summarizes individuals' rights for their PHI, but then also provide the longer, more detailed, full version of the notice as an attachment or addendum to the brief summary. The brief summary is in effect similar to an executive summary, and the full details provide elaboration and expand on the summary points. By using a layered approach you may get more individuals to read the summary page, realize the importance of their rights regarding their PHI, and then continue to read on to discover the details of their full rights.

It is important to understand that you will *not* satisfy the HIPAA Privacy Rule requirements by providing individuals with only the summary of the notice, and not also including the full details of the NPP. CEs are not required to provide layered notices; it is an allowable option that they can choose to do to help facilitate individuals' understanding of their privacy rights. However, if you want individuals to actually ready your notice and help to ensure their understanding, we encourage you to use a layered notice.

When writing your notice, be very careful to sufficiently detail your organization's uses and disclosures of PHI. The uses and disclosures will vary, often dramatically, from CE to CE, so do not depend on getting a copy of another CE's notice and using it verbatim. Not only could you be making some promises that your actual procedures do not support, you could also be opening your organization to some potentially nasty legal actions.

### Before You Post or Distribute Your Notice

If you are the person responsible for HIPAA compliance within your organization, you probably know more about your organization's privacy policies and practices than other co-workers. So, you are also most likely the best person to write the NPP and detail the uses and disclosures of PHI. However, upon finishing the document, do not post or publish the notice until you have been in touch with your legal counsel! This notice is a form of legal contract, and as such you want a lawyer to review it to ensure you have not inadvertently worded something in a way that could be misinterpreted or lead to litigation against your organization. After your lawyer has reviewed and expressed any concerns, make the necessary changes, get approval from the lawyer and any other necessary executives and personnel within your organization, and *then* post and publish.

### Example Notice

We cannot stress enough that your organization's notice of privacy practices must be based on your actual practices, as documented within your policies, procedures, standards, etc., prior to publishing your notice. You should not write a notice indicating you are performing procedures and practices that do not exist.

Also, this is strictly an example within which virtually all possible uses and disclosures are listed and explained. Please do not use this notice verbatim; chances are your organization would not be in compliance. The intent is to give you an idea of what your NPP will look like, and make your job a little easier by giving you a model to build on. Some points to keep in mind when using this example:

- This is *not* an example of a layered notice, but an example of a fully detailed notice.
- In the example shown in Exhibit 1, you will need to change the descriptions of the uses and disclosures if your state law further limits or prohibits any of the described uses and disclosures.

### Organizational Privacy Policies

You must formally document, communicate, and maintain the policies and procedures you implement to comply with the HIPAA Privacy Rule requirements. At a minimum you must create a privacy policy for your organization that directs personnel how to handle and process PHI, and what practices are allowed and disallowed. Your policy will set the boundaries around which your personnel activities occur with respect to PHI. It is likely you will need multiple policies to adequately address and communicate your organization's requirements with regard to protecting health information. How many policies you have will depend on what type of covered entity you are, the size of your organization, and how widely dispersed your offices are geographically.

# HIPAA PRIVACY RULE

## Exhibit 1. Notice of Privacy Practices

THIS NOTICE DESCRIBES HOW MEDICAL INFORMATION ABOUT YOU MAY BE USED AND DISCLOSED AND HOW YOU CAN GET ACCESS TO THIS INFORMATION. PLEASE REVIEW IT CAREFULLY.

Company XYZ is required by law to protect the privacy of your health information and to provide you with notice of its legal duties and privacy practices with respect to your health information. If you have questions about any part of this notice, or if you want more information about the privacy practices at Company XYZ, please contact:

Joe Doe, HIPAA Compliance Director
Street XXX
City, State 99999
Phone: (000) 000-0000

**Effective Date of This Notice:** April 14, 2003 (*Note: Use the date applicable to your organization; it may initially be different than the compliance date, and it will be different after you change your notice.*)

### I. How Company XYZ May Use or Disclose Your Health Information

Company XYZ collects health information from you and stores it on printed paper and on electronic computer systems. The collection of your health information is considered your medical record. The medical record is the property of Company XYZ, but the information within the medical record containing information about you belongs to you. Company XYZ cares about and protects the privacy of your health information. Law allows Company XYZ to use or disclose your health information for the following purposes:

1. *Treatment.* Put a description here of the provision, coordination, or management of healthcare and related services. Also include, as appropriate, a description of consultation between healthcare providers that relates to patients, and referrals of patients from one healthcare provider to another. Include at least one example of a treatment.
2. *Payment.* Describe the activities to obtain premiums and to determine or fulfill responsibility for coverage and provision of benefits, or to obtain or provide reimbursement for providing healthcare, whichever is appropriate. The activities may include such things as determinations of eligibility of coverage, risk adjusting amounts, billing, claims management, review of healthcare services with respect to medical necessity, utilization review activities, disclosure of PHI to consumer reporting agencies, etc. Include at least one example applicable to your organization.
3. *Regular Healthcare Operations.* Describe the healthcare operations your organization provides, if applicable. For example, you may conduct quality assessment and improvement activities, review the competence or qualifications of healthcare professionals, underwriting, premium rating, conducting, or arranging for medical reviews, legal services, auditing functions, fraud and abuse detection, business planning and development, business management and general administrative activities, etc. Include at least one example.
4. *Information provided to you.* Describe the type of information you provide to the individual, if applicable. Include at least one example.

**Exhibit 1. Notice of Privacy Practices (Continued)**

5. *Directory.* Describe what personal information your organization may list within facility directories, such as the patient's name, location, religious affiliation, and medical condition, if appropriate. Indicate what your organization will provide to other people who ask for the patient by name. State that the individual must request your organization not to list his information if he objects. Include at least one example.

6. *Notification and communication with family.* Describe how you may disclose an individual's health information to family members, friends, or personal representatives, and the individual's rights to agree or object to such disclosures. Include at least one example.

7. *Required by law.* If required to do so, Company XYZ will disclose your health information as required by law.

8. *Public health.* Company XYZ may disclose your health information as required by law to public health authorities for purposes related to preventing or controlling disease, injury, or disability; reporting child abuse or neglect; reporting domestic violence; reporting to the Food and Drug Administration problems with products and reactions to medications; and reporting disease or infection exposure.

9. *Health oversight activities.* Company XYZ may disclose your health information to health agencies during the course of audits, investigations, inspections, licensure, and other proceedings.

10. *Judicial and administrative proceedings.* Company XYZ may disclose your health information in the course of any administrative or judicial proceeding.

11. *Law enforcement.* Company XYZ may disclose your health information to a law enforcement official for purposes such as identifying or locating a suspect, fugitive, material witness, or missing person; complying with a court order or subpoena; and other law enforcement purposes.

12. *Deceased person information.* Company XYZ may disclose your health information to coroners, medical examiners, and funeral directors.

13. *Organ donation.* Company XYZ may disclose your health information to organizations involved in procuring, banking, or transplanting organs and tissues.

14. *Research.* Company XYZ may disclose your health information to conduct research that has been approved by an Institutional Review Board or Company XYZ's privacy board.

15. *Public safety.* Company XYZ may disclose your health information to appropriate persons in order to prevent or lessen a serious and imminent threat to the health or safety of a particular person or the general public.

16. *Specialized government functions.* Company XYZ may disclose your health information for military, national security, prisoner, and government benefits. (*Note: Government benefits are applicable only for health plans purposes.*)

17. *Workers' compensation.* Company XYZ may disclose your health information as necessary to comply with workers' compensation laws.

18. *Marketing.* If applicable, indicate how your organization may contact individuals for marketing-related activities, such as appointment reminders or to give information about other treatments or health-related benefits and services that may be of interest. Include at least one example.

19. *Fundraising.* If applicable, indicate that your organization may contact individuals to participate in fundraising activities. Include at least one example.

20. *Health plan.* If applicable to your organization, indicate that your organization may disclose PHI to the sponsor of the individual's health plan. Include at least one example.

## Exhibit 1. Notice of Privacy Practices (Continued)

21. *Change of ownership.* In the event that Company XYZ is sold or merged with another organization, your health information will become the property of the new owner. (*Note: Be sure your lawyer reviews and approves of this statement; its applicability is based on a wide range of differing state laws.*)

### II. When Company XYZ May Not Use or Disclose Your Health Information

Company XYZ will not use or disclose your health information without your written authorization, except as described in this Notice of Privacy Practices. If you authorize Company XYZ to use or disclose your health information for another purpose, you may revoke your authorization in writing at any time.

### III. Your Health Information Rights

(*Note: Be sure you make the explanation of these rights appropriate for your organization. An individual reading your notice needs to understand that these rights are subject to certain unavoidable limitations and conditions, as are most legal rights, so that each "right" is not an absolute. Also, be sure you have procedures in place to support these activities.*)

1. You have the right to request restrictions on certain uses and disclosures of your health information. Company XYZ is not required to agree to the restriction that you requested.
2. You have the right to receive your health information through a reasonable alternative means or at an alternative location. You may request your information to be given to you in writing, add other methods as is applicable for your organization.
3. You have the right to inspect and copy your health information.
4. You have a right to request that Company XYZ amend your health information that is incorrect or incomplete. Company XYZ is not required to change your health information and will provide you with information about Company XYZ's denial and how you can disagree with the denial.
5. You have a right to receive an accounting of disclosures of your health information made by Company XYZ. However, Company XYZ does not have to account for disclosures for treatment, payment, healthcare operations, information provided to you, directory listings, and certain government functions.
6. You have a right to a paper copy of this Notice of Privacy Practices.

If you would like to have a more detailed explanation of these rights or if you would like to exercise one or more of these rights, contact:

Joe Doe, HIPAA Compliance Director
Street XXX
City, State 99999
Phone: (000) 000-0000

### IV. Changes to this Notice of Privacy Practices

Company XYZ reserves the right to amend this Notice of Privacy Practices at any time in the future, and to make the new provisions effective for all information that it maintains, including information that was created or received prior to the date of such amendment. Until such amendment is made, Company XYZ is required by law to comply with this Notice.

**Exhibit 1. Notice of Privacy Practices (Continued)**

Company XYZ will send updates of this Notice by (*add a description of the update distribution methods here.*)

### V. Complaints

Complaints about this Notice of Privacy Practices or how Company XYZ handles your health information should be directed to:

Joe Doe, HIPAA Compliance Director
Street XXX
City, State 99999
Phone: (000) 000-0000

If you are not satisfied with the manner in which this office handles a complaint, you may submit a formal complaint to:

Department of Health and Human Services
Office of Civil Rights
Hubert H. Humphrey Bldg.
200 Independence Avenue, S.W.
Room 509F HHH Building
Washington, D.C. 20201

You may also address your compliant to one of the regional Offices for Civil Rights. A list of these offices can be found online at http://www.hhs.gov/ocr/regmail.html.

---

First create your privacy policies draft. An example is provided here to give you a basis from which to work. Each organization is unique, so you must create policies based on your unique situation, business, and legal requirements. Italicized notes are provided where you need to pay particular attention to modifying the text to fit your organization's requirements. However, you may need to also change some of the other text that is not italicized as well. Please review the example carefully and only use what you can. It is likely your policies will look completely unlike the example!

When you have created your privacy policy you will then need to work with the appropriate members of your organization to create procedures that support the policies. The details of *how* to achieve compliance will be found within the procedures. The details of *what* needs to be the result must be described within the policy. Policy statements should not contain many, if any, "how to" statements; those belong in procedure documents.

Be sure to include "sanctions," or disciplinary consequences, within your policy. Besides being a Privacy Rule requirement, personnel must understand what actions they can expect if they do not comply with the policies, and your organization must follow through with these documented sanctions for personnel to take the policies seriously. Some organizations like to have a separate sanctions policy; however, including sanction descriptions with each privacy policy is generally more effective.

After you have finished your privacy policies, you need to have your executive management, legal department, human resources department, and any other appropriate management review them and give their approval. The personnel must know that your organizational leaders support the policies. Your leaders should communicate to the organization personnel that they support the policies and they will ensure sanctions are enforced for those who break the policies. Exhibit 2 is a sample policy.

### Exhibit 2. Example Organizational Privacy Policies

**Purpose:** Company XYZ personnel must comply with the following privacy policies to ensure the privacy of the information Company XYZ processes and handles, and also to ensure that Company XYZ complies fully with all applicable federal and state privacy protection laws and regulations. Protecting customer and patient information is of utmost importance to Company XYZ. Personnel violating this policy are subject to disciplinary action up to and including possible termination of employment and possible criminal prosecution.

**Effective Date: This policy is in effect as of April 14, 2003.** (*Note: Put whatever date is applicable to your organization.*)

**Expiration Date:** This policy has no expiration date. This policy will remain in effect until personnel are notified otherwise.

**Policy Owner:** (*Name*) owns and maintains this policy. Please direct questions regarding this policy to (*name and contact information*).

#### Assigning Privacy and Security Responsibilities

Specific positions within Company XYZ are assigned the responsibility of implementing and maintaining the HIPAA Privacy Rule requirements. These positions will be provided sufficient resources and authority to fulfill their responsibilities. There will be one individual or job position designated as the Privacy Officer. There will also be one individual or job position designated as the HIPAA Compliance Manager.

#### Uses and Disclosures of Protected Health Information

Company XYZ customer and patient information may only be used or disclosed in the following situations:

1. The individual who is the subject of the information has authorized the use or disclosure.
2. The individual who is the subject of the information has received the Company XYZ Notice of Privacy Practices and has acknowledged receipt of the Notice. This allows use or disclosure for treatment, payment, or healthcare operations.
3. The individual who is the subject of the information agrees or does not object to the disclosure to persons involved in the healthcare of the individual.
4. The disclosure is to the individual who is the subject of the information or to HHS for compliance-related purposes.
5. The use or disclosure is for a HIPAA "public purposes" exception.

## Exhibit 2. Example Organizational Privacy Policies (Continued)

### Deceased Individuals

Company XYZ privacy protections and procedures apply to information concerning deceased individuals.

### Notice of Privacy Practices

Company XYZ will publish a Notice of Privacy Practices and provide it to all individuals at the earliest practicable time. All uses and disclosures of protected health information will be done according to the Company XYZ Notice of Privacy Practices. Company XYZ will attempt to gain written acknowledgment of the receipt of the Notice from all individuals to whom we provide the Notice of Privacy Practices. Company XYZ will document our attempts to gain this acknowledgment if we cannot successfully obtain written receipt of the Notice.

### Restriction Requests

Company XYZ will give serious consideration to all requests for restrictions on uses and disclosures of protected health information as published in the Notice of Privacy Practices and follow Company XYZ procedures for addressing such requests. When Company XYZ agrees to a restriction, personnel with Company XYZ must observe and comply with the restriction.

### Minimum Necessary Disclosure of Protected Health Information

Except for disclosures made for treatment purposes, all disclosures of protected health information must be limited to the minimum amount of information necessary to accomplish the purpose of the disclosure. All requests for protected health information (except requests made for treatment purposes) will be limited to the minimum amount of information needed to accomplish the purpose of the request.

### Access to Protected Health Information

Company XYZ will grant access to protected health information to each employee or contractor based on the assigned job functions. The access privileges will not exceed those necessary to accomplish the assigned job function.

### Access to Protected Health Information by the Individual

Company XYZ will provide access to protected health information to the person who is the subject of such information when the individual requests access within the timeframes required by the HIPAA Privacy Rule. Company XYZ will inform the person requesting access of the location of their protected health information if Company XYZ does not physically possess the PHI but knows where it is located.

### Amendment of Incomplete or Incorrect Protected Health Information

Company XYZ will respond to all requests for amendment of protected health information in a timely manner following Company XYZ's procedures for updating PHI. If requests reveal the PHI is incorrect, Company XYZ will amend the PHI appropriately within the timeframe dictated by the HIPAA Privacy Rule and will document the amendment. A notice of corrections will be given to any organization with which the PHI has been shared.

## Exhibit 2. Example Organizational Privacy Policies (Continued)

### Access by Personal Representatives

Company XYZ will grant access to PHI to personal representatives of individuals in the same manner as if they were the individuals themselves, except in cases of abuse where granting the access could endanger the individual or someone else. We will observe the relevant state, local, and other applicable laws when disclosing information about minors to parents.

### Confidential Communications Channels

Company XYZ will use confidential communications channels if possible when requested by individuals.

### Disclosure Accounting

Company XYZ will provide an accounting of all disclosures of PHI subject to HIPAA Privacy Rule requirements to an individual upon the individual's request.

### Marketing Activities

Company XYZ will use or disclose PHI for marketing activities only after obtaining a valid authorization. Company XYZ considers marketing as any communication to purchase or use a product or service where an arrangement exists in exchange for direct or indirect payment, or where Company XYZ encourages purchase or use of a product or service. Company XYZ does not consider the communication of alternate forms of treatment, or the use of products and services in treatment to be marketing. Company XYZ will not obtain an authorization when a face-to-face communication is made by us to the patient, or when giving an individual a promotional gift of nominal value.

### Judicial and Administrative Proceedings

Company XYZ will disclose PHI for judicial or administrative proceedings only when:

- Accompanied by a court or administrative order or grand jury subpoena.
- Accompanied by a subpoena or discovery request that includes either the authorization of the individual to whom the information applies, documented assurances that good faith effort has been made to adequately notify the individual of the request for their information and there are no outstanding objections by the individual, or a qualified protective order issued by the court.

If a subpoena or discovery request is submitted to Company XYZ without one of these requirements, we will seek to notify the individual, obtain his or her authorization, or obtain a qualified protective order before disclosing any information. We will not disclose information other than that required by the court order, subpoena, or discovery request.

### De-Identified Data and Limited Data Sets

Company XYZ will disclose de-identified data only after it has been properly de-identified. Limited data sets will be used only after the relevant identifying data has been removed, and released only to organizations that have signed adequate data-use agreements. Limited data sets will be used only for research, public health, or healthcare operations purposes.

**Exhibit 2. Example Organizational Privacy Policies (Continued)**

### *Authorizations*

Company XYZ will obtain a valid authorization for all disclosures, other than those for treatment, payment, healthcare operations, to the individual or their personal representative, to persons involved with the individual's care, to business associates in their legitimate duties, to facility directories, or for public purposes. The authorization will include all the HIPAA required statements. Authorizations from outside this organization will be checked to confirm validity.

### *Complaints*

Company XYZ will investigate and resolve all complaints relating to the protection of health information within the time limits required by the HIPAA Privacy Rule. The Privacy Officer will investigate all complaints made to Company XYZ related to privacy practices and implement resolutions as appropriate.

### *Prohibited Activities*

No Company XYZ employee or contractor may engage in any intimidating or retaliatory acts against persons who file complaints or otherwise exercise their rights under HIPAA regulations. No Company XYZ employee or contractor may condition treatment, payment, enrollment, or eligibility for benefits on the provision of an authorization to disclose protected health information.

### *Responsibility*

The Privacy Officer is responsible for designing and implementing procedures to comply with the Company XYZ privacy policies.

### *Verification of Identity*

Company XYZ will verify the identity of all persons who request access to protected health information before such access is granted.

### *Mitigation*

Company XYZ will follow mitigation procedures to minimize the effects of any unauthorized use or disclosure of protected health information that may occur.

### *Safeguards*

Company XYZ will implement security procedures to appropriately safeguard physical and electronic PHI from intentional or unintentional use or disclosure that is in violation of the HIPAA Privacy Rule. The security procedures will include directives for physically protecting Company XYZ facilities and PHI, establishing technical security for electronic PHI, and establishing administrative security and access control protection. These procedures will include safeguarding the oral communication of PHI to the greatest extent possible.

### *Business Associates*

Company XYZ business associates will be contractually required to protect health information to the same degree as Company XYZ personnel. Company XYZ will deal with business associates who violate their agreement by first attempting to correct the situation; if the situation cannot be resolved, the business associate agreement will be terminated, and the services provided by the business associate will be discontinued.

**Exhibit 2. Example Organizational Privacy Policies (Continued)**

*Training and Awareness*

Company XYZ will train all personnel in the policies and procedures related to HIPAA Privacy Rule requirements. New personnel will receive training within 2 weeks of their start date. Existing personnel will receive ongoing awareness messages covering the privacy and security requirements for customer and patient information, and must attend formal training soon after the Company XYZ privacy policies are changed, and at least once a year. Company XYZ will document the training in which each personnel member participates, including the date and topic of the training.

*Sanctions*

Company XYZ will apply disciplinary sanctions to any personnel member who violates these policies, or any procedures implemented to support these policies. Sanctions include disciplinary actions up to and possibly including termination of employment and possible criminal prosecution.

*Retention of Records*

Company XYZ will retain, secure, and maintain all records identified within the HIPAA Privacy Rule for at least 6 years using procedures that allow for access when necessary within a reasonable amount of time as determined by the Privacy Officer. Company XYZ will extend the records retention time requirement as necessary to comply with other governmental regulations, laws, or requirements made by the Company XYZ professional liability carrier.

*Cooperation with Privacy Oversight Authorities*

Company XYZ will fully support and cooperate with oversight agencies such as the Office for Civil Rights of the Department of Health and Human Services during investigations and other efforts to ensure the protection of health information. All Company XYZ personnel will cooperate fully with all privacy compliance reviews and investigations.

## Chapter 7: Practical Checklist

- Does the NPP you give to your customers or patients contain all the sections required by the HIPAA Privacy Rule?
- Have you decided whether to use a layered NPP?
- Has your lawyer reviewed and approved your NPP?
- Have you communicated your NPP to your personnel?
- Do you have procedures established to support the promises made within the NPP?
- Have you created internal privacy policies for your personnel and BAs that cover the HIPAA Privacy Rule requirements?
- Has your lawyer reviewed your organizational privacy policies and signed off on them?
- Do you have the visible support of your executive management and other organization leaders for the policies?

# Chapter 8
# State Preemption

Covered entities (CEs) will not only need to be in compliance with the HIPAA Privacy Rule requirements, but also with the privacy and confidentiality state laws that are not preempted by the Privacy Rule. The Privacy Rule does not replace federal, state, or other laws that grant greater privacy protections than are stipulated within the Rule. Additionally, CEs are free to retain or adopt more protective privacy policies and practices. The HIPAA Privacy Rule defines "state law" to include statutes, regulations, case law, and other state action having binding legal effect. Preemption of state law is addressed in Part 160, sub-part B of the Privacy Rule. It is interesting to note that this section of the regulation was constructed not only to address the privacy issues, but also the preemption issues in the already-issued Transactions Rule, which did not cover this issue.

During the comment period for the 2002 Privacy Rule Notice of Proposed Rulemaking (NPRM), many healthcare plans and providers expressed concern that the preemption provision would be overly burdensome, ineffective, and that without a complete preemption of all the various and sundry state privacy laws, they would be hard to implement and enforce. Many commenters expressed concern that the proposed preemption provisions would result in litigation. It was feared that the exception determination process as outlined would be very costly and result in inconsistent handling from state to state. The Department of Health and Human Services (HHS) noted that many commenters asked to have the wording changed so that the rule would preempt all state privacy laws. On the other end of the spectrum, there were also many commenters that recommended there should be no exceptions granted to the federal standards, with the opinion that such exceptions defeat the goal of promoting uniform transactions.

**What Is Contrary?**

A state law is considered "contrary to" a HIPAA privacy standard, requirement, or implementation specification in one of two situations (45 CFR § 160.202), where:

---

The information and opinions provided in this book do not constitute or substitute for legal or other professional advice.

- The CE cannot possibly comply with both the state and federal requirements. So, compliance with a state requirement would prevent compliance with the HIPAA requirement.
- A provision of state law stands as "an obstacle" to the accomplishment and execution of the full purposes of the HIPAA legislation related to Administrative Simplification. This language is far from clear cut but anticipates situations in which state and federal law do not directly conflict, but state and federal requirements nevertheless compete with one another.
- Other situations that imply there may be a contrary situation, but upon further analysis reveals there is not, includes:
  - When state law privacy requirements are not contrary to the Privacy Rule, a CE must abide by both laws.
  - When the state imposes a requirement for which there is no analogous federal requirement, then the state law applies.

For example, when the HIPAA Privacy Rule allows, but does not require, a specific disclosure that is prohibited by state law, the state law is considered not contrary to HIPAA because the decision can be made to comply with both by not disclosing the information.

State laws are considered to be in agreement with or not contrary to HIPAA standards, requirements, and implementation specifications in the following situations:

- When both a state law and the Privacy Rule permit, or both require the same use or disclosure.
- When both a state law and the Privacy Rule prohibit, expressly or implicitly, the same use or disclosure.
- When both a state law and the Privacy Rule permit, both require, or both prohibit the same use or disclosure, but the state law is more restrictive or detailed in its requirements, or vice versa.
- When a use or disclosure is required by state law and permitted by the Privacy Rule, or vice versa.

State laws are considered to be in opposition to or contrary to HIPAA standards, requirements, and implementation specifications in the following situations:

- When a state law expressly or implicitly prohibits a use or disclosure that is permitted by a HIPAA standard, requirement, or implementation specification, or vice versa.
- When a state law requires a use or disclosure, but it is prohibited by the Privacy Rule, or vice versa. Preemption criteria that must be considered includes:
  - What criteria must be used to determine the state's laws that need to be reviewed?

- Is it the state in which the Group Health Plan is registered?
- Is it the state in which medical treatment was obtained?
- Is it the state in which the patient resides?
- Is it to the state in which the patient resides, and whose laws provide the privacy protection to the patient?

The answer is a definite "it depends!" In some states, the jurisdiction of the Department of Insurance is based on the membership covered under the master contracts used in that state, and also covered under master contracts used in out-of-state trusts. There is the need to have federal law, such as HIPAA, control competing state and local laws with respect to the specifications for the use of certain health transactions and associated information. The HIPAA rules for information transactions and the security of health information override any contrary provision of state law unless expressly excluded by the Secretary of HHS.

The Privacy Rule is treated slightly differently than the Security Rule and Transactions and Code Sets Standards. The Privacy Rule does not fully preempt state privacy laws. The Privacy Rule does not supercede a contrary provision of state law, if the state law imposes requirements, standards, or implementation specifications that are more stringent than the requirements, standards, or implementation specifications imposed under the Privacy Rule. The Privacy Rule sets the minimum privacy requirements that must be met by CEs in all states. Any Privacy Rule standard, requirement, or implementation guideline that is contrary to state law will preempt that state law unless one of the exceptions to preemption applies. (See 45 CFR § 160.203).

**Exceptions to Preemption**

Some state laws that may be contrary to HIPAA and the Privacy Rule may not be preempted if the law falls under an exception established within the HIPAA legislation or Privacy Rule. The following are the state law HIPAA and Privacy Rule preemption exception categories:

- *Public health and vital statistics.* This allows providers to report diseases or injuries, child abuse, births, or deaths, or those that authorize public health surveillance, or public health investigation or intervention.
- *Health plan regulation and monitoring.* This allows for the application of state laws that require a health plan to report or provide access to information for regulatory management audits, financial audits, program monitoring and evaluation, facility licensure or certification, or individual licensure and certification.
- *Determination by the Secretary of HHS.* The Secretary has the discretion to determine that HIPAA will not preempt contrary state laws that are necessary to prevent fraud and abuse related to healthcare payment; to ensure appropriate state regulation of insurance and health plans;

to permit state reporting on healthcare delivery or cost; or to serve a compelling need related to public health, safety, or welfare.

- *More stringent health privacy protections.* HIPAA does not preempt provisions of state law covering the privacy of individually identifiable health information and impose requirements that are more stringent than the requirements, standards, or specifications imposed under HIPAA privacy rule.

Requests for an exception may be submitted to the Secretary with information indicating, among other things, the specific state law and corresponding HIPAA privacy standard, requirement, or implementation specification for which the exception is requested. A request by a state must be submitted through its chief elected official or that person's designated representative. Until the Secretary makes a determination, the HIPAA rule will continue to preempt state law (see 45 CFR § 160.204).

## Preemption Analysis

Thousands of questions were posed during the public comment period regarding the interpretation, implications, and consequences of the preemption directives. Organizations will need to obtain significant advice and technical assistance about all of the regulatory requirements on an ongoing basis as they strive to maintain continued compliance.

HHS does not have the statutory authority under HIPAA to preempt state laws that impose more stringent privacy requirements on CEs. HIPAA provides that the rule promulgated by the Secretary may not preempt state laws that are in conflict with the regulatory requirements and that provide greater privacy protections.

So it becomes imperative for CEs to conduct a preemption analysis for the laws of the states in which they have or process PHI. Such an analysis will identify the state law requirements for which continued compliance is necessary along with the HIPAA requirements. As with any law or regulation that impacts your organization, be sure to discuss this issue thoroughly with your legal counsel. It will be important for you to identify and discuss with your legal counsel the technical, operational, and procedural issues related to the handling of PHI so the most applicable interpretation of state law can be made.

How do you approach this state preemption analysis? There are a few ways to accomplish this, but it will probably be easiest for you to decide first which states you can eliminate as having privacy laws that are in direct opposition with, or that have less restrictive privacy laws than the HIPAA laws. In these cases, the HIPAA requirements will take precedence. In general there are four broad situations within which state privacy laws may fall. These include when the state laws:

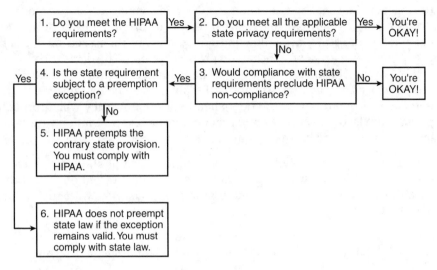

**Exhibit 1. HIPAA State Preemption Decision Tree**

1. Have been identified by the Secretary of HHS as specifically not being preempted by the HIPAA Privacy Rule
2. Are more stringent with regard to privacy and confidentiality requirements than the corresponding HIPAA requirement, standard, or implementation specification
3. Allow disease, injury, child abuse, birth, death, or public health surveillance, investigation, or intervention to be reported
4. Govern the access to or how to report the information health plans possess

Generally you can now disregard from analysis the state laws that fall into situations 1, 3, and 4; these generally are exceptions to preemption. Now you are ready to perform your preemption analysis. For each HIPAA requirement, use the decision tree shown in Exhibit 1.

### *Framework for Analyzing HIPAA Preemption Issues*

- Prepare an inventory of applicable state law requirements and the Privacy Rule.
- Review policies, procedures, and operations in relation to both state law and the Privacy Rule.
- Use the decision tree shown in Exhibit 1.

### Conclusion

State preemption issues are extremely complex. The laws in each state are worded vastly differently, and each part must be analyzed and compared to the Privacy Rule. It is often difficult to determine which law, state or federal Privacy Rule, is more stringent with regard to privacy protections. For example, some state laws allow patients copies of their records with no exceptions. The Privacy Rule has several exceptions. The decision of what actions to take in such a situation, perhaps hinging on the life or death of the patient vs. the general welfare of the public, can be extremely hard to determine. It is up to CEs to know ahead of time how they will approach preemption issues in general, and then to address each situation with their legal counsel, based on the unique factors involved.

Use the sites in Exhibit 2 as beginning points for your state law preemption research. Not all will have specific preemption information, but at the time this book was written, all had pointers to other sites with such information.

**Exhibit 2. State-by-State HIPAA Preemption-Related Information Web Sites**

1. General information
   - Government Information Value Exchange for States (GIVES); http://www.hipaagives.org/
   - Southern HIPAA Administrative Regional Process (SHARP); http://www.sharpworkgroup.com
2. Alabama
   - Alabama Medicaid; http://www.medicaid.state.al.us/HIPAA/
3. Alaska
   - Department of Health and Social Services; http://health.hss.state.ak.us/das/is/hipaa/
4. Arizona
   - Arizona Health Care Cost Containment System; http://www.ahcccs.state.az.us/HIPAA/
5. Arkansas
   - Arkansas Department of Human Services; http://www.hipaa.state.ar.us/
6. California
   - Southern California HIPAA Forum; http://www.hipaausa.com/socal/forum.html
   - Department of Health Services; http://www.dhs.ca.gov/hipaa/
   - Medi-CAL; http://files.medi-cal.ca.gov/pubsdoco/pubsframe.asp?hURL = /pubsdoco/Publications/bulletins/HIPAA/hipaa_m.htm
   - Office of HIPAA Implementation; http://www.ohi.ca.gov/
   - Department of Developmental Services; http://www.dds.ca.gov/hipaa/hipaa_main.cfm
   - Department of Mental Health; http://www.dmh.ca.gov/hipaa/
7. Colorado
   - Department of Health Care Policy and Financing; http://www.chcpf.state.co.us/HIPAA/hipaaindex.htm
   - Division of Insurance; http://www.dora.state.co.us/insurance/consumer/hipaa1.htm
   - Colorado Department of Human Resources, Alcohol and Drug Abuse Division; http://www.cdhs.state.co.us/ohr/adad/hipaafinall.htm

**Exhibit 2.  State-by-State HIPAA Preemption-Related Information Web Sites (Continued)**

8. Connecticut
   - Department of Information Technology; http://www.doit.state.ct.us/HIPAA/HIPAA.htm
   - Department of Social Services; http://www.ctmedicalprogram.com/hipaa.html
9. Florida
   - State Technology Office; http://www.myflorida.com/myflorida/sto/hipaa/
10. Georgia
   - Georgia Department of Community Health; http://www.communityhealth.state.ga.us/
11. Hawaii
   - Hawaii HIPAA Readiness Collaborative; http://www.hhic.org/hipaa
12. Idaho
   - Idaho HIPAA Coordinating Council; http://www2.state.id.us/dhw/hipaa/cc/council_home.htm
   - Department of Health and Welfare; http://www2.state.id.us/dhw/hipaa
13. Illinois
   - Department of Public Aid; http://www.state.il.us/dpa/hipaa.html
14. Indiana
   - Indiana Health Coverage Programs; http://www.indianamedicaid.com/ihcp/ProviderServices/hipaa.asp
   - Department of Insurance; http://www.ai.org/idoi/health/hipaa.html
15. Iowa
   - Iowa SNIP; http://www.iowasnip.org/iowasnip/nonScripts/ipa.asp
   - HIPAA Compliance Project; http://www.state.ia.us/government/hipaa/
16. Kansas
   - HIPAA Awareness and Readiness for Kansas; http://www.hark.info/
17. Kentucky
   - Department for Mental Health and Mental Retardation; http://dmhmrs.chr.state.ky.us/hipaa.asp
   - Department for Medicaid Services; http://chs.state.ky.us/dms/HIPAA/default.htm
18. Louisiana
   - Department of Health and Hospitals; http://www.dhh.state.la.us/HIPAA/index.htm
19. Maine
   - Department of Human Services; http://www.state.me.us/bms/hipaainfo.html
20. Maryland
   - Maryland Health Care Commission; http://www.mhcc.state.md.us/edi/hipaa/_hipaa.htm
   - Department of Health and Mental Hygiene; http://dhmh.state.md.us/HIPAA/
21. Massachusetts
   - Massachusetts Health Data Consortium; http://www.mahealthdata.org/
   - New England HIPAA Workgroup; http://www.hipaausa.com/NEHW.html
   - Executive Office for Administration and Finance; http://www.state.ma.us/itd/spg/publications/bulletins/ITBulletinWinter2001/hipaa.html
22. Michigan
   - Department of Community Health; http://www.michigan.gov/mdch/0,1607,7-132-2945-36737 — ,00.html

## Exhibit 2. State-by-State HIPAA Preemption-Related Information Web Sites (Continued)

23. Minnesota
    - Minnesota Center for Healthcare Electronic Commerce (MCHEC); http://www.mhdi.org/mchec/index.html
    - Department of Human Services; http://www.dhs.state.mn.us/hipaa/
24. Mississippi
    - Department of Information Technology Services; http://www.hipaa.state.ms.us/
25. Missouri
    - Department of Health and Senior Services; http://www.health.state.mo.us/HIPAA/
    - Department of Mental Health; http://www.modmh.state.mo.us/homeinfo/hipaa/index.htm
26. Montana
    - Department of Public Health and Human Services; http://www.dphhs.state.mt.us/hpsd/medicaid/hipaa/index.htm
27. Nevada
    - Department of Insurance; http://doi.state.nv.us/
28. New Hampshire
    - New Hampshire and Vermont Strategic HIPAA Implementation Plan (NHVSHIP); http://www.nhvship.org/
    - Developmental Disabilities Service System; http://www.nhdds.org/nhddsit/HIPAA/overview.html
29. New York
    - Preemption Charts; http://www.health.state.ny.us/nysdoh/hipaa/hipaa_preemption_charts.htm
    - NYS Central HIPAA Coordination Project; http://www.oft.state.ny.us/hipaa/index.htm
30. North Carolina
    - North Carolina HIPAA Strategic Plan; http://dirm.state.nc.us/hipaa/hipaa2002/statewide/doc/01%20Executive%20SummaryP.pdf
    - North Carolina Healthcare Information Communications Alliance (NCHICA); http://www.nchica.org/
    - Department of Health and Human Services; http://dirm.state.nc.us/hipaa/
31. North Dakota
    - Department of Health; http://www.health.state.nd.us/ndhd/admin/hipaa/
32. Ohio
    - HIPAA Statewide Project; http://www.state.oh.us/hipaa/index.htm
33. Oregon
    - Department of Human Services; http://www.hr.state.or.us/hipaa/
34. Pennsylvania
    - e-Pennsylvania Alliance; http://www.e-paalliance.org/
    - Department of Public Welfare; http://www.dpw.state.pa.us/omap/hipaa/omaphipaa.asp
    - Public School Employees' Retirement System; http://www.psers.state.pa.us/Publications/newsletters/Updates/2003/p4.htm
    - Department of Insurance; http://www.insurance.state.pa.us/html/hipaa.html
    - Governor's Office of Administration; http://www.emanager.state.pa.us/bmc/cwp/view.asp?a=234&q=168122
35. Rhode Island
    - Department of Human Services; http://www.dhs.state.ri.us/dhs/dhipaa.htm

**Exhibit 2. State-by-State HIPAA Preemption-Related Information Web Sites (Continued)**

36. South Carolina
    - South Carolina HIPAA Office; http://www.hipaa.state.sc.us/
37. South Dakota
    - Department of Health; http://www.state.sd.us/doh/rural/tehipaa.htm
38. Texas
    - Texas Health and Human Services Commission;
      http://www.hhsc.state.tx.us/NDIS/NDISTaskForce.html
39. Utah
    - Utah Health Information Network; http://www.uhin.com/
40. Vermont
    - New Hampshire and Vermont Strategic HIPAA Implementation Plan (NHVSHIP);
      http://www.nhvship.org/
41. Virginia
    - Department of Medical Assistance; http://www.dmas.state.va.us/hpa-home.htm
    - Department of Health and Human Resources;
      http://www.hhr.state.va.us/Initiatives/hippa.cfm
42. Washington
    - Washington State HIPAA Partnership; http://maa.dshs.wa.gov/dshshipaa/
    - Department of Social and Health Services; http://maa.dshs.wa.gov/
43. West Virginia
    - Department of Health and Human Resources;
      http://www.wvdhhr.org/bms/hipaa/hipaa.htm
    - Department of Insurance; http://www.state.wv.us/insurance/new_law.htm
44. Wisconsin
    - HIPAA Collaborative of Wisconsin (COW); http://www.hipaacow.org/
    - Department of Health and Family Services; http://www.dhfs.state.wi.us/HIPAA/
45. Wyoming
    - Department of Health; http://wdh.state.wy.us/hipaa.htm

## Chapter 8: Practical Checklist

- Identify state laws applicable to your organization that have laws that are contrary to, but more stringent than portions of the HIPAA Privacy Rule requirements. These laws are generally not preempted.
- Identify state laws applicable to your organization that have laws that are contrary to, but are less stringent than portions of the HIPAA Privacy Rule requirements. These laws will generally be preempted.
- Identify state laws applicable to your organization that have requirements that are not contrary to the HIPAA Privacy Rule requirements. These laws are generally not preempted.
- Incorporate noncontrary laws into your HIPAA Privacy Rule authorization, privacy notice practices, and policies and procedures of your organization.
- *Very important:* Discuss the state preemption issues with your legal counsel to determine how this issue affects your particular organization.

# Chapter 9
# Crafting a Privacy Implementation Plan

Preparing for HIPAA compliance is complex and must be thoroughly planned. Planning should involve the entire organization; it is not just an information technology issue, nor just a business application issue. It certainly involves these issues, but also much more. HIPAA compliance is both a project to be implemented, as well as an ongoing practice to oversee. Most organizations will already meet some of the HIPAA requirements. Other requirements will still need to be addressed. Organizations must accurately review their state of HIPAA compliance, identify the outstanding requirements, and create a functional plan for implementation. A baseline compliance assessment (Chapter 6) needs to occur to determine where the organization is presently at with regard to HIPAA compliance. A successful assessment will have the beneficial side effect of creating an information flow document.

Many organizations struggle with the initial approach to creating an implementation plan. Exhibit 1 shows a plan to help you get started; modify it to best meet your organization's business environment.

### Some Points to Keep in Mind

Here are some Privacy Rule compliance facts related to common questions and concerns you need to keep in mind when creating and applying your Privacy Rule implementation plan:

- Physicians and nurses can discuss protected health information (PHI). They need to take care not to discuss PHI in locations outside their facilities where others can hear. However, discussing within their facilities (such as in a hospital room shared by patients) is considered acceptable even if the possibility exists that someone may overhear their discussion.
- Covered entities (CEs) are not required to monitor or oversee how business associates (BAs) apply safeguards to the PHI they are processing. However, they must include safeguard requirements in

their BA contracts, and must discontinue the associations (if possible) if they notice a BA is in violation of the safeguards and does not correct the violation.

- The Privacy Rule does not prevent the use of sign-in sheets or calling names of patients in the waiting room.
- The Privacy Rule does not require the use of specific technologies or operating systems.
- The Privacy Rule does not prohibit faxing PHI. However, CEs must use appropriate administrative, technical, and physical safeguards to protect the PHI in the faxes. Also keep in mind that many organizations now use eFax, which delivers the faxes to servers and e-mail accounts.
- The Privacy Rule permits a disclosure of PHI that is required by other applicable laws.
- The Privacy Rule permits disclosures to researchers and law enforcement; however, it does not require the disclosures. In some cases (such as for research), authorization may be required. Even when an authorization is not required and the Privacy Rule permits a disclosure, there may be other limitations or laws preventing such disclosures, as well as the discretion of the CE.
- Unless a patient objects, a physician can discuss a patient's condition with family or friends involved with the patient's care.
- The Privacy Rule allows hospitals and disaster relief agencies to notify family members that a family member has been admitted to a hospital or has been involved in a disaster.
- An organization cannot and is not expected to be "perfect." Organizations are expected to identify mistakes and correct them as best as possible to meet HIPAA compliance. Noncompliance issues arise when an organization recognizes it has problem or noncompliance areas and does not take corrective action.

## Conclusion

The HIPAA compliance plan will require ongoing maintenance. Unlike a project such as Y2K compliance, when the project was essentially finished shortly after January 1, 2000, HIPAA compliance does not have a termination point. HIPAA requirements will impose strict penalties for noncompliance from the compliance date forward. You cannot expect to meet all the HIPAA compliance requirements upon one date and be done; this must be a long-term commitment your organization makes.

**Exhibit 1. Privacy Rule Implementation Plan**

1. Determine your covered entity status.
   - Are you a covered entity? What kind? A healthcare provider? A health plan? A healthcare clearinghouse? A hybrid entity?
   - Are you a BA?
   - See Chapter 1, as well as Chapters 16 through 20, to help you make these determinations. Then, discuss with your legal counsel.
2. Establish a HIPAA Privacy Project. Start planning for your compliance activities.
   - Determine who will sponsor the project.
   - Establish a steering committee to oversee and guide the HIPAA compliance effort.
   - Organize a team of people to track and manage the HIPAA activities. Develop a project management environment.
   - Assign a HIPAA compliance team.
   - Develop a strategic plan so that everyone in the organization understands the mission, goals, and objectives of the effort.
   - Confirm your scope and establish your due diligence documentation method and repository.
   - Develop initiative-level roles and responsibilities so that each major component of the organization knows who is doing what in the effort.
   - Develop detailed work plans for at least the next phase of your effort and a master plan for the initiative.
   - Establish a HIPAA compliance budget and timeline.
3. Understand the activities covered by HIPAA.
   - Read and understand the HIPAA regulations (see Chapters 5 and 6).
   - Analyze the requirements as they relate to your organization.
   - Know the compliance timelines and penalties (see Chapter 5).
   - Analyze the HIPAA regulations against potentially preemptive, superceding, or conflicting privacy regulations with which you must comply (see Chapter 8):
     – State
     – Other federal
     – International
   - Identify which parts of your organization are impacted by the regulations.
   - Is your organization a covered entity or a hybrid entity under HIPAA?
     – If a hybrid entity, identify the covered functions are within your organization.
   - Obtain regulatory guidance materials (see Appendix C).
   - Make top management aware of the issues and obtain their documented commitment to compliance.
4. Identify a Privacy Officer and privacy contact for HIPAA questions and complaints.
   - Identify and appoint a qualified Privacy Officer to address HIPAA and other privacy-related issues if you are a covered entity.
   - Identify privacy and security officers within each healthcare component of a hybrid-covered entity.
   - Identify a contact person to receive complaints about policies, privacy, and HIPAA compliance, to provide information about the Notice of Privacy Practices (NPP), and to answer general related questions.
   - Train the Privacy Officer(s) and privacy contact(s).

## Exhibit 1. Privacy Rule Implementation Plan (Continued)

- Visit Web sites often to obtain new and updated HIPAA privacy information (see Appendix C).
- Assign members of the HIPAA compliance team with specific responsibilities for addressing each of the HIPAA gap analysis action items.

5. Perform a gap analysis and determine the baseline compliance status for the organization.
    - Develop an assessment method. You will likely need a different method for each regulation area (see Chapter 6).
    - Collect and review printed documentation.
    - Conduct interviews to collect unwritten methods and procedures.
    - Review electronic information.
    - Create an inventory of all current policies, procedures, and documentation related to HIPAA privacy requirements.
    - Analyze the HIPAA regulations against your existing organizational policies, rules, procedures, directives, etc.
    - Create an inventory of all information that is considered individually identifiable health information (see Chapter 5). Classify the information that is PHI under HIPAA definitions.
    - Create an inventory of all your medical devices that store individually identifiable health information.
    - Create an inventory of all your BAs (vendors, contractors, etc.) and electronic trading partners with whom your organization shares health information.
    - Identify all BAs who have remote access capabilities to your facilities (for example, dial-in, VPN, etc.) for support purposes.
    - Map data flows with BAs:
        – Identify paper systems and forms.
        – Identify information systems.
        – Identify all BA contracts.
        – Identify all BAs policies and procedures related to health information.
        – Determine existing responsibilities within BAs for the privacy function.
    - Document the uses and disclosures for PHI within your organization and by your BAs.
    - Test information systems to determine if access controls are implemented.
    - Conduct assessment activities to establish baseline HIPAA compliance and a risk assessment summary.
    - Analyze the HIPAA regulations against existing organization-specific rules, directives, enterprise policies, etc.
    - Analyze gaps between the existing organizational (human) environment and HIPAA requirements.
    - Analyze gaps between the existing technical and networking environment and HIPAA requirements.
    - Analyze gaps between the existing information policies and procedures and HIPAA requirements.
    - Document and date all identified gaps.
    - Create a compliance plan for closing gaps and meeting compliance.
    - Maintain the compliance plan and gap analysis for future reference.
    - Document potential impacts the gaps present to your organization.

**Exhibit 1. Privacy Rule Implementation Plan (Continued)**

6. Planning remediation strategies.
   - Document your business compliance strategy and implementation plan.
   - Document your technical compliance strategy and implementation plan.
   - Refine your budget estimates as necessary.
   - Seek additional funding commitment if necessary.
   - Organize or recruit the staff necessary to close the gaps.
   - Determine if you can meet HIPAA Privacy Rule compliance on your own, or if you will need outside help. Consider hiring temporary workers or outside consultants experienced with HIPAA remediation if you do not have the staff, resources, or experience available in-house.
   - Consider using other resources as well:
     - Professional associations
     - Software
     - Forms
7. Remediate the organization.
   - Update existing policies and procedures and develop new policies and procedures as necessary.
   - Update organizational procedures, systems, and documentation to match policy and procedure requirements.
   - Develop training to give to the workforce covering HIPAA and privacy requirements.
   - Conduct appropriate levels of training for implementation staff as well as designated privacy and security officers.
   - Give all personnel awareness training.
   - Document privacy training and the personnel who attended.
   - Establish and update BA contracts as necessary to provide directive for protecting PHI.
   - Modify business processes, business application systems, and technical infrastructure as necessary to comply.
   - Test information systems; modify as necessary and pilot modifications.
   - Conduct training relating to modifications or specific compliance issues.
   - Implement and install changes.
   - Transition the maintenance of new processes and products to the responsible parties.
   - Determine the appropriate administrative, physical, and technical security measures to apply to medical devices.
   - Create operating procedures for secure medical equipment use.
   - Develop privacy notices and any necessary accompanying forms and documents.
   - Develop consent forms and documents (if applicable for your organization). Consent forms are not required by HIPAA; however, some state or international regulations may require them, and your organization may choose to use them based on your legal counsel advice.
   - Develop authorization forms and documents.
   - Develop accounting for disclosure forms and documents.
   - Develop formal documentation procedures and standards to ensure information is adequately maintained for the appropriate time limits.
   - Implement and maintain the use of notice, consent (if applicable), and authorization forms.

**Exhibit 1. Privacy Rule Implementation Plan (Continued)**

- Get the new and updated BA agreements signed.
- Perform due diligence on your business relationships.
- Create or update your NPP appropriately.
- Communicate your NPP to your patients and health plan members.
- Establish compliance systems and a plan for ongoing compliance.
- Create and maintain HIPAA compliance activities documentation.

8. Monitor progress and changes in HIPAA rules and update your organizational policies, procedures, and technologies appropriately.
   - Keep current with changes in the HIPAA regulations.
   - Keep current with new and updated state, federal, and international regulations related to privacy.
   - Update policies and procedures as necessary to meet new requirements and to reflect organizational changes.
   - Monitor organizational procedures and follow up on activities falling out of compliance.
   - Manage BAs and other relationships related to processing and handling health information.
   - Perform periodic gap analysis (at least annually and following major organizational and systems changes).
   - Perform regular privacy risk assessments to discover and address new risks.
   - Review audit and activity logs for health information.
   - Perform regular internal audits for each aspect of Privacy Rule compliance.
   - Ongoing training and awareness.
   - Document all your activities related to HIPAA compliance and maintain the documentation in a central location.

## Chapter 9: Practical Checklist

- Determine your covered entity status.
- Establish a HIPAA compliance project.
- Understand your HIPAA obligations.
- Assign privacy responsibilities.
- Perform a gap analysis and identify risks.
- Create a remediation plan.
- Implement the plan.
- Monitor ongoing compliance.

# Chapter 10
# Privacy Rule Compliance Checklist

When striving for HIPAA Privacy Rule compliance, keep all the information in the previous chapters in mind. To make your efforts a little easier to keep track of, use the following checklist to identify the HIPAA activities you have fulfilled and those that you still need to address. To help you determine specific regulatory requirements, the corresponding location within the regulatory text is noted, and the wording from within the text has been preserved as much as possible, with some modification for clarification.

### A. Prohibited Disclosures

\_\_\_\_ 1. Privacy Protection
**§ 164.502(a):** A covered entity may not use or disclose protected health information (PHI) except as provided in the HIPAA privacy rule. Those provisions include uses and disclosures to the individual himself or herself; for treatment, payment, and operations; as authorized by the individual; for research, public health or healthcare operations in the form of limited data sets; for listings in facility directories or disclosures to those involved in the individual's care provided that the individual does not object; to business associates; as required by law for health oversight activities, compliance investigations, or other public purposes.

\_\_\_\_ 2. Deceased Individuals
**§ 164.502(f):** HIPAA privacy protections include the protection of information for deceased individuals.

\_\_\_\_ 3. Consistency with Notice
**§ 164.502(i):** A covered entity may not use or disclose protected health information in a manner that is inconsistent with its notice of information practices.

---

   \_\_\_\_ 4. Physician–Patient Privilege

§ **164.512(j)(2):** A covered entity may not disclose protected health information to reduce the possibility of harm caused by a criminal act if the information is obtained as part of treatment to reduce the possibility for the criminal activity to occur.

   \_\_\_\_ 5. Underwriting Disclosures

§ **164.514(g):** A health plan that receives protected health information for the purposes of underwriting, premium rating, etc., may not use or disclose this information for any other purpose.

   \_\_\_\_ 6. Access Locked by Agency or Official

§ **164.528(a)(2)(i):** A covered entity (CE) must temporarily suspend an individual's right to receive an accounting of disclosures for the duration specified by the agency or official if a health oversight agency or law enforcement official provides a written statement that an accounting of the disclosures a CE made to such agency or official about an individual (patient or health plan member) would interfere with official business.

## B. Disclosures Requiring Opportunity to Agree or Object

   \_\_\_\_ 7. Listings in Facility Directories

§ **164.510(a)(2):** A covered entity must inform an individual that protected health information relating to them may be listed in a facility directory and provide the individual with the ability to object, except in emergencies or if the individual is incapacitated.

§ **164.510(a)(1)(i):** A facility directory may contain name, location, general condition, and religious affiliation.

§ **164.510(a)(1)(ii)(A):** A covered entity may disclose religious affiliation only to members of the clergy.

§ **164.510(a)(1)(ii)(B):** A covered entity may disclose facility directory information only to persons who ask for the individual by name, with certain exceptions (for example, clergy members).

   \_\_\_\_ 8. Disclosures to Persons Involved with the Individual

§ **164.510(b):** A covered entity must provide an individual with an opportunity to object prior to revealing protected health information to family, friends, or others involved with the care of the individual.

§ **164.510(b)(3):** If a covered entity (CE) uses professional judgment to disclose information to a person involved in the individual's care when the individual is not present, then the CE may disclose only the protected health information directly relevant to the person's involvement with the individual's care.

## C. Disclosures for treatment, payment, and operations (TPO)

_____ 9. Healthcare Operations Disclosures

**§ 164.506(c)(4):** A covered entity (CE) may disclose protected health information to another CE only under certain allowed conditions; for example, when each has a relationship with the individual, the information disclosed must pertain to that relationship.

_____ 10. Restrictions on Use and Disclosure for Treatment, Payment, and Healthcare Operations

**§ 164.522(a)(1)(i):** A covered entity (CE) must permit an individual to request restriction of uses and disclosures of protected health information for treatment, payment, and operations or to family, friends, or others involved in the healthcare of the individual. The CE is not required to agree to the requested restriction.

**§ 164.502(c):** If a covered entity (CE) agrees to a restriction on the use of protected health information, the CE is bound by that restriction, except in emergency situations.

**§ 164.522(a)(2):** A covered entity may terminate its agreement to a restriction request only under certain circumstances. For example, the individual agrees, termination applies only to information collected after the termination, etc.

## D. Disclosures Requiring Authorization

_____ 11. Disclosures Must Be Consistent with Authorizations

**§ 164.508(a)(1):** When a covered entity uses or discloses protected health information for a purpose that requires authorization, the information must be used or disclosed in a way that is consistent with the terms of the authorization.

_____ 12. Authorization Is Required for Disclosure of Psychotherapy Notes

**§ 164.508(a)(2):** Authorization is required for any use or disclosure of psychotherapy notes, with certain exceptions (for example, by the originator of the psychotherapy notes for treatment, for the covered entity's mental health student training under supervision, or for the covered entity to defend itself in a legal action brought by the corresponding individual).

_____ 13. Mandatory Contents of Authorization

**§ 164.508(c):** An authorization must have certain elements in it, for example, it must be in plain language, it must describe the information to be used or disclosed, contain an expiration date or expiration event, etc.

**§ 164.508(a)(3)(ii):** The authorization must state that remuneration is involved if the covered entity receives any form of payment from a third party resulting from marketing activity allowed by the authorization.

_____ 14. Individual Retains a Copy of the Authorization

**§ 164.508(c)(4):** If the covered entity seeks an authorization from an individual, the individual must be given a copy of the authorization.

_____ 15. Authorizations May Be Defective

**§ 164.508(b)(2):** A covered entity may not use or disclose protected health information (PHI) using a defective authorization. Authorization is defective if it has expired, it is incomplete, it has been revoked, it is known to be false, it is part of a compound authorization, or treatment, or if payment, enrollment or eligibility has been conditioned on obtaining the individual's signature.

_____ 16. Compound Authorizations Not Allowed

**§ 164.508(b)(3):** An authorization may not be combined with another document to create a compound authorization with certain exceptions. Two examples: for the use or disclosure of protected health information for a research study combined with any other type of written permission for the same research study; or the use or disclosure of psychotherapy notes combined with another authorization for a use or disclosure of psychotherapy notes.

_____ 17. Revocation

**§ 164.508(b)(5):** An individual may revoke an authorization at any time with certain exceptions. For example, if the covered entity has already taken action based on the authorization, or if the authorization was obtained as a condition of obtaining insurance coverage.

## E. Minimum Necessary Disclosure

_____ 18. Disclosure Limitations

**§ 164.502(b):** A covered entity must make reasonable efforts to limit the amount of protected health information used or disclosed to the minimum necessary to accomplish the purpose of the use or disclosure with certain exceptions. For example, disclosures to or requests by a healthcare provider for treatment, or uses or disclosures made pursuant to an authorization.

**§ 164.512(j)(3):** A covered entity that discloses information to law enforcement about an individual who admits participation in a violent crime may reveal only the admission and certain specified information.

**§ 164.514(d)(3)(i):** A covered entity must implement policies and procedures for routine disclosures to limit the information disclosed to that needed to accomplish the purpose of the disclosure.

**§ 164.514(d)(3)(ii):** A covered entity (CE) must develop criteria for nonroutine disclosures to limit the information disclosed to the minimum necessary to accomplish the purpose of the disclosure. The CE must review nonroutine requests for disclosure on an individual basis.

**§ 164.514(d)(5):** A covered entity may not use, disclose, or request an entire medical record unless the entire medical record is specifically justified as the amount of information needed to accomplish the purpose of the use, disclosure, or request.

____ 19. Minimum Necessary Requests for Disclosure

**§ 164.514(d)(4)(i):** A covered entity must limit its own requests for protected health information to the minimum necessary to accomplish the purpose for which the request is made.

**§ 164.514(d)(4)(ii):** A covered entity must implement policies and procedures for its own routine requests for protected health information to ensure that it requests the minimum information needed to accomplish the intended purpose.

**§ 164.514(d)(4)(iii):** A covered entity must develop criteria to limit each of its nonroutine requests for information to the minimum information necessary to accomplish the purpose of the request. The entity must review each of its own nonroutine requests for protected health information with respect to those criteria.

____ 20. Minimum Necessary Access Privileges

**§ 164.514(d)(2):** A covered entity (CE) must identify classes of persons who need access to protected health information to carry out their duties and must establish the levels of access needed by each. A CE must make reasonable efforts to limit access to the minimum information required to perform an assigned job function.

## F. Notice

____ 21. Individual's Right to Notice

**§ 164.520(a)(1):** A covered entity, with certain exceptions, must provide a notice of information practices. An example of an exception is providing notice to an inmate.

**§ 164.520(a)(2)(ii):** A group health plan that provides benefits through an insurance issuer or HMO and that creates or receives protected health information, must maintain a notice of information practices and provide it to any person who requests it.

____ 22. Timeliness

**§ 164.520(c)(1)(i):** A health plan must provide notice no later than the compliance date for the health plan to individuals covered by the plan, to new enrollees at the time of enrollment, and to all individuals covered by the plan within 60 days of a material revision to the notice.

**§ 164.520(c)(1)(ii):** A health plan must notify all individuals covered by the plan at least once every 3 years that the notice of information practices is available. The health plan must also advise them of how to obtain a copy of the notice of information practices.

**§ 164.520(c)(2)(i):** A healthcare provider that has a direct treatment relationship with an individual must provide notice of information practices no later than the date of the first service delivery following the compliance date for the provider or as soon as possible after an emergency treatment situation.

____ 23. Location of Notice

**§ 164.520(c)(2)(iii):** A healthcare provider that maintains a physical service delivery site must have copies of the notice of information practices available that individuals may take with them. The provider must also post the notice where individuals seeking service may read it.

____ 24. Notice of Revised Practices

**§ 164.520(c)(2)(iv):** A healthcare provider must make a revised Notice of Privacy Practices available on request on or after the effective date of the revision. If the covered entity maintains a physical service delivery site, it must prominently post the notice where patients may see it and make copies of the notice available.

____ 25. Electronic Notice

**§ 164.520(c)(3)(i):** A covered entity that maintains a Web site providing information about the entity's services must post its Notice of Privacy Practices on the Web site.

**§ 164.520(c)(3)(ii):** If a covered entity (CE) attempts to provide a Notice of Privacy Practices electronically and knows that the transmission has failed, then the CE must provide a paper copy.

**§ 164.520(c)(3)(iii):** If the first service to an individual is delivered electronically, a copy of the Notice of Privacy Practices must be delivered, and an attempt must be made to gain a written acknowledgment that it has been received, at the same time in response to the request for service.

**§ 164.520(c)(3)(iv):** A covered entity must honor a request for a paper copy of the notice of information practices when the notice has previously been delivered electronically.

____ 26. Mandatory Content of Notice

§ **164.520(b):** The Notice of Privacy Practices that a covered entity provides must contain certain mandatory elements.

____ 27. Acknowledgment

§ **164.520(c)(2)(ii):** A covered entity must make a good faith effort to obtain a written acknowledgment of receipt of the notice except in an emergency situation and must document the efforts to obtain the acknowledgment if it cannot get the acknowledgment itself.

## G. Access

____ 28. Individual's Right to Access and Copy Protected Health Information (PHI)

§ **164.524(a)(1):** A covered entity (CE) must grant access to protected health information to the corresponding individual with certain exceptions. One example of an exception is a CE that is a correctional institution or a covered healthcare provider acting under the direction of the correctional institution.

§ **164.524(c)(1):** A covered entity must provide access to protected health information to the individual in designated record sets.

§ **164.524(c)(2)(i):** A covered entity must provide access to protected health information to the individual in the form requested by the individual, if it is readily producible in such form.

____ 29. Denial of an Individual's Request for Access

§ **164.524(d)(1):** If a covered entity (CE) denies an individual's request to access certain protected health information, the CE must allow access to all information for which the reason for the rejection does not apply.

§ **164.524(d)(2):** If a covered entity denies an individual's request to access certain protected health information, the denial must be in writing and must contain: the basis for the denial; a statement of the individual's rights; and a description of how the individual may appeal the decision.

§ **164.524(a)(4):** If a covered entity (CE) has denied access to protected health information to the individual, the CE must allow review of the denial by a licensed healthcare professional and must abide by the reviewer's decision.

____ 30. Miscellaneous Rules Governing Access by the Individual

§ **164.524(d)(3):** If a covered entity (CE) does not possess the protected health information requested by an individual, but knows where it is, the CE must inform the individual of where to direct the request.

§ **164.524(b)(2)(i):** A covered entity (CE) must act on a request for access to protected health information (PHI) by the individual within 30 days, with certain exceptions. For example, if the request for access is for PHI that is not maintained or accessible to the CE on-site, the CE must take an action by no later than 60 days from the receipt of such a request.

§ **164.524(c)(4):** A covered entity may not charge fees for granting access to protected health information to the individual in excess of the cost of copying, postage, and preparation of summaries or explanations.

## H. Amendment

_____ 31. Individual's Right to Request Amendment

§ **164.526(a)(1):** A covered entity (CE) must honor an individual's request to amend incorrect or incomplete protected health information (PHI), with certain exceptions. For examples, if the CE determines that the PHI or record that is the subject of the request is accurate and complete.

_____ 32. Timeliness

§ **164.526(b)(2)(i):** A covered entity (CE) must act on an individual's request for amendment of protected health information within 60 days of the submission of the request. The CE is entitled to one 30-day extension if it provides the individual with the reasons for the delay.

_____ 33. Denial of Individual's Request for Amendment

§ **164.526(b)(2)(i)(B):** A covered entity that denies a request for amendment of protected health information must notify the requestor in writing.

§ **164.526(d):** If a covered entity denies a request for amendment, the denial must have certain mandatory elements.

_____ 34. Acceptance of Request

§ **164.526(c)(1):** If a covered entity accepts a request for amendment of protected health information, it must make the appropriate amendment or provide a link to the amendment in the designated record set.

§ **164.526(c)(2):** If a covered entity accepts a request for amendment of protected health information, it must inform the individual and obtain a list of persons with whom the amendment needs to be shared.

**§ 164.526(c)(3):** If a covered entity (CE) accepts a request for amendment of protected health information, it must make reasonable efforts to provide the amendment to all persons identified by the individual. The CE must also inform business associates known to have a copy of the inaccurate or incomplete information.

____ 35. Transitivity

**§ 164.526(e):** A covered entity (CE) that is informed by another CE of an amendment to an individual's health information must make the same amendment to its own copies of the information.

## I. Personal Representatives

____ 36. Personal Representative Rights to Access or Amend Protected Health Information (PHI)

**§ 164.502(g)(1):** A covered entity must treat a personal representative of an individual as the individual for the purposes of protecting health information concerning that individual, with certain exceptions.

**§ 164.502(g)(2):** A covered entity must treat a person as a personal representative of an individual (such as an adult or emancipated minor) if that person has the authority to act on behalf of the individual in making healthcare decisions.

____ 37. Parents and Guardians Are Personal Representatives

**§ 164.502(g)(3):** A covered entity (CE) must treat a parent, guardian, or person acting with parental rights of an unemancipated minor as a personal representative of that minor, unless the minor may lawfully obtain the healthcare without parental consent. If the minor may lawfully obtain the healthcare without parental consent, then the CE must follow state law with respect to disclosures to parents, guardians, and persons acting with parental rights. If state law is unclear on this matter a licensed healthcare professional may exercise his or her professional judgment.

____ 38. Executors Are Personal Representatives

**§ 164.502(g)(4):** A covered entity must treat a representative of a deceased person as a personal representative for the purposes of health information protection.

## J. Confidential Communications Channels

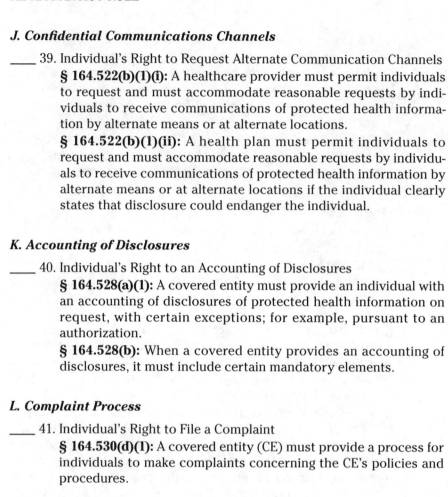

____ 39. Individual's Right to Request Alternate Communication Channels

**§ 164.522(b)(1)(i):** A healthcare provider must permit individuals to request and must accommodate reasonable requests by individuals to receive communications of protected health information by alternate means or at alternate locations.

**§ 164.522(b)(1)(ii):** A health plan must permit individuals to request and must accommodate reasonable requests by individuals to receive communications of protected health information by alternate means or at alternate locations if the individual clearly states that disclosure could endanger the individual.

## K. Accounting of Disclosures

____ 40. Individual's Right to an Accounting of Disclosures

**§ 164.528(a)(1):** A covered entity must provide an individual with an accounting of disclosures of protected health information on request, with certain exceptions; for example, pursuant to an authorization.

**§ 164.528(b):** When a covered entity provides an accounting of disclosures, it must include certain mandatory elements.

## L. Complaint Process

____ 41. Individual's Right to File a Complaint

**§ 164.530(d)(1):** A covered entity (CE) must provide a process for individuals to make complaints concerning the CE's policies and procedures.

## M. Prohibited Activities

____ 42. Intimidation

**§ 164.530(g):** A covered entity may not engage in any intimidating or retaliatory acts against persons who file complaints or otherwise exercise their rights under HIPAA regulations.

____ 43. Conditioning

**§ 164.530(h):** A covered entity may not require an individual to waive the right to file a complaint as a condition of the provision of treatment, payment, enrollment, or eligibility for benefits.

**§ 164.508(b)(4):** A covered entity may not condition treatment, payment, enrollment or eligibility for benefits on the provision of an authorization to disclose protected health information (PHI) by the individual, with certain exceptions. For example, a covered healthcare provider may condition the provision of research-related treatment on provision of an authorization for the use or disclosure of PHI for such research.

**§ 164.522(b)(2)(iii):** A covered healthcare provider may not require an individual to explain their reasons for requesting communications be done in a confidential manner.

___ 44. Employment-Related Disclosures

**§ 164.504(f)(3)(iv):** A group health plan may not disclose protected health information to a plan sponsor for the purpose of employment-related actions.

## N. Safeguards

___ 45. Specific Actions Must Be Taken to Implement HIPAA Regulations

**§ 164.530(c)(1):** A covered entity must have in place appropriate administrative, technical, and physical safeguards to protect the privacy of protected health information.

**§ 164.530(i)(1):** A covered entity must implement policies and procedures with respect to protected health information to comply with all HIPAA standards.

**§ 164.530(i)(2):** A covered entity must promptly change its policies and procedures to comply with changes in the law and document such changes.

___ 46. Responsibility Assignment

**§ 164.530(a)(1)(i):** A covered entity must designate a privacy official who is responsible for development and implementation of privacy policies and procedures.

**§ 164.530(a)(1)(ii):** A covered entity must designate a contact person responsible for receiving and addressing complaints.

## O. Training

___ 47. Workforce Training

**§ 164.530(b)(1):** A covered entity must train all members of its workforce on its policies and procedures with respect to protected health information.

### P. Authentication

_____ 48. Requestor Identity and Authority Verification

**§ 164.514(h)(1)(i):** A covered entity must verify the identity of a person who requests protected health information and the authority of the person to have access to the information they request.

**§ 164.514(h)(1)(ii):** A covered entity must obtain from the requestor any documents, statements, or representations required before disclosing protected health information.

### Q. Mitigation

_____ 49. Policy or Procedure Violation

**§ 164.530(f):** A covered entity must mitigate to the extent possible the harmful effects of a violation of its privacy policies and procedures.

_____ 50. Emergency Disclosures

**§ 164.522(a)(1)(iv):** If a covered entity (CE) discloses protected health information for emergency treatment, the CE must request that the healthcare provider not further use or disclose the information.

**§ 164.512(c)(2):** A covered entity (CE) that discloses protected health information to a government authority concerning a victim of abuse must promptly notify the individual, with certain exceptions. For example, if the CE believes informing the individual would place the individual at risk of serious harm, or if the CE would be informing a personal representative, and the CE believes the personal representative is responsible for the abuse, neglect, or other injury, and that informing such person would not be in the best interests of the individual.

### R. Mandatory Documentation

_____ 51. General

**§ 164.530(j)(1)(ii):** A covered entity is required to keep copies of all communications that are required to be in writing.

**§ 164.530(j)(1)(iii):** A covered entity is required to keep records of all actions, activities, and designations that are required to be documented.

_____ 52. Personnel

**§ 164.524(e)(2):** A covered entity must maintain documentation on the titles and offices of personnel responsible for receiving requests to access protected health information.

**§ 164.526(f):** A covered entity must maintain documentation on the titles of persons or offices responsible for processing requests for amendment of protected health information.

**§ 164.528(d)(3):** A covered entity must retain records of the titles of persons or offices responsible for receiving and processing requests for an accounting of disclosures.

**§ 164.530(b)(2)(ii):** A covered entity must maintain records of training that has been provided.

**§ 164.530(e)(2):** A covered entity must maintain records of sanctions that are applied to members of its workforce who have failed to comply with its privacy and security policies and procedures.

____ 53. Access

**§ 164.524(e)(1):** A covered entity must maintain documentation of the designated record sets (information used to make decisions about the individual) for which an individual may submit a request for access.

____ 54. Disclosures

**§ 164.528(d)(1):** A covered entity must retain documentation on each disclosure of protected health information that could be the subject for a request for an accounting of disclosures. The information maintained must include all items that are required to be part of a disclosure accounting.

**§ 164.528(d)(2):** A covered entity must maintain a record of written accountings of disclosures provided to individuals.

**§ 164.508(b)(6):** A covered entity must document and retain all signed authorizations.

**§ 164.522(a)(3):** A covered entity that agrees to restrictions on the use or disclosure of protected health information for treatment, payment, and operations must maintain written records of such agreements.

____ 55. Notice History

**§ 164.520(e):** A covered entity must maintain copies of all published Notice of Privacy Practices and acknowledgments, and attempts to gain acknowledgment, of the receipt of such notices as part of the required documentation.

____ 56. Complaints

**§ 164.530(d)(2):** A covered entity must maintain records of all complaints received and the disposition of each complaint.

**§ 164.530(j)(1)(i):** A covered entity must document all policies and procedures adopted to protect the privacy of protected health information.

____ 57. Retention

§ **164.530(j)(2):** A covered entity must maintain all required documentation for a period of at least 6 years following its creation date or last date in effect.

____ 58. Business Associate Agreements

§ **164.502(e)(2):** A covered entity must document the satisfactory assurances given by a business associates in the form of a contract, agreement, or other arrangement.

§ **164.504(e)(2):** A business associate's agreement with a covered entity describing their satisfactory assurances must contain certain mandatory elements, including permitted uses and disclosures, appropriate safeguards, etc.

____ 59. Hybrid and Affiliated Entities

§ **164.504(c)(3)(iii):** A hybrid entity is responsible for designating the healthcare components of the organization.

§ **164.504(d)(2):** If two covered entities are designated as affiliated (i.e., acting as a single covered entity), documentation of this designation must be maintained.

## S. Demonstrating Compliance

____ 60. Mandatory Disclosure

§ **164.502(a)(2)(ii):** A covered entity must disclose protected health information if required to do so as part of a compliance review or investigation.

____ 61. Record Keeping

§ **160.310(a):** A covered entity must keep appropriate records and submit appropriate reports to demonstrate HIPAA compliance, as directed by the Department of Health and Human Services.

____ 62. Cooperation

§ **160.310(b):** A covered entity must cooperate with compliance reviews and investigations.

§ **160.310(c)(1):** A covered entity (CE) must permit HHS to inspect its facilities, books and records, and other information, including protected health information, that are pertinent to determining whether or not the CE is in compliance with HIPAA regulations.

### T. Business Associate Agreements

____ 63. Formal Agreements Required for Shared Protected Health Information (PHI)

**§ 164.502(e)(1)(i):** A covered entity (CE) must not disclose protected health information (PHI) to business associates (BAs) unless it first obtains satisfactory assurance from the BAs that the associate will appropriately safeguard the information, with certain exceptions. For example, this standard does not apply to disclosures by a CE to a healthcare provider concerning the treatment of the individual; to disclosures by a group health plan or a health insurance issuer or HMO with respect to a group health plan to the plan sponsor, to the extent that the HIPAA requirements apply and are met; or to uses or disclosures by a health plan that is a government program providing public benefits, if eligibility for, or enrollment in, the health plan is determined by an agency other than the agency administering the health plan, or if the PHI used to determine enrollment or eligibility in the health plan is collected by an agency other than the agency administering the health plan, and such activity is authorized by law, with respect to the collection and sharing of individually identifiable health information for the performance of functions by the health plan and the agency other than the agency administering the health plan.

____ 64. Agreement Is Binding

**§ 164.502(e)(1)(iii):** A covered entity (CE) that acts as a business associate (BA) of another CE may not use or disclose protected health information except as provided by the BA agreement.

____ 65. Breaches of Agreements

**§ 164.504(e)(1)(ii):** A covered entity (CE) that is aware of a breach of a business associate's contract is out of compliance unless the CE takes reasonable steps to cure the breach. If these steps are unsuccessful the CE must either terminate the contract or notify the Secretary of the Department of Health and Human Services.

### U. Disclosures for Research, Marketing, and Fundraising

____ 66. Institutional Review Board Waiver

**§ 164.512(i)(1):** A covered entity may not use or disclose protected health information for research without individual authorization unless a privacy board or an Institutional Review Board has approved a waiver.

**§ 164.512(i)(2):** A privacy board or Institutional Review Board may authorize a waiver of authorization to release protected health information for research purposes only if it contains certain provisions.

\_\_\_\_ 67. Mandatory Notice Content for Fundraising

**§ 164.514(f)(2)(i):** If a covered entity (CE) uses protected health information for fundraising, where authorization is not required, its Notice of Privacy Practices must state that the individual may be contacted by the CE to raise funds.

\_\_\_\_ 68. Opt-Out Feature

**§ 164.514(f)(2)(ii):** If a covered entity uses protected health information for fundraising where authorization is not required, the fundraising material must state how the individual may opt-out of future fundraising communications.

**§ 164.514(f)(2)(iii):** A covered entity must make reasonable efforts to ensure that individuals who opt-out of receiving fundraising communications are not sent such material.

\_\_\_\_ 69. Authorization Required for Marketing

**§ 164.508(a)(3)(i):** A covered entity must obtain an authorization to use protected health information for marketing activities, with certain exceptions. For example, except if the communication is in the form of a face-to-face communication made by a covered entity to an individual; or a promotional gift of nominal value provided by the covered entity.

### V. Hybrid Entities

\_\_\_\_ 70. Wall between Regulated and Unregulated Business Components

**§ 164.504(c)(2):** A hybrid entity must ensure that healthcare components do not disclose protected health information to non-healthcare components of the organization.

## W. Group Health Plans

____ 71. Disclosures to Plan Sponsors

**§ 164.504(f)(1)(i):** A group health plan must ensure that the plan documents restrict uses and disclosures of protected health information by plan sponsors before such information may be disclosed to the plan sponsor, with certain exceptions. For example, the group health plan may disclose summary health information to the plan sponsor, if the plan sponsor requests the summary health information for the purpose of obtaining premium bids from health plans for providing health insurance coverage under the group health plan; or modifying, amending, or terminating the group health plan.

**§ 164.504(f)(2):** Plan documents of group health plans must contain certain mandatory elements.

**§ 164.504(f)(3)(iii):** A group health plan may not disclose protected health information to a plan sponsor unless its notice of information practices contains a separate statement to that effect.

## X. Healthcare Clearinghouses

____ 72. Compliance Requirements

**§ 164.500(b)(1):** A healthcare clearinghouse that is a business associate (BA) of a covered entity may use or disclose protected health information only as permitted in the BA's agreement. Additionally, it must comply with sections of the privacy rule specific to clearinghouses.

**§ 164.500(b)(2):** A healthcare clearinghouse that creates or receives protected health information other than as a business associate of another covered entity must comply with all HIPAA standards and requirements.

## Y. Public Interest Disclosures

____ 73. Disclosures for Law Enforcement Purposes

**§ 164.512(f):** A covered entity may disclose only certain kinds of protected health information for law enforcement purposes to law enforcement officials.

____ 74. Disclosures about Victims of Abuse

**§ 164.512(c)(1):** A covered entity may disclose protected health information concerning suspected victims of abuse, neglect, or domestic violence to appropriate government authority only if the individual agrees to the disclosure, the disclosure is required by law, or the disclosure is authorized by state statute and is necessary to prevent harm.

____ 75. Judicial and Administrative Proceedings

§ **164.512(e)(1):** A covered entity may disclose protected health information in the course of a judicial or administrative proceeding only in certain circumstances.

§ **164.512(e)(1)(i):** A covered entity that discloses protected health information in response to a court order may disclose only that information expressly authorized by the order.

§ **164.512(e)(1)(ii):** A covered entity may disclose protected health information in response to a subpoena or discovery request only when accompanied by certain satisfactory assurances that contain certain mandatory elements.

____ 76. Disclosures about Decedents

§ **164.512(g):** A covered entity may disclose protected healthcare information to coroners, medical examiners, and funeral directors only as necessary to carry out their duties.

____ 77. Averting a Serious Threat to Health or Safety

§ **164.512(j):** A covered entity may disclose information to avert a serious threat to health or safety only if the disclosure is necessary and is made to a person able to prevent or reduce the threat.

## Z. De-Identified Data Disclosures

____ 78. De-Identified Data

§ **164.514(b):** A covered entity may disclose de-identified information only if the de-identification procedure meets certain basic requirements.

____ 79. Limited Data Sets

§ **164.514(e)(2):** A covered entity may disclose information contained in a limited data set only if certain data identifiers are removed.

§ **164.514(e)(3):** A covered entity may disclose information contained in a limited data set only for specific purposes.

§ **164.514(e)(4):** A covered entity may disclose information contained in a limited data set only if it at first obtains a data use agreement with certain mandatory provisions.

## AA. Organized Healthcare Arrangements

___ 80. Joint Notice

**§ 164.520(d)(1):** Covered entities that participate in an organized healthcare arrangement must publish a joint Notice of Privacy Practices.

**§ 164.520(d)(2):** The notice provided by an organized healthcare arrangement (OCHA) must include a description of the entities or classes of entities to which the notice applies. It must also contain a description of the service delivery sites and state that the covered entities in the OCHA will share protected health information with each other.

# Section 2: HIPAA Privacy Rule Quiz

1. Which of the following is an intention of the Privacy Rule?
   A. Remove limitations on the use and disclosure of health records
   B. Enable patients to learn how their information can be used along with the disclosures of other information
   C. Give employers the right to examine their employees' personal health records
   D. Give individual patients complete control in deciding who gets access to their information, regardless of the situation

2. Which of the following best describes what "use" of PHI means?
   A. The sharing, employment, application, utilization, examination, or analysis of individually identifiable health information within a covered entity
   B. The release, transfer, provision of access to, or divulging of information outside the entity holding the information
   C. The utilization of health information to assist with investigations related to public health issues
   D. The sharing, utilization, or examination of individually identifiable health information with a third party

3. In which of the following situations may PHI be used without authorization?
   A. To publish the names of people who have been admitted to a hospital, and their accompanying malady, in the local newspaper
   B. To send names and addresses to a company marketing a birth announcement service
   C. For including PHI within a research study
   D. For treatment activities of a healthcare provider

4. An incidental use or disclosure is not permitted if it results from a violation of the Privacy Rule. What is an incidental use or disclosure?
   A. A primary use or disclosure that is too expensive to address adequately
   B. A secondary use or disclosure that cannot reasonably be prevented as a result of an acceptable use or disclosure, and is limited in nature
   C. A secondary use or disclosure that occurs within a business associate network
   D. A primary use or disclosure that results as a result of lack of privacy training

5. When can a covered entity deny an individual's PHI amendment request?
   A. If the individual has not kept their health insurance coverage premiums paid to date
   B. If the cost of updating the PHI would cause financial hardship for the covered entity
   C. If the PHI is in actuality accurate and complete
   D. If the PHI was created more than 3 years prior to the amendment request

6. What is the best way for you to determine where HIPAA compliance requirements must be addressed within your organization?
   A. Perform a penetration test
   B. Perform a gap analysis
   C. Perform a cost analysis
   D. Perform a social engineering test

7. Which of the following is the header that must appear in your Notice of Privacy Practices?
   A. THIS NOTICE DESCRIBES HOW MEDICAL INFORMATION ABOUT YOU MAY BE USED AND DISCLOSED AND HOW YOU CAN GET ACCESS TO THIS INFORMATION. PLEASE REVIEW IT CAREFULLY.
   B. THIS NOTICE ADVISES YOU OF YOUR LEGAL RIGHTS WITH RESPECT TO HOW MEDICAL INFORMATION ABOUT YOU MAY BE USED. PLEASE REVIEW THIS CAREFULLY.
   C. THIS NOTICE DESCRIBES YOUR OBLIGATIONS TO ENSURE THE PROTECTION OF YOUR OWN MEDICAL INFORMATION THAT IS PROCESSED BY THIS ORGANIZATION. PLEASE REVIEW THIS INFORMATION CAREFULLY.
   D. THIS NOTICE DETAILS YOUR RIGHTS, OBLIGATIONS, AND COURSE OF ACTIONS RELATED TO YOUR HEALTH INFORMATION. REVIEW THIS CAREFULLY.

8. There are three requirements related to the content of a Notice of Privacy Practices. Which of the following is one of these three requirements?
   A. A listing of your business associates
   B. Your organization's legal duties for handling PHI
   C. The technical safeguards you have in place to protect PHI
   D. The background check practices you follow for your personnel

9. Which of the following describes a situation in which a state law is considered "contrary to" a HIPAA privacy standard, requirement, or implementation specification?
   A. Where the penalties for the state requirements are more excessive than those for the HIPAA requirements
   B. Where the state law is similar in all respects to the HIPAA requirements
   C. Where the state law has an expiration date
   D. Where the covered entity cannot comply with both the state and HIPAA requirements

10. Which of the following is a state preemption category?
    A. Health plan regulation and monitoring
    B. International requirements
    C. Litigation activities
    D. Determination by the HIMSS president

11. Which of the following should be included within your HIPAA Privacy Rule implementation plan?
    A. Planning remediation strategies
    B. Implementing PKI
    C. Upgrading all your systems
    D. Creating consents for all individuals to sign

12. When is an authorization defective?
    A. If it was obtained within a provider's facility
    B. If it was signed just prior to April 14, 2003
    C. When it contains the names of hybrid entities
    D. If it has expired

13. Which of the following is an example of when a covered entity is applying the minimum necessary requirement?
    A. A covered entity denies an individual's request to amend PHI
    B. A covered entity identifies classes of persons who need access to PHI to carry out job responsibilities
    C. A covered entity permits an individual to opt-out of having certain pieces of their PHI used in the facility directory
    D. A covered entity does not give law enforcement access to the PHI they want to see

14. When may a CE choose not to treat a parent as a personal represen-
    tative of a minor?
    A. When the parent has a criminal record
    B. When the minor signs an authorization
    C. When the parent lives in a different state as where the treatment
       occurs
    D. When the minor may lawfully obtain healthcare without parental
       consent

15. Access controls are fundamentally what kind of mechanisms?
    A. Legal
    B. Security
    C. Technology
    D. Administrative

# Section 3
# HIPAA
# Security Rule

# Chapter 11
# Security Rule Requirements Overview

### Introduction to the Security Rule

The HIPAA Security Rule was originally published in a proposed form on August 12, 1998. Approximately four-and-a-half years later, the long-anticipated final Security Rule made its way to the Federal Register on February 20, 2003. The Security Rule covers all protected health information (PHI) that a covered entity (CE) creates, receives, maintains, or transmits in an electronic format. In the text of the final Security Rule, the Department of Health and Human Services (HHS) summarizes the Security Rule as follows:

> *This final rule adopts standards for the security of electronic protected health information to be implemented by health plans, healthcare clearinghouses, and certain healthcare providers. The use of the security standards will improve the Medicare and Medicaid programs, and other federal health programs and private health programs, and the effectiveness and efficiency of the healthcare industry in general by establishing a level of protection for certain electronic health information.* *

Overall, the Security Rule can be characterized as:

- A set of information security "best practices" that make good business sense
- A minimum security baseline that is intended to help prevent unauthorized use and disclosure of PHI
- An outline of what to do

*Department of Health and Human Services HIPAA Security Rule, available at http://www.cms.hhs.gov/hipaa/hipaa2/regulations/security/default.asp

---

The information and opinions provided in this book do not constitute or substitute for legal or other professional advice.

- Something that encourages healthcare organizations to embrace E-business and leverage the benefits that an improved technology infrastructure can provide
- Standards to reduce the threats, vulnerabilities, and overall risks to PHI along with their associated costs and negative impact on the organization

On the other hand, the Security Rule is not:

- A set of how-to instructions covering exactly how to secure PHI
- A set of rules that must be implemented the same way for every organization
- New, magical, or all that complicated

The overall goals of the Security Rule revolve around the confidentiality, integrity, and availability of electronic PHI. These terms are defined as:

- *Confidentiality:* The requirement that data stored or transmitted is revealed only to those authorized to see it
- *Integrity:* The requirement that data remains free from unauthorized creation, modification, or deletion
- *Availability:* The requirement that data is available when it is needed

When the proper policies, procedures, and technologies are in place, PHI can be reasonably protected against known threats and vulnerabilities. This will allow CEs to protect against unauthorized uses and disclosures of PHI — a main consideration of the HIPAA Privacy Rule. We go into detail on some of the specific policies, procedures, and technologies that CEs should consider implementing in Chapters 13 and 21.

The Security Rule was designed to be:

- *Technology neutral:* Focuses on what needs to be done rather than how to do it or what technologies to use
- *Scalable:* Does not require all organizations to implement the same exact policies, procedures, and technologies — a CE's information systems' complexity will define its Security Rule implementation complexity
- *Flexible:* Allows CEs to take their size, capabilities, risks, and costs into consideration when trying to determine whether or not to implement certain security systems
- *Comprehensive:* Covers the technical, business, and behavioral issues related to securing PHI

The Security Rule, like all other HIPAA Administrative Simplification rules, has a set of effective dates and compliance deadlines. The effective date for the Security Rule was April 21, 2003. Most CEs have 2 years to implement and comply with the rule, which makes the effective deadline April 21, 2005. The exception to this is small health plans with annual receipts of $5M or less. They must be in compliance by April 21, 2006. Technically speaking, the majority of the Security Rule requirements were to be in place by April 14, 2003 to meet the Privacy Rule requirements of having certain administrative, physical, and technical safeguards in place to protect PHI.

### What's New in the Final Security Rule

Numerous changes were integrated to the Security Rule in its final form. The proposed rule contained several terms that were unclear and there were several areas of overlap among the four different safeguard sections. HHS clarified these confusing terms and removed the redundancies so that there are now 18 standards in the final rule instead of the original 24. HHS has also made the following additional changes to the Security Rule of which you should be aware:

- It now more closely parallels the Privacy Rule including its terminology, treatment of business associates, and the three major safeguard sections.
- A new concept of required and addressable implementation specifications for each standard has been introduced providing more rule flexibility.
- Encryption is no longer required on open networks — this is now an addressable implementation specification that depends on the results of the risk analysis.
- The electronic signatures requirement was removed.
- The former concept of "certification" has been incorporated into the evaluation standard that mandates periodic testing and reassessment of compliance.
- Chain of trust partner agreements are now part of the overall HIPAA BA contracts.
- The term "breach" was replaced with the term "security incident" throughout the rule because it better describes the types of situations that were referred to as breaches.
- The term "open network" was removed because it was considered too broad.

### *Key Terms Referenced in the Security Rule*

HHS references several key terms in the Security Rule that deserve mentioning. As defined in the Security Rule, these terms are as follows:

- *Facility:* The physical premises and interior and exterior of a building.
- *Security incident:* The attempted or successful unauthorized access, use, disclosure, modification, or destruction of information or interference with system operations in an information system.

- *System:* An interconnected set of information resources under the same direct management control that shares common functionality. A system normally includes hardware, software, information, data, applications, communications, and people.
- *Workstation:* An electronic computing device; for example, a laptop or desktop computer or any other device that performs similar functions, and electronic media stored in its immediate environment.

## General Rules for Security Rule Compliance

In § 164.306 of the Security Rule, there are various general rules to which every CE must adhere:

- Ensure the confidentiality, integrity, and availability of all electronic PHI that the CE creates, receives, maintains, or transmits
- Protect against any reasonably anticipated threats or hazards to the security or integrity of PHI
- Protect against any reasonably anticipated uses or disclosures of PHI
- Ensure that its workforce complies with the Security Rule
- Comply with the Security Rule standards with respect to all electronic PHI
- Review and modify security measures as needed to ensure reasonable and appropriate protection of electronic PHI

In addition, as outlined in § 164.316 of the Security Rule, CEs must consider the security policy, procedure, and documentation requirements:

- CEs must implement reasonable and appropriate policies and procedures to comply with the standards, implementation specifications, or other requirements of the Security Rule.
- CE may change their policies and procedures at any time provided that they document the changes and implement them in accordance with the Security Rule.
- CEs must maintain their Security Rule policies and procedures in written or electronic form.
- CEs must maintain a written or electronic record of any actions, activities, or assessments related to the Security Rule.
- CEs must retain all of this documentation for at least 6 years from the date it was created or 6 years from the date when it last was in effect, whichever is longer.
- CEs must make this documentation available to anyone responsible for implementing the documentation's associated procedures.
- CEs must review this documentation periodically, and update as needed based on any environmental or operational changes that may affect the security of electronic PHI.

In addition, regarding the flexible characteristic of the Security Rule, CEs may use any security measures that allow them to reasonably and appropriately implement the standards and implementation specifications of the Security Rule. When deciding which security measures to use, a CE must consider the following factors:

- Their size, complexity, and capabilities
- Their geographic locations
- Their technical infrastructure, hardware, and software security capabilities
- The cost of security measures
- The probability and criticality of potential risks to electronic PHI

**Required vs. Addressable**

Another general rule that deserves closer attention is that of required vs. addressable implementation specifications. The 18 Security Rule standards contain a total of 42 implementation specifications that are either required or addressable. There are a total of 20 required implementation specifications that must be implemented by all CEs regardless of the outcome of their risk analysis. There are a total of 22 addressable implementation specifications that must be considered based solely on the outcome of their risk analysis. These factors include the CE's size, existing security controls in place, and the cost to mitigate the risks that are discovered.

CEs have the options listed in Exhibit 1 when handling these addressable implementation specifications.

The steps in Exhibit 1 have been a considerable source of confusion and discussion within the industry. The addressable option does not imply that CEs can simply make their own rules or ignore the implementation specifications altogether if an implementation specification simply does not seem like a good fit or may be an inconvenience. It means that CEs have the flexibility to make their own choices based on their risks, but there must be genuine and documented business reasons behind these decisions.

Our take on handling addressable implementation specifications is that CEs should consider treating every implementation specification as if it is required yet scalable and flexible. The time spent trying to determine whether or not something should be implemented based on the results of a risk analysis may very well be more difficult than implementing the specification itself. The key here is to document everything to support your decisions.

**Insight into the Security Rule**

The Security Rule is broken down into three major sections, as shown in Exhibit 2.

**Exhibit 1. Scenarios**

**Scenario 1**

IF:

• The implementation specification is reasonable and appropriate for the CE

THEN:

• It must be implemented

**Scenario 2**

IF:

• The specification is unreasonable and inappropriate for the CE, but the overall standard cannot be met otherwise

THEN:

• The CE must:

1. Implement an alternate security measure to accomplish the same goal

AND

2. Document the decision not to implement the specification

AND

3. Document why it is unreasonable and inappropriate

AND

4. Document how the overall standard is being met otherwise

**Scenario 3**

IF:

• The specification is unreasonable and inappropriate for the CE, but the overall standard can be met without alternate measures

THEN:

• The CE must:

1. Document the decision to not implement the specification

AND

2. Document why it is unreasonable and inappropriate

AND

3. Document how the overall standard is being met otherwise

As you will see in Exhibit 3, HHS outlines what needs to be done, but does not give specifics on how to do it. In the information in Exhibit 3, we outline the actual Security Rule verbiage for each standard and implementation specification, whether each implementation specification is required or addressable, and some tips on what you can use to meet each standard or specification. Keep in mind these are not the only possible solutions to meet each particular standard or implementation specification — just some information security best practices that have worked for us and others in the past. Also, just because we list it does not mean you should use it. We will not go into technical detail in these tips, so be sure to refer to Chapter 21 for more specific technical information and practical

**Exhibit 2. Major Sections of the Security Rule and Their Locations in the Regulation Text**

**Administrative Safeguards: § 164.308**
- Approximately 55 percent of total rule
- 9 standards
- 12 required implementation specifications
- 11 addressable implementation specifications

**Physical Safeguards: § 164.310**
- Approximately 24 percent of total rule
- 4 standards
- 4 required implementation specifications
- 6 addressable implementation specifications

**Technical Safeguards: § 164.312**
- Approximately 21 percent of total rule
- 5 standards
- 4 required implementation specifications
- 5 addressable implementation specifications

advice on certain technologies you can implement in your HIPAA compliance efforts. In addition, Appendix C contains a listing of some vendors and products that you may be able to use and benefit from as well.

## Other Organizational Requirements

The Security Rule outlines specific organizational requirements in addition to the overall administrative, physical, and technical safeguards we outlined above. These requirements are for hybrid entities, affiliated covered entities, and governmental entities, and are covered in Security Rule sections § 164.105 and § 164.314. If your organization is considered as, or does business with, one of the three types of entities listed above, we recommend that you review these specific sections of the Security Rule with your legal counsel to see how it may affect your organization.

## Reasons to Get Started on Security Rule Initiatives

If you have followed the Privacy Rule requirements, you are probably well on your way to achieving Security Rule compliance. As if you do not have enough other issues to worry about outside of HIPAA, if you have not started working toward Security Rule compliance it may be time to take that leap. You may already have a lot of the policies, procedures, or technologies in place that it will take to become compliant. Regardless of your situation, here are a few reasons to consider moving forward:

- You do not need perfection; just perform a risk analysis, create a good plan, and show that you are working on it.
- Security Rule compliance is more about culture and business processes than anything else. The sooner you get started, the sooner your workforce will be working with a security-aware state of mind.
- The sooner you get started doing just a few small things at a time to become compliant, the easier and cheaper it will be.
- The Security Rule is all about well-known (and well-documented) best practices and common sense — nothing more and nothing less.
- Your PHI is at risk now. You should not wait to protect it until the compliance deadlines come around.
- Security compliance does not have to be that expensive or complicated — keep things simple.

The bottom line is that if you get started now, you can integrate your Security Rule compliance efforts with your Privacy Rule compliance efforts and kill two huge birds with one stone.

**Exhibit 3. Interpretation of Security Rule**

**Administrative Safeguard Requirements**
1. Security Management Process
   **Defined in the rule as:**
   "Implement policies and procedures to prevent, detect, contain, and correct security violations."

   **Implementation Specifications**
   a. Risk Analysis (Required)
      **What the rule says**
      "Conduct an accurate and thorough assessment of the potential risks and vulnerabilities to the confidentiality, integrity, and availability of electronic protected health information held by the covered entity."
      **What can be used to assist in meeting this specification**
      - Chapter 12 of this book
      - CERT's OCTAVE or similar methodology
      - Risk analysis automation and management software
      - Network and application vulnerability assessment software
      - War dialing software
   b. Risk Management (Required)
      **What the rule says**
      "Implement security measures sufficient to reduce risks and vulnerabilities to a reasonable and appropriate level to comply with § 164.306(a)."
      **What can be used to assist in meeting this specification**
      - Chapter 12 of this book
      - CERT's OCTAVE or similar methodology
      - Risk analysis automation and management software
      - Security policy management software

**Exhibit 3. Interpretation of Security Rule (Continued)**

    c. Sanction Policy (Required)

       *What the rule says*

       "Apply appropriate sanctions against workforce members who fail to comply with the security policies and procedures of the covered entity."

       *What can be used to assist in meeting this specification*

- Chapter 13 of this book
- Security policy management software to store and help train everyone on the policy
- Various books and Internet resources on security policy development

    d. Information System Activity Review (Required)

       *What the rule says*

       "Implement procedures to regularly review records of information system activity, such as audit logs, access reports, and security incident tracking reports."

       *What can be used to assist in meeting this specification*

- Intrusion Detection Systems (IDS)
- Logging capabilities built into your operating systems (OSs) and/or applications

2. Assigned Security Responsibility

   *Defined in the rule as:*

   "Identify the security official who is responsible for the development and implementation of the policies and procedures required by this sub-part for the entity."

   *Implementation Specifications*

   None

   *What can be used to assist in meeting this specification*

   The Security Officer job description found in Appendix B of this book

3. Workforce Security

   *Defined in the rule as:*

   "Implement policies and procedures to ensure that all members of its workforce have appropriate access to electronic protected health information, as provided under paragraph (a)(4) of this section, and to prevent those workforce members who do not have access under paragraph (a)(4) of this section from obtaining access to electronic protected health information."

   *Implementation Specifications*

    a. Authorization and/or Supervision (Addressable)

       *What the rule says*

       "Implement procedures for the authorization and/or supervision of workforce members who work with electronic protected health information or in locations where it might be accessed."

       *What can be used to assist in meeting this specification*

- Certain OS and application access controls
- Standard user IDs and passwords
- Biometrics, tokens, or other authentication devices
- System logging software
- HR, supervisor, and manager education on this matter

    b. Workforce Clearance Procedure (Addressable)

       *What the rule says*

       "Implement procedures to determine that the access of a workforce member to electronic protected health information is appropriate."

**Exhibit 3. Interpretation of Security Rule (Continued)**

*What can be used to assist in meeting this specification*
- Workforce member job descriptions
- HR, supervisor, and manager education on this matter

c. Termination Procedures (Addressable)

*What the rule says*

"Implement procedures for terminating access to electronic protected health information when the employment of a workforce member ends or as required by determinations made as specified in paragraph (a)(3)(ii)(B) of this section."

*What can be used to assist in meeting this specification*
- HR, supervisor, and manager education on this matter
- Strong line of communication between HR and IT

4. Information Access Management

*Defined in the rule as:*

"Implement policies and procedures for authorizing access to electronic protected health information that are consistent with the applicable requirements of sub-part E of this part."

*Implementation Specifications*

a. Isolating Healthcare Clearinghouse Functions (Required)

*What the rule says*

"If a healthcare clearinghouse is part of a larger organization, the clearinghouse must implement policies and procedures that protect the electronic protected health information of the clearinghouse from unauthorized access by the larger organization."

*What can be used to assist in meeting this specification*
- Network perimeter devices such as firewalls, routers, and switches that can be configured to segment the network
- OS or application access controls.

b. Access Authorization (Addressable)

*What the rule says*

"Implement policies and procedures for granting access to electronic protected health information, for example, through access to a workstation, transaction, program, process, or other mechanism."

*What can be used to assist in meeting this specification*
- HR, supervisor, and manager education on this matter
- Strong line of communication between HR and IT
- Security policy management software to store the policies and procedures

c. Access Establishment and Modification (Addressable)

*What the rule says*

"Implement policies and procedures that, based upon the entity's access authorization policies, establish, document, review, and modify a user's right of access to a workstation, transaction, program, or process."

*What can be used to assist in meeting this specification*
- HR, supervisor, and manager education on this matter
- Strong line of communication between HR and IT
- Security policy management software to store the policies and procedures

5. Security Awareness and Training

*Defined in the rule as:*

"Implement a security awareness and training program for all members of its workforce (including management)."

**Exhibit 3. Interpretation of Security Rule (Continued)**

*Implementation Specifications*

a. Security Reminders (Addressable)

   *What the rule says*

   "Periodic security updates."

   *What can be used to assist in meeting this specification*

   - Screen savers
   - Periodic e-mails
   - Log-in banners
   - Periodic classroom training
   - Lunch and learns
   - Newsletter or magazine articles
   - Pamphlets and brochures
   - Posters around the office
   - Promotional items such as coffee mugs, mouse pads, sticky notes, etc.
   - Intranet Web site

b. Protection from Malicious Software

   *What the rule says*

   "Procedures for guarding against, detecting, and reporting malicious software."

   *What can be used to assist in meeting this specification*

   - Antivirus software
   - Pest control software to protect against spyware and adware
   - Personal firewall/IDS software

c. Log-in Monitoring (Addressable)

   *What the rule says*

   "Procedures for monitoring log-in attempts and reporting discrepancies."

   *What can be used to assist in meeting this specification*

   - Logging capabilities into your operating systems (OSs) and/or applications
   - HR, supervisor, and manager education on this matter
   - Strong line of communication between HR and IT

d. Password Management (Addressable)

   *What the rule says*

   "Procedures for creating, changing, and safeguarding passwords."

   *What can be used to assist in meeting this specification*

   - Password features built into OSs and/or applications
   - Directory services software
   - Single sign-on management software
   - User education on this matter

6. Security Incident Procedures

   *Defined in the rule as:*

   "Implement policies and procedures to address security incidents."

   *Implementation Specifications*

   a. Response and Reporting (Required)

      *What the rule says*

      "Identify and respond to suspected or known security incidents; mitigate, to the extent practicable, harmful effects of security incidents that are known to the covered entity; and document security incidents and their outcomes."

      *What can be used to assist in meeting this specification*

      - IDS
      - Miscellaneous forensics tools

**Exhibit 3. Interpretation of Security Rule (Continued)**

7. Contingency Plan
   *Defined in the rule as:*
   "Establish (and implement as needed) policies and procedures for responding to an emergency or other occurrence (for example, fire, vandalism, system failure, and natural disaster) that damages systems that contain electronic protected health information."

   *Implementation Specifications*
   a. Data Backup Plan (Required)
      *What the rule says*
      "Establish and implement procedures to create and maintain retrievable exact copies of electronic protected health information."
      *What can be used to assist in meeting this specification*
      - Chapter 22 of this book
      - Tape backup
      - CD-ROM or other optical backup
      - Internet-based backup
      - Redundant computer system(s)
   b. Disaster Recovery Plan (Required)
      *What the rule says*
      "Establish (and implement as needed) procedures to restore any loss of data."
      *What can be used to assist in meeting this specification*
      - Chapter 22 of this book
      - Offsite failover facilities
      - Uninterruptible power supplies
      - Backup generators
   c. Emergency Mode Operation Plan (Required)
      *What the rule says*
      "Establish (and implement as needed) procedures to restore any loss of data."
      *What can be used to assist in meeting this specification*
      - Chapter 22 of this book
      - Offsite failover facilities
      - Uninterruptible power supplies
      - Backup generators
   d. Testing and Revision Procedure (Addressable)
      *What the rule says*
      "Establish (and implement as needed) procedures to enable continuation of critical business processes for protection of the security of electronic protected health information while operating in emergency mode."
      *What can be used to assist in meeting this specification*
      - Chapter 22 of this book
   e. Applications and Data Criticality Analysis (Addressable)
      *What the rule says*
      "Assess the relative criticality of specific applications and data in support of other contingency plan components."
      *What can be used to assist in meeting this specification*
      - Chapters 12 and 22 of this book
      - The results of your risk analysis
      - CERT's OCTAVE or similar methodology
      - Risk analysis automation and management software

**Exhibit 3. Interpretation of Security Rule (Continued)**

8. Evaluation

*Defined in the rule as:*

"Perform a periodic technical and nontechnical evaluation, based initially on the standards implemented under this rule, and subsequently, in response to environmental or operational changes affecting the security of electronic protected health information, which establishes the extent to which an entity's security policies and procedures meet the requirements of this sub-part."

*Implementation Specifications*

None

*What can be used to assist in meeting this specification*

- Chapter 12 of this book
- The results of your initial risk analysis
- CERT's OCTAVE or similar methodology
- Risk analysis automation and management software
- Network and application vulnerability assessment software
- War dialing software
- Security policy management software to store the policies and procedures

9. Business Associate Contracts and Other Arrangement

*Defined in the rule as:*

"A covered entity, in accordance with § 164.306, may permit a business associate to create, receive, maintain, or transmit electronic protected health information on the covered entity's behalf only if the covered entity obtains satisfactory assurances, in accordance with § 164.314(a), that the business associate will appropriately safeguard the information. This standard does not apply with respect to:

(i) The transmission by a covered entity of electronic protected health information to a healthcare provider concerning the treatment of an individual;

(ii) The transmission of electronic protected health information by a group health plan or an HMO or health insurance issuer on behalf of a group health plan to a plan sponsor, to the extent that the requirements of § 164.314(b) and § 164.504(f) apply and are met; or

(iii) The transmission of electronic protected health information from or to other agencies providing the services at § 164.502(e)(1)(ii)(C), when the covered entity is a health plan that is a government program providing public benefits, if the requirements of § 164.502(e)(1)(ii)(C) are met.

A covered entity that violates the satisfactory assurances it provided as a business associate of another covered entity will be in noncompliance with the standards, implementation specifications, and requirements of this paragraph and § 164.314(a)."

*Implementation Specifications*

a. Written contract or other arrangement (Required)

*What the rule says*

"Document the satisfactory assurances required by paragraph (b)(1) of this section through a written contract or other arrangement with the business associate that meets the applicable requirements of § 164.314(a)."

*What can be used to assist in meeting this specification*

- Chapter 20 of this book
- Outside consulting or legal counsel

**Exhibit 3. Interpretation of Security Rule (Continued)**

**Physical Safeguard Requirements**

1. Facility Access Controls
   *Defined in the rule as:*
   "Implement policies and procedures to limit physical access to its electronic information systems and the facility or facilities in which they are housed, while ensuring that properly authorized access is allowed."

   *Implementation Specifications*
   a. Contingency Operations (Addressable)
      *What the rule says*
      "Establish (and implement as needed) procedures that allow facility access in support of restoration of lost data under the disaster recovery plan and emergency mode operations plan in the event of an emergency."
      *What can be used to assist in meeting this specification*
      - Chapters 13 and 22 of this book
      - Offsite failover facilities
      - Uninterruptible power supplies
      - Backup generators
   b. Facility Security Plan (Addressable)
      *What the rule says*
      "Implement policies and procedures to safeguard the facility and the equipment therein from unauthorized physical access, tampering, and theft."
      *What can be used to assist in meeting this specification*
      - Chapters 13 and 21 of this book
      - Various books and Internet resources on security policy development
      - ID badges, biometrics, locks, and other physical security devices
      - Security policy management software to store the policies and procedures
   c. Access Control and Validation (Addressable)
      *What the rule says*
      "Implement procedures to control and validate a person's access to facilities based on their role or function, including visitor control, and control of access to software programs for testing and revision."
      *What can be used to assist in meeting this specification*
      - Chapters 13 and 21 of this book
      - ID badges, biometrics, locks, and other physical security devices
   d. Maintenance Records (Addressable)
      *What the rule says*
      "Implement policies and procedures to document repairs and modifications to the physical components of a facility which are related to security (for example, hardware, walls, doors, and locks)."
      *What can be used to assist in meeting this specification*
      - Chapter 13 of this book
      - Various books and Internet resources on security policy development
      - Security policy management software to store the policies and procedures
2. Workstation Use
   *Defined in the rule as:*
   "Implement policies and procedures that specify the proper functions to be performed, the manner in which those functions are to be performed, and the physical attributes of the surroundings of a specific workstation or class of workstation that can access electronic protected health information."

## Exhibit 3.  Interpretation of Security Rule (Continued)

*Implementation Specifications*

None

***What can be used to assist in meeting this specification***

- Chapters 13 and 21 of this book
- The results of your risk analysis
- Various books and Internet resources on security policy development
- Security policy management software to store the policies and procedures

3. Workstation Security

***Defined in the rule as:***

"Implement physical safeguards for all workstations that access electronic protected health information, to restrict access to authorized users."

*Implementation Specifications*

None

***What can be used to assist in meeting this specification***

- Chapter 21 of this book
- The results of your risk analysis
- Moving computers or monitors
- Secured rooms
- Curtains
- Partitions
- Standard user ID and passwords
- Biometrics, tokens, or other authentication devices
- OS or application access controls

4. Device and Media Controls

***Defined in the rule as:***

"Implement policies and procedures that govern the receipt and removal of hardware and electronic media that contain electronic protected health information into and out of a facility, and the movement of these items within the facility."

*Implementation Specifications*

a. Disposal (Required)

***What the rule says***

"Implement policies and procedures to address the final disposition of electronic protected health information, and/or the hardware or electronic media on which it is stored."

***What can be used to assist in meeting this specification***

- Chapters 13 and 21 of this book
- Media cross shredder
- Bulk eraser or degausser
- Physical destruction
- Various books and Internet resources on security policy development
- Security policy management software to store the policies and procedures

b. Media Reuse (Required)

***What the rule says***

"Implement procedures for removal of electronic protected health information from electronic media before the media are made available for reuse."

***What can be used to assist in meeting this specification***

- Bulk eraser
- Degausser
- Disk wiping tools

**Exhibit 3. Interpretation of Security Rule (Continued)**

   c. Accountability (Addressable)

     *What the rule says*

     "Maintain a record of the movements of hardware and electronic media and any person responsible therefore."

     *What can be used to assist in meeting this specification*

     • Chapter 13 of this book

     • Various books and Internet resources on security policy development

     • Security policy management software to store the policies and procedures

   d. Data Backup and Storage (Addressable)

     *What the rule says*

     "Create a retrievable, exact copy of electronic protected health information, when needed, before movement of equipment."

     *What can be used to assist in meeting this specification*

     • Chapter 22 of this book

     • Tape backup

     • CD-ROM or other optical backup

     • Internet-based backup

     • Redundant computer system(s)

**Technical Safeguard Requirements**

1. Access Control

   *Defined in the rule as:*

   "Implement technical policies and procedures for electronic information systems that maintain electronic protected health information to allow access only to those persons or software programs that have been granted access rights as specified in § 164.308(a)(4)."

   *Implementation Specifications*

   a. Unique User Identification (Required)

     *What the rule says*

     "Assign a unique name and/or number for identifying and tracking user identity."

     *What can be used to assist in meeting this specification*

     • User ID management built into OSs and/or applications

     • Directory services

     • Single sign-on software

   b. Emergency Access Procedure (Required)

     *What the rule says*

     "Establish (and implement as needed) procedures for obtaining necessary electronic protected health information during an emergency."

     *What can be used to assist in meeting this specification*

     • Chapter 22 of this book

     • Offsite failover facilities

     • Uninterruptible power supplies

     • Backup generators

   c. Automatic Log-off (Addressable)

     *What the rule says*

     "Implement electronic procedures that terminate an electronic session after a predetermined time of inactivity."

     *What can be used to assist in meeting this specification*

     • Screen savers built into OSs or applications

**Exhibit 3. Interpretation of Security Rule (Continued)**

- Timeout configuration settings built into OSs or applications
- Proximity sensors

d. Encryption and Decryption (Addressable)

***What the rule says***

"Implement a mechanism to encrypt and decrypt electronic protected health information."

***What can be used to assist in meeting this specification***

- Chapter 21 of this book
- Encryption software
- PKI systems
- S/MIME support built into e-mail applications
- E-mail firewalls with encryption support

2. Audit Controls

***Defined in the rule as:***

"Implement hardware, software, and/or procedural mechanisms that record and examine activity in information systems that contain or use electronic protected health information."

***Implementation Specifications***

None

***What can be used to assist in meeting this specification***

- Chapter 21 of this book
- Logging capabilities into your operating systems (OSs) and/or applications

3. Integrity

***Defined in the rule as:***

"Implement policies and procedures to protect electronic protected health information from improper alteration or destruction."

***Implementation Specifications***

Mechanism to Authenticate Electronic PHI (Addressable)

***What the rule says***

"Implement electronic mechanisms to corroborate that electronic protected health information has not been altered or destroyed in an unauthorized manner."

***What can be used to assist in meeting this specification***

- Chapter 21 of this book
- Encryption software
- PKI systems
- S/MIME support built into e-mail applications
- E-mail firewalls with encryption support

4. Person or Entity Authentication

***Defined in the rule as:***

"Implement procedures to verify that a person or entity seeking access to electronic protected health information is the one claimed."

***Implementation Specifications***

None

***What can be used to assist in meeting this specification***

- Chapter 21 of this book
- Standard user IDs and passwords
- Biometrics, tokens, or other authentication devices

**Exhibit 3. Interpretation of Security Rule (Continued)**

5. Transmission Security

   ***Defined in the rule as:***

   "Implement technical security measures to guard against unauthorized access to electronic protected health information that is being transmitted over an electronic communications network."

   ***Implementation Specifications***

   a. Integrity Controls (Addressable)

      ***What the rule says***

      "Implement security measures to ensure that electronically transmitted electronic protected health information is not improperly modified without detection until disposed of."

      ***What can be used to assist in meeting this specification***

      - Chapter 21 of this book
      - SSL/TLS protocol
      - PGP
      - PKI systems
      - S/MIME support built into e-mail applications
      - E-mail firewalls with encryption support

   b. Encryption (Addressable)

      ***What the rule says***

      "Implement a mechanism to encrypt electronic protected health information whenever deemed appropriate."

      ***What can be used to assist in meeting this specification***

      - Chapter 21 of this book
      - Encryption software
      - PKI systems
      - S/MIME support built into e-mail applications
      - E-mail firewalls with encryption support

## Chapter 11: Practical Checklist

- The Security Rule is nothing more than best practices that are intended to protect the confidentiality, integrity, and availability of PHI.
- The Security Rule requires both technical and nontechnical systems, policies, and procedures to be in place.
- Perform a risk analysis as your first step.
- The flexibility characteristic of the Security Rule does not absolve you of reasonable efforts to comply and protective measures for PHI, regardless of your organization's size.
- Seriously consider treating all implementation specifications as required so you do not have to explain why you did not implement a particular specification when a security incident occurs.
- Remember to document all of your decisions.
- Get started on Security Rule compliance as soon as possible to save time, effort, and future stress once the rule is enforced.

# Chapter 12
# Performing a Security Rule Risk Analysis

## Background

Security Rule compliance is only possible when an appropriate risk analysis (sometimes referred to as a risk assessment) is performed on your information systems. Stated another way, you must know what you are trying to protect and what you are trying to protect against before you can actually protect anything. The Department of Health and Human Services (HHS) states in the Security Rule that:

> The most appropriate means of compliance for any covered entity can only be determined by that entity assessing its own risks and deciding upon the measures that would best mitigate those risks.

In fact, the first step listed and recommended by HHS in the Security Rule is a required risk analysis. We must say they are right on target with this. A risk analysis needs to be done before starting any of your HIPAA security compliance efforts.

It is no secret that you have got to ensure the confidentiality, integrity, and availability of PHI, but you have got to get more specific than that. A risk analysis will help you determine:

- What PHI your organization has
- Where the PHI is stored and transmitted
- Who has access to the PHI
- Where PHI enters your network, and where it leaves your network
- What the specific threats and vulnerabilities are associated with the PHI
- What could happen to the PHI if unauthorized uses or disclosures occur
- How confidential the PHI needs to be
- When and how the PHI needs to be protected
- Whether or not encryption is needed

---

The information and opinions provided in this book do not constitute or substitute for legal or other professional advice.

- What security policies need to be developed
- What areas of security need to be audited on an ongoing basis
- Specific access controls that need to be in place
- How detailed security incident and contingency plans should be
- What physical security controls are necessary to ensure the protection of PHI

This information can be used to supplement an existing information security infrastructure or to create a new one from scratch.

Part of this overall process is determining where you currently stand vs. where you need to be — analyzing your gaps — with regard to HIPAA compliance. We encourage you to refer to Chapter 6, where we have detailed questions that must be answered as part of your overall risk analysis and gap analysis for Privacy Rule compliance — most of this applies to the Security Rule as well. Chapter 14 also outlines some specific areas to focus on to come up with a solid implementation plan for Security Rule compliance. In this chapter we provide an overview of the risk analysis process and the steps involved with managing information risks.

### Risk Analysis Requirements According to HIPAA

The Security Rule requires CEs to perform an initial risk analysis to determine specific unauthorized uses, disclosures, and data integrity losses that could occur to PHI if certain systems are not in place. This is part of the Security Management standard that falls under the Administrative Safeguards. In fact, a risk analysis is a required implementation specification that all CEs must perform. As we covered in Chapter 11, the Security Rule is flexible and scalable based on what is derived from the risk analysis. What this means is that a risk analysis must be used to determine whether or not all of the other addressable implementation specifications must be implemented. Depending on the results, a CE may come to the conclusion that:

- The PHI threats and vulnerabilities are not significant enough to worry about.
- The cost to mitigate those threats and vulnerabilities is too high.
- Their capabilities are not sufficient to warrant security measures.

Not so fast though — we cannot imagine any scenario where a CE would come to the conclusion that its PHI is at no risk whatsoever. There are bound to be certain threats and vulnerabilities that exist that just may not be so obvious. Hopefully, the threats and vulnerabilities to PHI we list in this chapter will make you aware of just how easily PHI can be at risk. On another note, the Security Rule does not apply to information in any risk analysis documentation unless it specifically contains PHI. Just make sure that you secure these records as you would any other critical business document.

**Exhibit 1. Common PHI Threats and Vulnerabilities**

**Threats**
- Viruses and other malicious software
- Hackers
- Disgruntled employees
- Untrained users
- Fires, earthquakes, tornados, etc.

**Vulnerabilities**
- Computer systems with default configurations and passwords
- No data backup system
- No security policies
- Careless business associates
- Weak passwords

## Risk Analysis Essentials

Before we get started, we need to define some key terms associated with information risk in the context of HIPAA, as follows:

- *Threat:* An indication or intent to cause disturbance or harm to PHI.
- *Vulnerability:* An information system weakness or flaw that can be exploited to cause disturbance or harm to PHI.

There is an indefinite number of threats and vulnerabilities associated with PHI. We have listed some of the more common ones in Exhibit 1 of which you should be aware.

Next, we will define risk as

> *The likelihood that the confidentiality, integrity, or availability of PHI will be adversely affected if a threat occurs and a vulnerability is exploited.*

There are various levels of risk that need to be taken into consideration when analyzing risks to your PHI:

- *Inherent Risk:* Built-in risks that do not consider any security measures taken to protect PHI.
- *Present Risk:* Risk that includes security measures taken to protect PHI.
- *Residual Risk:* Risk that is left over after all existing and recommended security measures have been taken to protect PHI; this will always be greater than zero.

## Stepping through the Process

The process of performing a risk analysis can be made quite complex, but it does not necessarily have to be. There are various popular risk analysis methodologies and software applications that can be used during this process. See Appendix C for a listing of some of our favorites. We highly recommend using these as resources whenever possible. We could dedicate an entire book to performing a risk analysis, but we will spare you all those details for now! Instead, we have outlined in Exhibit 2 the high-level steps involved with performing a risk analysis so you will know where to get started and what to expect.

When moving forward with your risk analysis, several factors will affect your approach and how detailed you will need to get. This includes:

- The various business processes your organization has
- Your information systems complexity
- The number of business partners your organization deals with
- Your level of perceived risks
- Whether or not you have an Internet connection
- How you store PHI on medical devices such as ultrasound, cardiogram, and other equipment
- Whether or not you use wireless or dial-up connections (or both)
- Whether or not you allow remote processing of PHI
- Whether or not you use PDAs and laptops outside your facility to store or process PHI
- The number of employees in your organization

### Calculating Risk

There are several formulas for calculating risk. We will introduce you to a couple of the common ones here and show you an example of how to calculate risk. In general terms, risk is defined in the following formula:

$$\text{Risk} = \text{Threat} \times \text{Vulnerability} \times \text{Cost}$$

This essentially requires a numeric value to be assigned to both the threats and vulnerabilities for a given situation and those values to be multiplied by the cost of the occurrence. Obviously, this is not a highly scientific formula. It is more of a guideline to show that the calculation of risk is dependent on how high or low the threat, vulnerability, and cost is for a particular scenario. For instance, in a given situation, imagine that the latest and greatest operating system (OS) is installed on one of your computers but no security patches are applied. This in itself is considered a high vulnerability. However, if you choose to only use the computer as a stand-alone word processing station with no network or Internet connection and no PHI stored on it, the threats to that computer are going to be pretty low. In addition, the costs associated with any sort of compromise of that computer are going to be low as well. Worst-case scenario, you will lose your word processing documents or perhaps have to replace the computer and its software. Overall, using the above formula, the risk will be low, and therefore you will not have to implement many security measures, if any, to ensure its viability.

**Exhibit 2. High Level Steps in Performing a Risk Analysis**

1. Identify your PHI and other supporting information systems and business assets
   - What PHI and associated systems is your organization dependent on?
     - Interview key personnel
     - Take an inventory of all your hardware, software, and information
     - Document your information flows
   - Review existing policies and procedures
   - Review your exiting technology infrastructure supporting the privacy and security of PHI
   - Prioritize your findings based on criticality to the business

2. Determine both tangible and intangible costs associated with your PHI and its supporting systems
   - Cost to originally acquire or create
   - Cost to replace
   - Cost to maintain and repair
   - Cost to completely rebuild from scratch
   - Costs associated with any liabilities (such as the HIPAA penalties)

3. Identify the threats and vulnerabilities
   - Use automated tools and manual assessments to determine the specific threats and vulnerabilities associated with PHI — see Appendix C for a listing of some of these tools

4. Calculate the specific risks
   - Determine the actual risk factor involved (see the section on calculating risk, later)

5. Analyze your actual results
   - Identify and prioritize the specific risks that were discovered and determine:
     - How certain are you of your calculations?
     - What could happen if the risk became a reality?
     - How often could it occur?
     - What security measures are currently in place to mitigate those risks?

6. Complete a cost–benefit analysis
   - Determine how willing your organization is to accept those risks
   - Decide whether or not the PHI you are trying to protect is as valuable as the costs, time, and effort it would require to protect it

7. Make upper management aware of the risks involved

8. Determine your risk mitigation plan — you have a few options
   - Accept the risks — be sure to get it in writing from upper management that the risks are being accepted — just make sure you have warned them of the HIPAA penalties involved
   - Reduce your risks through specific policies, procedures, and technologies
   - Transfer your risks to another entity or via a contract or an insurance policy
     - Be careful with this one! Transferring risks this way still might not keep you from getting in trouble with the law

On the other hand, if you have that same OS installed on a practice management computer that stores and transmits PHI via the Internet or a dial-up connection, and the same security patches are not applied — you have got a pretty serious situation on your hands. This is a high-threat, high-vulnerability, and potentially high-cost situation if that computer is compromised. Therefore, the risk is going to be much higher, and this system will in turn need to be much more secure in order to prevent unauthorized uses and disclosures of PHI. Keep in mind that there are thousands of possible scenarios and calculations you can make using this formula, depending on your particular situation. If you choose to use this qualitative method to calculate your risks, just be sure to come up with a standard scale for rating your threats (for example, 1 = lowest risk and 10 = highest risk), document how you came to your conclusions, and prioritize your risks that need to be addressed based on your findings.

Another commonly used formula for calculating risk is the annual loss expectancy (ALE) formula. The formula for this quantitative method is as follows:

$$\text{Annual Loss Expectancy (ALE)} = \text{SLE} \times \text{ARO}$$

where:
SLE (Single Loss Expectancy) = value of the asset ($) × impact of the threat (percent)
ARO (Annual Rate of Occurrence) = frequency that a threat is expected to occur in a year

We will not go into specific details on this calculation, but you can see how the SLE and ARO can drive up the risk in certain situations. For example, if you have PHI, or even just a critical information system that is worth a lot of money to your organization combined with a specific virus or worm outbreak that you know will wreak havoc so many times a year on your systems that are not protected, you can calculate the ALE or specific risk involved. Regardless of how you calculate your risks, whether they are scientifically calculated using these formulas or unscientifically calculated using your experience or good old common sense, just pick a method and stick with it if it works for you and your organization. If you document how you have calculated your risks and provided reasonable supporting evidence that you can explain, you will be off to a great start with your Security Rule compliance efforts.

**Managing Risks Going Forward**

A risk analysis can be a complicated process from both a business and technical perspective, so make sure you have the right person(s) for the job. Refer to Chapter 23 for more tips on outsourcing information technology services related to HIPAA. Keep in mind that you have got to balance the value of the PHI and systems you are protecting with how much it costs to protect them. Also remember that not implementing security simply because it costs money that you do not want to spend is *not* considered a reasonable or acceptable justification for not having the security. The best you can do is to reduce the window of exposure and minimize your vulnerabilities. Some solid efforts combined with some common sense will enable to you to determine what is best for your organization.

Keep in mind that the final Security Rule requires CEs to reassess and update their security measures as needed on a regular basis. It specifically states that

> *Security measures implemented must be reviewed and modified as needed to continue provision of reasonable and appropriate protection of electronic protected health information.*

We go into more detail on this subject in Chapter 25.

The outcome of your risk analysis depends on the results you want in return. Moving forward, you must manage your risks, not avoid the threats and vulnerabilities — they will always exist and most likely keep getting worse. As long as you try, in good faith, to reasonably balance cost effectiveness with HIPAA compliance and maintain reasonable security measures on an ongoing basis, there is no reason you should not be successful in your HIPAA efforts.

## Chapter 12: Practical Checklist

- You must determine what you are trying to protect before you can protect it.
- Threats are an indication of intent to inflict harm or damage.
- Vulnerabilities are weaknesses or flaws that can be exploited by a threat.
- Risk is the likelihood of threat occurring.
- Perform a thorough analysis of your business processes, information systems, and PHI to identify your assets.
- Make sure your costs do not outweigh the benefits of mitigating your risks.
- A risk analysis should not be a one-time deal — every day new information systems threats and vulnerabilities crop up that must be addressed on a regular basis.

# Chapter 13
# Writing Effective Information Security Policies

## Introduction to Security Policies

There are many policies specific to the Security Rule that must be written so your organization can be in compliance with HIPAA. These security policies are such a critical staple item for your overall information security infrastructure that we decided to dedicate an entire chapter to the topic. So, what are security policies? Security policies basically define the framework around which your information security program is managed. They are the core of any successful information security initiative.

Security policies are documents that define the final "what" that must be accomplished with regard to your organization's information protection strategy. You will need to create supporting documents. These supporting documents will provide the "who, how, why, when, and where" information necessary to meet these required accomplishments. These supporting documents will outline:

- Information systems roles and responsibilities
- Who has access to what information
- Acceptable usage for your employees
- Standards to which all employees must adhere
- Procedures to actually carry out the specific policies, standards, and guidelines

Some people might say, "We know what our security needs and technologies are so we do not need formal policies." This could not be further from the truth. Security policies should come first. Technically they come second, after your formal risk analysis, but they should be a top priority nonetheless. Security technologies are merely a way to enforce your policies and should not be seen as the only requirement for adequate security.

---

What people typically refer to as "security policies" are actually more than just policies. They usually also define security standards, guidelines, and procedures. In this chapter, although we will mostly refer to these documents as security policies, keep in mind that we are referring to the complete set of policies, standards, guidelines, and procedures. Before we go any further, we will take a look at the definitions of each of these terms as used in the context of security policy development:

- *Policy:* The overall definition of your organization's position on specific security topics. Policies state "this is what we do here."
- *Standard:* Specific information on technology, business, and systems criteria that provide supporting details for meeting policy requirements. A standard might use words such as "will," or "shall," or "must."
- *Guideline:* Provides supporting details for a policy, but is less specific than a standard. A guideline might use words such as "should" or "consider."
- *Procedure:* Outlines the specific details of how a security policy will be implemented. These are often technical and very specific to a particular system, department, or organization.

We will not go into specific details on security procedures as they depend on specific technologies and will differ greatly among organizations. However, we have included a few tips for you to consider when developing your security procedures:

- Make sure they are thoroughly documented and stored in a safe and secure place.
- Make them detailed and succinct.
  - Document every step in the process.
  - A nontechnical person should be able to implement well-written procedures.
- Ensure they are tested on a regular basis.
- Update them as needed along with your security policies.
- Assign broad responsibilities for your procedures to the smallest number of people possible to ensure that the overall business objective of each policy is met without having too many people involved.
- Given their technical details, they should not require the formal approval of upper management.

Well-written security policies are fairly high level and thus easy to manage over time. In addition, security policies should generally not be one large document. Instead, they should be short, individual documents that cover a specific security topic. Most policy documents should not be more than 1 to 2 pages in length. This might hold true for most of your policies even if you choose to document your standards, guidelines, and procedures along with them. The Security Officer should "own" and maintain the full set of information security policies in one location.

To simplify your policies, it is common (and preferable) to summarize each of them in a few sentences and have a reference back to the more detailed documentation. This is helpful for use in employee handbooks, etc., where you do not want to inundate your employees with a lot of details that they may not understand and probably will not read. We go into detail on how to handle this issue in Chapter 24 when we discuss HIPAA training, education, and awareness.

There are three main categories of policies:

1. *Organizational Policies:* These cover specific organizations, departments, or offices within a company.
2. *Issue-Specific Policies:* These cover specific issues such as passwords and employee termination.
3. *System-Specific Policies:* These cover specific information systems, computers, or applications.

To be compliant with the HIPAA Security Rule, your organization will need several policies in each category. One of the most important factors you will want to consider is relating your security policies to specific business functions whenever possible. This will help with the integration of your security policies into everyday business processes as well as ensure that everyone has a fair chance of understanding how the policies apply to everyday business needs.

**Critical Elements of Security Policies**

On average, security policies either do not exist or are not enforced in today's healthcare environment. The first major hurdle that must be addressed to ensure security policies are implemented and managed properly is that of upper management support. Even though HIPAA compliance is federal law, healthcare organizations still need buy-in from their upper management if security policies are to be successfully developed and embraced. If you have reached the point of communicating the value and requirements of HIPAA to upper management and are already working toward compliance, this should not be a major issue for you as it is in other nonregulated environments.

Beyond upper management buy-in, there are several other critical factors that will determine whether or not security policies are effective. In no particular order, these factors are as follows:

- *People must be aware of security policies.* Perhaps the greatest mistake in handling security policies is to create them and then put them on a shelf without making anyone aware of them. The organization would be just as well off without security policies in this case. Refer to Chapter 24 for details on the best ways to get the word on your security policies out to everyone involved.

- *Create a committee to develop security policies.* You do not want to develop security policies all by yourself. This could be misconstrued as one-sided or biased, and this is certainly not the position any one individual wants to be in. Additionally, you must consider the expertise of your business leaders to ensure the security policies you create are feasible. Get other people involved. It is preferable to get HR, Legal, and applicable business unit representatives to help with this.

- *Security policies must be specific to your organization.* You cannot simply buy a security policies book or download sample policies off the Internet and apply them verbatim to your immediate needs. Do not get us wrong; these policies are a great place to start — they can definitely save you a lot of time, money, and effort. Just remember to tailor these policies to your organization's specific needs and requirements. In fact, try to relate your security policies to your various privacy policies whenever possible. Tailoring these policies should not take a lot of work, and it is absolutely necessary to make sure your information systems and protected health information (PHI) are properly protected in your particular environment.

- *Security policies must be readable and understandable.* Make sure you know your intended audience before you start writing your policies. Regardless of who will be reading them, use the legal and technical jargon sparingly. All of your employees, independent of their knowledge and intellect, need to be able to read any and all of your organization's security policies and completely understand them. This is not just an education or awareness issue. It also depends on how well written the policies are in the first place.

- *Security policies must be fair, reasonable, and legal.* Put yourself in your end users' position. Do the policies seem fair and reasonable in order to get the job done? If security policies are not fair and reasonable, people will break them, and that is the last thing anyone needs to have happen with their HIPAA policies. It really is possible to balance security, HIPAA compliance, and convenience. Make sure your organization is doing that. Also, do not forget to run your security policies by your legal counsel before you publish them to make sure they are legal from an HR and employees' rights perspective.

- *Security policies must be enforced.* It is not enough for security policies to be fair, reasonable, and legal. They must also be enforced within the organization for all users, including upper management. Sure, HIPAA mandates security policies, but similar to the awareness issue discussed previously, if security policies are not enforced by the security policy committee, HIPAA Officer(s), or upper management, then it is probably not worth the time, money, and effort to develop them in the first place. Not only this, but HIPAA also mandates sanction policies and requires documentation that you are actually enforcing the policies.

**Sample Security Policy Framework**

The following framework should be considered when developing security policies to ensure all the essential areas are covered. Even the most basic set of policies and supporting documents needs to have a structure such as this to ensure consistency, proper coverage, and ease of readability. Remember to create a separate policy for each issue you need to cover.

- *Introduction:* One or two sentences describing the policy. This may also include any background information.
- *Purpose:* One or two sentences describing why the policy exists. This may also include specific policy objectives.
- *Related documents:* Any other documentation that might play a role in this policy, including any documents that the policy relies on and any documentation that the policy replaces or outdates.
- *Scope:* What and who is actually covered by this policy.
- *Statement of policy:* The actual policy statement itself (examples are given in Appendix B).
- *Responsibilities:* What is expected by people or systems covered by the policies.
- *Standards and guidelines:* Any criteria that provide supporting details to successfully implement the policy. Consider documenting these separately to keep your policy simple.
- *Procedures:* How the specific policy will be implemented. Consider documenting these separately to keep your policy simple.
- *Compliance:* How policy compliance will be measured and what the repercussions will be if the policy is not adhered to.
- *Revisions:* Any changes to the policy along with the date of the change and who made the change.

**Security Policies You May Need for HIPAA Security Rule Compliance**

Depending on the results of your risk assessment, your organization will need various security policies in place to become compliant with the Security Rule. Exhibit 1 contains a list of security policies you may need organized by the three major Security Rule safeguards sections. Emphasis here is on the word "may" because every organization's needs are different. This is not intended to be a comprehensive list, but should be a good starting point in your security policy development process. Keep in mind that security incident procedures, contingency plans, and evaluation methods are not listed here, as they are covered in depth in Chapters 14 and 25.

**Managing Your Security Policies**

As part of your ongoing HIPAA compliance initiatives, you will need to ensure that your security policies are kept up to date. You should perform an annual review of your policies to ensure they are still appropriate for

**Exhibit 1. Possible HIPAA-Related Information Security Policies**

| Administrative Safeguard Policies | Physical Safeguard Policies | Technical Safeguard Policies |
|---|---|---|
| **Security Management Process**<br>Risk assessment requirements<br>Sanction/discipline for violation<br>System logging requirements<br>System monitoring requirements<br>System auditing requirements<br>System maintenance requirements<br>Policy review and maintenance | **Facility Access Controls**<br>Building access and validation controls<br>Emergency operation instructions<br>Locks and other controls<br>Facility maintenance record controls | **Access Control**<br>Unique user IDs<br>Emergency operation instructions<br>Automatic log-off time limits<br>Systems or controls to ensure data<br>  confidentiality<br>Server security settings<br>Workstation security settings |
| **Assigned Security Responsibility**<br>Security Officer roles and responsibilities<br>Workforce security<br>User authorization controls<br>Administrative supervision methods<br>Employee termination methods<br>Background check requirements<br>Outside consultant/vendor access controls | **Workstation Use**<br>Permitted workstation uses<br><br>**Workstation Security**<br>Computer location and physical controls<br><br>**Device and Media Controls**<br>Information disposal instructions<br>Media reuse controls<br>Physical hardware accountability controls<br>Data backup and storage controls | **Audit Controls**<br>Technical methods used to enable system<br>  auditing<br><br>**Integrity**<br>Systems or controls to ensure data is not<br>  tampered with<br><br>**Person or Entity Authentication**<br>Requirement to ensure a user or entity is known<br>  and trusted |
| **Information Access Management**<br>System usage controls<br>Instructions for privileged use of systems<br>Isolation of clearinghouse functions<br>User authorization controls<br>User access establishment/review controls | | **Transmission Security**<br>Systems or controls to ensure data in transit is<br>  not tampered with<br>Systems or controls to ensure data in transit is<br>  kept confidential |
| **Security Awareness and Training**<br>Security reminders<br>Antivirus protection<br>Log-in monitoring and reporting<br>Password management controls<br>Software installation controls | | |

your information systems and business needs, as well as update them to reflect major organizational or technology changes as necessary. You may need to create new policies or revise or remove outdated ones. Staying abreast of your information security and policy needs will not be a simple task. We will talk more about this in Chapter 25 when we discuss performing HIPAA compliance reviews and audits.

With today's more advanced security infrastructure applications, many policies can be directly enforced by defining specific systems settings. For example, you can "program" some of your specific policies directly into firewalls, intrusion-detection systems, and centrally managed antivirus products for automated enforcement. In addition, with our modern software, everything from enterprise directory services to workstation operating systems has the ability to configure and enforce specific policies for items such as passwords, authentication, and logging. We cover HIPAA technology infrastructures in more detail in Chapter 21, but wanted to note this point here to remind you that many technologies you may already have in place can assist you with your security policy efforts. Keep in mind these programmable policies still must be documented and maintained as described earlier.

For larger organizations where information systems and security policies are extremely complex, there are various third-party products that can assist in the ongoing management of them. These applications can help:

- Store policies and track changes
- Centrally host policies for easy access by everyone
- Get the word out on policies through online tutorials and training sessions
- Assess everyone's understanding of the policies via quizzes

See Appendix C for more information on specific vendors and products that can assist you with the ongoing management of your security policies.

### Chapter 13: Practical Checklist

- What most of us refer to as security "policies" can be more than just policies. Depending on how you structure your documentation, security policies may also include standards, guidelines, and procedures.
- Have you formed your security policy development committee?
- Consider reviewing potential third-party products and Internet resources that can assist in your security policy development.
- Ensure that your policies are enforceable by making them fair and reasonable.
- Ensure that your policies are enforced by obtaining upper management support and buy-in up front.
- Remember that your current technologies may be able to assist in security policy enforcement.

# Chapter 14
# Crafting a Security Implementation Plan

## Background

Preparing for Security Rule compliance is very similar to preparing for Privacy Rule compliance in that it can be very complex and must be thoroughly planned out, utilizing virtually every department in your organization. A large portion of the Privacy Rule standards requires a solid information security infrastructure to be in place. Chapter 4 discussed the issue of how the rules are related. Many covered entities (CEs) may already be well ahead of the Security Rule curve because of their Privacy Rule initiatives or simply because they have been following information security best practices as part of their daily business operations.

From a high-level perspective, Security Rule compliance requires determining where your organization stands compared to the HIPAA requirements, what protected health information (PHI) risks are present, what information security mechanisms can be put in place to reduce those risks, and how you will go about implementing those information security mechanisms. To reduce the overall burden of Security Rule compliance, the Department of Health and Human Services (HHS) has made the final Security Rule as scalable and flexible as possible. This means that you can tailor your implementation plan based on your specific circumstances. According to the final Security Rule documentation, it is "focused more on what needs to be done and less on how it should be accomplished." This will allow small CEs to reasonably comply without breaking the bank, and larger CEs to integrate the specific requirements into their current systems.

Exhibit 1 contains a plan to help you get started with your information security initiatives. You will, of course, have to modify it depending on your organization's needs, size, and information systems' complexity. Keep in mind that this is can be a complex subject, so we are keeping it fairly high level. For more detailed information and guidelines, you may consider referring to the ISO 17799 standard found at http://www.iso.ch or other similar framework.

---

The information and opinions provided in this book do not constitute or substitute for legal or other professional advice.

## Exhibit 1. A Security Rule Implementation Plan

1. Determine your covered entity status.
   - Is your organization a HIPAA CE? If so, what type:
     – Healthcare provider
     – Health plan
     – Healthcare clearinghouse
     – Hybrid entity (HIPAA covered functions are not the primary functions of the organization.)
   - Is your organization a business associate (BA) of a HIPAA CE? See Chapter 20 for more information on BA issues and Appendix B for a sample BA agreement.
   - We outline the steps to determine your HIPAA status in Section 4. Be sure to confirm your status with your legal counsel or other HIPAA expert.

2. Initiate your security project and start planning for your compliance activities.
   - Determine who will sponsor your HIPAA security initiatives (owner, executive management, board of directors, etc.), and document and communicate their commitment to your HIPAA compliance initiatives.
   - Establish a steering committee that will plan, oversee, and guide your HIPAA security efforts. You do not want to go at this alone. Even if you are a small CE, get at least one other person involved. This can be the same committee used for your HIPAA privacy initiatives.
   - Develop a high-level HIPAA strategic plan that involves all of your information security initiatives. Make this available to everyone in your organization so they understand the mission, goals, and objectives of your HIPAA security efforts.
   - Establish a HIPAA security compliance team that is responsible for project implementation. For small CEs, this could be the same people who are on the steering committee. This could be performed by internal personnel, external personnel, or a combination of both. See Chapter 23 for more information on outsourcing your information security initiatives.
   - Develop detailed roles and responsibilities for your HIPAA security compliance efforts. To help prevent a "not invented here" culture as well as to maximize quality and efficiency, keep the roles broad and responsibilities specific as there will be overlap in certain areas.
   - Organize people, processes, and methodologies to track and manage your HIPAA security initiatives. For small CEs, this could be the same people who are on the steering committee. Consider using a whiteboard or project management software to ensure everything is kept in line and addressed.
   - Develop a master HIPAA security plan and timeline for your overall goals and specific plans for each project phase (see Chapter 11 for specific information on what is required by the Security Rule).
   - Determine how you are going to measure and keep track of your project results.
   - Establish a HIPAA security compliance budget.

3. Understand the activities covered by the Security Rule.
   - Communicate the noncompliance penalties mentioned in Chapter 1 to everyone in the organization, especially upper management.
   - Read and understand the HIPAA Security Rule (see Chapter 11).
   - Associate the specific administrative, physical, and technical safeguards outlined in the Security Rule to what your organization is doing.

**Exhibit 1. A Security Rule Implementation Plan (Continued)**

4. Identify and prepare a Security Officer for the upcoming tasks.
   - Identify and appoint a qualified Security Officer to address HIPAA security-related issues. See Appendix B for a sample Security Officer job description.
   - Identify the Privacy Officer and other HIPAA compliance team members with whom the Security Officer will have to work closely.
   - If necessary, ensure that the Security Officer has received the proper training. Outside of this book, HIPAA workshops and conferences are a great place to start. There are also various information security classes and conferences held around the United States. See Appendix C for a list of organizations sponsoring these events.

5. Perform a Security Rule gap analysis and baseline the organization.
   - Develop an assessment methodology. There will be both technical and business issues to assess, so make sure you have the proper methodologies and resources. See Chapter 12 for detailed information on this.
   - Collect and review existing information security policies, procedures, and standards.
   - Collect and review existing network diagrams and network hardware and software inventory lists.
   - Conduct interviews to collect and document undocumented practices and procedures.
   - Identify all employees who have remote access capabilities to your information systems (dial-up, VPN, etc.).
   - Collect the inventory of the electronic PHI that you compiled for your Privacy Rule initiatives. Verify that this inventory is still accurate and comprehensive.
     – Be sure to include your network infrastructure devices that either store or transmit PHI such as storage area networks (SANs) and routers.
     – Be sure to include electronic devices such as personal digital assistants (PDAs) and medical equipment.
   - Create an inventory and sort all of the information you have collected based on its association with the HIPAA Security Rule standards and implementation specifications.
   - Determine which areas of your organization are affected by the Security Rule:
     – Where is PHI stored and transmitted within the organization?
     – Which departments or people are responsible for this PHI?
     – Which departments utilize or otherwise rely on your organization's information systems?
     – Which facilities will need to be protected by the physical safeguards?
   - Create an inventory of all your BAs (such as healthcare and IT vendors, lawyers, contractors, etc.) and electronic trading partners with whom your organization shares PHI.
   - Identify and diagram all BAs who have remote access to your information systems (dial-up, VPN, etc.) for support purposes, etc.
   - Diagram all other electronic information flows with all of your BAs.
   - Perform a risk analysis that includes vulnerability assessments and penetration tests to determine specific risks to your information systems.
   - Test all information systems to determine which authentication and access controls are currently being used.

## Exhibit 1. A Security Rule Implementation Plan (Continued)

- Compare existing organizational information security policies, procedures, and administrative functions with the Security Rule standards and document the differences.
- Compare existing organizational culture (the human environment) with the Security Rule standards and document the differences.
- Compare existing physical and technical security measures with the Security Rule standards and document the differences.
- Create a remediation/compliance plan for closing the gaps that were found and implement new systems to meet the Security Rule requirements.
- Document potential impacts the gaps present to your organization.

6. Plan remediation strategies.
   - Document your administrative (policy and procedure) compliance strategy, implementation plan, and timeline.
   - Document your technical compliance strategy, implementation plan, and timeline.
   - Refine your Security Rule compliance budget as needed and seek additional funding commitment if necessary.
   - Organize the teams necessary to close the gaps found. This can be performed by internal personnel, external personnel, or a combination of both. See Chapter 23 for more information on outsourcing your information security initiatives.

7. Remediate the organization.
   - Update existing security policies and procedures or develop new security policies and procedures as necessary.
   - Update organizational policies and procedures to match your HIPAA security policy and procedure requirements.
   - Develop or outsource information security training for all personnel, including upper management. Be sure to document this training, including who was in attendance.
   - Update existing BA contracts or develop new ones as necessary to include verbiage ensuring the protection of PHI.
   - Execute these BA agreements.
   - Modify business processes, technical systems, and physical facilities or create new ones as necessary to comply with the Security Rule standards.
   - Transition the responsibility and maintenance of new processes and systems to the appropriate parties.
   - Establish and document ongoing compliance procedures and implement the appropriate systems. See Chapter 25 for information on ongoing HIPAA compliance reviews and audits.

8. Monitor progress and changes in HIPAA rules and update your organizational policies, procedures, and technologies appropriately.
   - Keep current with changes to the HIPAA regulations.
   - Keep current with new and updated state, federal, and international regulations related to information security.
   - Keep current with various information security standards and best practices.
   - Update policies and procedures as necessary to meet new regulatory requirements and to reflect organizational and business process changes.

**Exhibit 1. A Security Rule Implementation Plan (Continued)**

- Monitor organizational procedures and follow up on areas of information security falling out of compliance.
- Regularly review information systems activity logs. With a few exceptions, this is the only way you will find out if any inappropriate computer activity is occurring.
- Manage business associates and other relationships related to the electronic storage or transmission of PHI.
- Perform periodic risk analyses and gap analyses annually, at a minimum, to ensure PHI is protected against newly discovered information threats and vulnerabilities. Perform these immediately after any major information systems or businesses process changes to ensure that no new threats or vulnerabilities were introduced with the changes.
- Perform regular internal audits for each aspect of Security Rule compliance. See Chapter 11 for the specific requirements on this.
- Perform ongoing information security training and awareness activities for all personnel, including upper management.
- Maintain documentation on your HIPAA compliance activities and store it securely for future reference.

## Some Points to Keep in Mind

Here are compliance facts related to common questions and concerns you need to keep in mind when creating and applying your Security Rule implementation plan:

- Security rule requirements are flexible and scalable depending on the size of a CE, its internal culture, the complexity of its information systems, and the number of business associates it deals with.
- Information security is more than just technical safeguards. It is more about business procedures, organizational culture, and ensuring that everyone involved with PHI knows what to look for and what (and what not) to do.
- The Security Rule does not require the use of specific technologies such as firewalls and operating systems that support access controls and logging; however, their use is implied.
- There is no such thing as 100-percent security. CEs are just expected to follow the Security Rule standards; implement the proper policies, procedures, and technologies; and reasonably show that the organization is making an effort to protect against common threats and vulnerabilities.

## Conclusion

As with the Privacy Rule requirements and implementation efforts, the Security Rule compliance initiatives will be an ongoing task that must be managed appropriately. You cannot simply implement new policies, procedures, and technologies expecting that to be sufficient and not need any ongoing management. There are newly discovered information threats and vulnerabilities almost every day. If you create your information security team, assess your gaps and risks, implement reasonable safeguards, document all of your compliance efforts, and manage your ongoing risks, you can in good conscience say that you have done everything you can to ensure that your PHI is as secure as possible.

**Chapter 14: Practical Checklist**

- Determine your CE status.
- Obtain Security Rule compliance sponsorship from upper management.
- Establish a Security Rule compliance project plan.
- Assign the appropriate responsibilities to your team.
- Perform a gap analysis and risk analysis to determine where your organization stands.
- Create a remediation plan consisting of the appropriate policies, procedures, and technical systems that meet the compliance requirements.
- Implement your security plan.
- Monitor ongoing Security Rule compliance.
- Remember that there's no such thing as 100-percent security.

# Chapter 15
# Security Rule Compliance Checklist

As with the Privacy Rule Compliance Checklist in Chapter 10, we have created a Security Rule Checklist for you as well. This is only high-level coverage, so be sure to refer to the other chapters on Security Rule compliance when moving forward. The corresponding location in the regulatory text is listed for your reference.

**Administrative Safeguard Requirements**

*A. Security Management Process*

____ 1. Risk Analysis (Required)

§ **164.308(1)(a):** "Conduct an accurate and thorough assessment of the potential risks and vulnerabilities to the confidentiality, integrity, and availability of electronic protected health information held by the covered entity."

____ 2. Risk Management (Required)

§ **164.308(1)(b):** "Implement security measures sufficient to reduce risks and vulnerabilities to a reasonable and appropriate level to comply with § 164.306(a)."

____ 3. Sanction Policy (Required)

§ **164.308(1)(c):** "Apply appropriate sanctions against workforce members who fail to comply with the security policies and procedures of the covered entity."

____ 4. Information System Activity Review (Required)

§ **164.308(1)(d):** "Implement procedures to regularly review records of information system activity, such as audit logs, access reports, and security incident tracking reports."

---

The information and opinions provided in this book do not constitute or substitute for legal or other professional advice.

## B. Assigned Security Responsibility

_____ 5. Assign a Security Official

§ **164.308(2):** "Identify the security official who is responsible for the development and implementation of the policies and procedures required by this sub-part for the entity."

## C. Workforce Security

_____ 6. Authorization and/or Supervision (Addressable)

§ **164.308(3)(a):** "Implement procedures for the authorization and/or supervision of workforce members who work with electronic protected health information or in locations where it might be accessed."

_____ 7. Workforce Clearance Procedure (Addressable)

§ **164.308(3)(b):** "Implement procedures to determine that the access of a workforce member to electronic protected health information is appropriate."

_____ 8. Termination Procedures (Addressable)

§ **164.308(3)(c):** "Implement procedures for terminating access to electronic protected health information when the employment of a workforce member ends or as required by determinations made as specified in paragraph (a)(3)(ii)(B) of this section."

## D. Information Access Management

_____ 9. Isolating Healthcare Clearinghouse Functions (Required)

§ **164.308(4)(a):** "If a healthcare clearinghouse is part of a larger organization, the clearinghouse must implement policies and procedures that protect the electronic protected health information of the clearinghouse from unauthorized access by the larger organization."

_____ 10. Access Authorization (Addressable)

§ **164.308(4)(b):** "Implement policies and procedures for granting access to electronic protected health information, for example, through access to a workstation, transaction, program, process, or other mechanism."

_____ 11. Access Establishment and Modification (Addressable)

§ **164.308(4)(c):** "Implement policies and procedures that, based upon the entity's access authorization policies, establish, document, review, and modify a user's right of access to a workstation, transaction, program, or process."

## E. Security Awareness and Training

____ 12. Security Reminders (Addressable)

§ **164.308(5)(a):** "Periodic security updates."

____ 13. Protection from Malicious Software

§ **164.308(5)(b):** "Procedures for guarding against, detecting, and reporting malicious software."

____ 14. Log-In Monitoring (Addressable)

§ **164.308(5)(c):** "Procedures for monitoring log-in attempts and reporting discrepancies."

____ 15. Password Management (Addressable)

§ **164.308(5)(d):** "Procedures for creating, changing, and safeguarding passwords."

## F. Security Incident Procedures

____ 16. Response and Reporting (Required)

§ **164.308(6)(ii):** "Identify and respond to suspected or known security incidents; mitigate, to the extent practicable, harmful effects of security incidents that are known to the covered entity; and document security incidents and their outcomes."

## G. Contingency Plan

____ 17. Data Backup Plan (Required)

§ **164.308(7)(a):** "Establish and implement procedures to create and maintain retrievable exact copies of electronic protected health information."

____ 18. Disaster Recovery Plan (Required)

§ **164.308(7)(b):** "Establish (and implement as needed) procedures to restore any loss of data."

____ 19. Emergency Mode Operation Plan (Required)

§ **164.308(7)(c):** "Establish (and implement as needed) procedures to restore any loss of data."

____ 20. Testing and Revision Procedure (Addressable)

§ **164.308(7)(d):** "Establish (and implement as needed) procedures to enable continuation of critical business processes for protection of the security of electronic protected health information while operating in emergency mode."

____ 21. Applications and Data Criticality Analysis (Addressable)

§ **164.308(7)(e):** "Assess the relative criticality of specific applications and data in support of other contingency plan components."

## H. Evaluation

____ 22. Security Evaluation

§ 164.308(8): "Perform a periodic technical and nontechnical evaluation, based initially upon the standards implemented under this rule and subsequently, in response to environmental or operational changes affecting the security of electronic protected health information, that establishes the extent to which an entity's security policies and procedures meet the requirements of this sub-part."

## I. Business Associate Contracts and Other Arrangement

____ 23. Written Contract or Other Arrangement (Required)

§ 164.308(b)(1)(4): "Document the satisfactory assurances required by paragraph (b)(1) of this section through a written contract or other arrangement with the business associate that meets the applicable requirements of § 164.314(a)."

## Physical Safeguard Requirements

## J. Facility Access Controls

____ 24. Contingency Operations (Addressable)

§ 164.310(2)(i): "Establish (and implement as needed) procedures that allow facility access in support of restoration of lost data under the disaster recovery plan and emergency mode operations plan in the event of an emergency."

____ 25. Facility Security Plan (Addressable)

§ 164.310(2)(ii): "Implement policies and procedures to safeguard the facility and the equipment therein from unauthorized physical access, tampering, and theft."

____ 26. Access Control and Validation (Addressable)

§ 164.310(2)(iii): "Implement procedures to control and validate a person's access to facilities based on their role or function, including visitor control, and control of access to software programs for testing and revision."

____ 27. Maintenance Records (Addressable)

§ 164.310(2)(iv): "Implement policies and procedures to document repairs and modifications to the physical components of a facility which are related to security (for example, hardware, walls, doors, and locks)."

## K. Workstation Use

____ 28. Workstation Use

**§ 164.310(b):** "Implement policies and procedures that specify the proper functions to be performed, the manner in which those functions are to be performed, and the physical attributes of the surroundings of a specific workstation or class of workstation that can access electronic protected health information."

## L. Workstation Security

____ 29. Workstation Safeguards

**§ 164.310(c):** "Implement physical safeguards for all workstations that access electronic protected health information, to restrict access to authorized users."

## M. Device and Media Controls

____ 30. Disposal (Required)

**§ 164.310(d)(1)(2)(i):** "Implement policies and procedures to address the final disposition of electronic protected health information, and/or the hardware or electronic media on which it is stored."

____ 31. Media Reuse (Required)

**§ 164.310(d)(1)(2)(ii):** "Implement procedures for removal of electronic protected health information from electronic media before the media are made available for re-use."

____ 32. Accountability (Addressable)

**§ 164.310(d)(1)(2)(iii):** "Maintain a record of the movements of hardware and electronic media and any person responsible therefore."

____ 33. Data Backup and Storage (Addressable)

**§ 164.310(d)(1)(2)(iv):** "Create a retrievable, exact copy of electronic protected health information, when needed, before movement of equipment."

## Technical Safeguard Requirements

### N. Access Control

____ 34. Unique User Identification (Required)

§ **164.312(2)(i):** "Assign a unique name and/or number for identifying and tracking user identity."

____ 35. Emergency Access Procedure (Required)

§ **164.312(2)(ii):** "Establish (and implement as needed) procedures for obtaining necessary electronic protected health information during an emergency."

____ 36. Automatic Log-Off (Addressable)

§ **164.312(2)(iii):** "Implement electronic procedures that terminate an electronic session after a predetermined time of inactivity."

____ 37. Encryption and Decryption (Addressable)

§ **164.312(2)(iv):** "Implement a mechanism to encrypt and decrypt electronic protected health information."

### O. Audit Controls

____ 38. Audit Mechanisms

§ **164.312(b):** "Implement hardware, software, and/or procedural mechanisms that record and examine activity in information systems that contain or use electronic protected health information."

### P. Integrity

____ 39. Mechanism to Authenticate Electronic PHI (Addressable)

§ **164.312(c)(1)(2):** "Implement electronic mechanisms to corroborate that electronic protected health information has not been altered or destroyed in an unauthorized manner."

____ 40. Person or Entity Authentication

§ **164.312(d):** "Implement procedures to verify that a person or entity seeking access to electronic protected health information is the one claimed."

## Q. Transmission Security

____ 41. Integrity Controls (Addressable)

**§ 164.312(e)(1)(2)(i):** "Implement security measures to ensure that electronically transmitted electronic protected health information is not improperly modified without detection until disposed of."

____ 42. Encryption (Addressable)

**§ 164.312(e)(1)(2)(ii):** "Implement a mechanism to encrypt electronic protected health information whenever deemed appropriate."

# Section 3: HIPAA Security Rule Quiz

1. Which of the following does *not* characterize the Security Rule?
   A. A set of information security best practices that make good business sense
   B. A minimum security baseline which is intended to help prevent unauthorized access of PHI
   C. An inflexible and unscalable set of rules that healthcare organizations must comply with
   D. An outline of what to do

2. The Security Rule was designed to be which of the following?
   A. Technology neutral
   B. Scalable
   C. Flexible
   D. All of the above

3. Have there been any changes to the Security Rule since it was first proposed?
   A. Yes, the entire original rule was scrapped and a new one was created
   B. No, the document was so comprehensive that no changes were needed
   C. Yes, numerous changes were made to the Security Rule before its final form
   D. There have not been any changes yet, but new ones are expected in the Fall of 2005

4. How many required implementation specifications does the Security Rule have?
   A. Over 300
   B. None
   C. 20
   D. Each CE must find out after doing a risk analysis

5. What can be used to assist meeting the Access Authorization (Addressable) specification in the Security Rule?
   A. HR, supervisor, and manager education on this matter
   B. Strong line of communication between HR and IT
   C. Internal employee to develop the specific procedures
   D. All of the above

6. What do security policies and supporting documents outline?
   A. Roles and responsibilities
   B. Standards for all employees to adhere to
   C. Both A and B
   D. None of the above

7. How often should you consider performing a review of your security policies?
   A. Never; once you finish, it should work forever
   B. Every 5 years
   C. Right before you are audited
   D. Annually

8. What should you establish that will plan, oversee, and guide your HIPAA security efforts?
   A. A Vendor-Neutral Task Force
   B. A Steering Committee
   C. A Yearly Calendar
   D. Rules and Regulations

9. What is helpful in performing a Security Rule gap analysis?
   A. Collecting the inventory of the electronic PHI that you compiled for your Privacy Rule initiatives
   B. Making sure that all computers on your network are using Windows 2000
   C. Deleting old transaction logs
   D. Compiling a list of all current and former patients

10. At what point can you achieve 100 percent security for your organization?
    A. Six months into the HIPAA Security Compliance Process
    B. After all recommended security measures have been taken
    C. Never
    D. When you have installed all necessary software

11. Security Rule compliance is only possible with which of the following?
    A. A large HIPAA compliance budget
    B. Outside help from HIPAA experts
    C. A complete copy of the Security Policy in hand
    D. An appropriate risk analysis is performed on your information systems

12. A risk analysis will help you determine which of the following?
    A. How confidential the PHI needs to be
    B. When and how the PHI needs to be protected
    C. Where the PHI is stored and transmitted
    D. All of the above

13. Is it possible for a CE to come to the conclusion that the PHI is not at risk whatsoever?
    A. Yes, if they already had the proper safeguards in place
    B. No
    C. Perhaps once the Risk Analysis is complete
    D. None of the above

14. The Security Rule requires CEs to perform an initial risk analysis to determine which of the following?
    A. Specific unauthorized uses
    B. Disclosures
    C. Data integrity losses that could occur to PHI
    D. All of the above

15. The Security Rule does not apply to information in any risk analysis documentation except in which of the following situations?
    A. It involves information stored on your computer
    B. The information is used to diagnose medical problems
    C. It specifically contains PHI
    D. None of the above

# Section 4
# Covered
# Entity Issues

# Chapter 16
# Healthcare Provider Issues

## Background

If you are a person, business, or agency that furnishes, bills, or receives payment for healthcare in the normal course of business, then it is likely you are a healthcare provider. A healthcare provider provides healthcare services or supplies related to the health of an individual. It includes, but is not limited to, the following:

*(1) Preventive, diagnostic, rehabilitative, maintenance, or palliative care, and counseling, service, assessment, or procedure with respect to the physical or mental condition, or functional status, of an individual or that affects the structure or function of the body; and (2) sale or dispensing of a drug, device, equipment, or other item in accordance with a prescription.*

See 45 CFR 160.103 of the Privacy Rule for a complete definition.

## Privacy Notices

Covered direct healthcare treatment providers must provide a Notice of Privacy Practices (NPP) to an individual on the date of first service delivery and, except in emergencies, attempt to obtain the individual's written acknowledgment of receipt of the notice. When an acknowledgment cannot be obtained, the provider must document the efforts to obtain the acknowledgment and provide an explanation why it was not obtained. If first service delivery to an individual is provided over the Internet through e-mail or using some other electronic method, the provider must send an electronic notice automatically at the same time of the individual's first request for service. The provider must try to obtain a return receipt or some other recognition from the individual in response to receiving the notice.

---

The information and opinions provided in this book do not constitute or substitute for legal or other professional advice.

There are many situations in which providers must provide an NPP, and some in which providing notice is not necessary. Here are some NPP pointers for providers:

- In emergencies, a provider must provide the notice to the individual as soon as possible after the emergency is over.
- Make the most recent notice available to individuals at their offices and facilities to allow individuals to obtain them there. Additionally, they must post the notice in a prominent location within the building.
- You may e-mail the notice if the individual agrees to receive it this way.
- You can develop more than one notice, such as when you perform different types of covered functions. You should provide the most appropriate version of the notice to the individual as applicable.
- If you participate in an organized healthcare arrangement (OHCA), you can create a single, joint notice following some specific conditions. For example, the joint notice must describe the covered entities (CEs) and the service delivery sites to which it applies.
- If you choose to use consents for the use or disclosure of protected health information (PHI), you must try to obtain an acknowledgment of the NPP.
- You do not need to obtain a new acknowledgment of receipt of notice from patients when your privacy policy changes.
- You can obtain an electronic acknowledgment of the privacy notice from an individual if it was delivered electronically. An acknowledgment for a notice given face-to-face can also be an electronic version of the individual's handwritten signature.
- If your first treatment of a patient is not face-to-face (for example, over the phone), you can mail the notice to the individual as soon as possible (the same day, if possible) and include some way for the individual to sign an acknowledgment and mail it back to you. Be sure to file a copy of the form sent to the patient to document the form and the accompanying acknowledgment.
- If the initial contact is simply to schedule an appointment, the notice may be given at the time the individual arrives for the appointment.
- For service provided electronically, the notice must be sent electronically automatically and contemporaneously in response to the individual's first request for service. In this situation, an electronic return receipt or other return transmission from the individual is considered a valid written acknowledgment of the notice.
- Healthcare providers and other covered entities that participate in an OHCA can use a single, joint notice that covers all of the participating covered entities, or each can use their own separate notice. Each direct treatment provider within the OHCA must make an effort to obtain the individual's acknowledgment of the notice provided.

- When an individual, such as a child, has a personal representative, you satisfy the notice distribution requirements by giving the notice to the personal representative (for example, the child's parent), and make an effort to get the personal representative's acknowledgment of the notice.
- You must post your entire notice at your healthcare facility in a clear and prominent location. You cannot post just a brief description of the notice.
- You are not required to mail revised notices to patients when the notice changes. However, when the patient next receives care, the new notice must be given to the individual.
- If you make the notice available on a customer service Web site, it must be kept current.
- If you have direct treatment relationships with individuals, you must give the NPP to every individual on the first date of service delivery and try as best as possible to obtain a written acknowledgment of the receipt of notice. This is in addition to posting the entire notice in a prominent location. The only exception to this is during an emergency situation.
- If the initial contact with a patient is to collect preoperative information over the phone or collect some other information in anticipation of an appointment or procedure, you may satisfy the notice requirement by giving the notice at the time the individual arrives for the appointment.
- Pharmacists can have customers provide their acknowledgment of receipt of notice in a log book if the individual is clearly told what they are acknowledging, and if their acknowledgment is not also used for some other permission that appears in the log book.
- Notices can be distributed as part of other mailings or distributions. However, the notice cannot be combined into a single form that is mailed at the same time, such as an authorization.
- E-mails containing the notice may also contain other information as well. However, you must keep the notice separate for the other e-mail attachments and still make an effort to obtain the individual's written acknowledgment of receipt of the notice.

## Fees for Record Review

Individuals must be given a copy of their corresponding PHI within a reasonable period of time after they request it. If the individual agrees to a summary or explanation of the information, you can request a reasonable fee based on the cost of providing that information. The fee must only consist of the costs involved in:

- Copying the PHI, including the cost of the supplies for the copy and the labor used for the copy

- Postage, if the individual has asked for the copy of PHI or the summary or explanation to be mailed
- Preparing the explanation or summary of the PHI, if the individual is told of this cost and agrees to it prior to preparing it

It is very important to understand that HIPAA makes no provision for providers or any other covered entity to charge the individual for the cost involved for personnel who supervise the patient while they are reviewing their PHI within the facilities. In most if not all cases, state laws allowing such charges do not preempt the HIPAA prohibition on such supervisory costs. Carefully study your applicable state laws and discuss with your legal counsel to determine if this is a practice you can implement within your facility.

**Mitigation Measures**

The Privacy Rule requires covered entities to follow mitigation procedures to address unauthorized use or disclosure of PHI. The description of what is adequate mitigation is purposely vague. In fact, HHS provided only one specific example of what is meant by appropriate mitigation: basically, to notify a patient immediately when inappropriate disclosure of his PHI occurs. Once the confidentiality of PHI has been breached, there is no way to make the information truly private again. So, to determine appropriate mitigation measures, consider what can be done to prevent further inappropriate unauthorized distribution of the PHI. For example, if PHI was mistakenly faxed to the wrong phone number, consider asking the inappropriate recipient to respect the corresponding person's privacy and destroy the faxed information. In fact, it is a good business practice to put a notice on all fax transmittals asking recipients to destroy misguided faxed information immediately.

**Fax Use**

Providers can fax PHI to another physician's office for treatment purposes. You must have reasonable and appropriate administrative, technical, and physical safeguards in place for these faxes to help ensure the privacy of the PHI. Besides putting a notice on the cover sheet of all faxes asking recipients to destroy misguided faxed information, you should also consider procedures to confirm the fax number is correct, physically locating the fax machine in a secured location, and other similar safeguards.

**Sign-In Sheets**

Physician offices can use patient sign-in sheets or call out the names of patients in their waiting rooms. Be careful that the information disclosed is limited. The Privacy Rule permits certain incidental disclosures, such as in waiting rooms when patient names are called. However, they are allowed only as long as your office has implemented reasonable safeguards to implement the minimum necessary standard. For example, consider calling out only the first name of the patient instead of the full name, and do not place medical information on the sign-in sheet that is not necessary for sign-in purposes.

## Patient Charts

The HIPAA Privacy Rule allows providers to place patient charts in the plastic box outside an exam room, as is customarily done, as long as the clinic takes reasonable and appropriate safeguards to protect the patient's privacy. The physician and other healthcare professionals typically use the patient charts for treatment purposes. Incidental disclosures to others that might occur as a result of the charts being left in the box are permitted as long as reasonable safeguards are in place. The minimum necessary requirement needs to be met. For example, it could be reasonable and appropriate to safeguard the patient chart by limiting access to the area from the public, by supervising the area, by escorting all nonemployees who are in the area, or by putting the patient information within a folder so the information cannot be viewed by anyone who happens to be passing by. Each provider needs to determine what safeguards, procedures, and measures are appropriate for his own unique situation and circumstances.

The situation is similar in hospital settings where patient names are often displayed by the doors. In this case, disclosure of patient names is permitted if the use or disclosure is for treatment, which it would be if the practice is to ensure that care is given to the correct individual, or for healthcare operations purposes such as providing a service to patients and their families. The disclosure of the patient name in this situation to other persons in the area would typically be considered an incidental disclosure. These incidental disclosures are allowed to the extent that the hospital has applied appropriate safeguards. By providing just the patient name by the door, it would likely seem the disclosure is the minimum necessary for the purposes described. Again, it is important for each covered entity to evaluate what measures are reasonable and appropriate in its particular circumstances. For more information, see the preamble to the final modifications to the Privacy Rule (67 Fed. Reg. 53182, 53193-95 (August 14, 2002)).

## Business Associates

Providers generally are not business associates of payers. When a provider is a member of a health plan network and the only relationship between the health plan and the provider is that the provider submits claims for payment to the plan, then the provider is not a BA of the health plan. However, a BA relationship could arise if the provider performs a function on behalf of or provides services to the health plan, such as in case management services. For more information about these situations, see 67 Fed. Reg. 14776, 14788 (March 27, 2002).

Hospitals do not need to actively monitor their BAs' activities with regard to PHI. However, they must have a written contract or some other formal arrangement for BAs to ensure they appropriately protect the privacy of the health information. If a covered entity finds out there is a violation of the BA contract or arrangement, and the BA does nothing to correct the situation, then it must terminate the BA contract. If the arrangement is such that termination is not possible, then the problem must be reported to the Office for Civil Rights. See 45 CFR § 164.504(e)(1) for more information.

BAs are contractors or other personnel, who are not part of the hospital workforce, hired to do work that involves the use or disclosure of PHI. Plumbers, electricians, photocopy repair technicians, and similar workers typically do not require access to PHI to perform work for a provider, so they do not meet the definition of a BA, and do not need a BA agreement. Janitorial services are typically not BAs either, because the work they perform usually does not involve the use or disclosure of PHI. Any disclosure of PHI that occurs in performing janitorial duties, such as when emptying trash cans, is likely limited in nature and is incidental to their janitorial functions.

When a service is hired to do work for a covered entity and the PHI disclosure is not limited, such as routine shredding of PHI documents, then the service would likely be considered a BA. If the work is performed under the direct control of the covered entity, for instance within the covered entity's facilities, then the covered entity treats the service as part of its workforce, and will typically not need a BA contract.

BAs do not need to create an NPP. However, a covered entity must contractually ensure the BA's use and disclosure of PHI is in compliance with the covered entity's NPP. This is a promise made within the covered entity's NPP. Covered entities may also use a BA to distribute the notices to individuals.

## Authorizations

A covered entity cannot bypass getting individuals' authorization for a use or disclosure that is not permitted by the HIPAA Privacy Rule merely by notifying individuals of the use or disclosure in the NPP. A notice is not a substitute for an individual's authorization. An individual's written authorization must be obtained for any use or disclosure of PHI that is not permitted or required by the Privacy Rule. The NPP must describe the permitted uses and disclosures a covered entity may make without the

218

individual's authorization, as well as state that any other uses or disclosures will be made only with the individual's written authorization.

## *Marketing*

Healthcare providers are increasingly performing more marketing activities to create revenue. The HIPAA Privacy Rule marketing requirements will have a significant impact on these providers. It is important for providers to thoroughly review and follow the HIPAA requirements for marketing. CEs generally cannot market health-related products and services without authorization from the patient. Providers need to review and assess their marketing plans to determine if current marketing activities or plans are in compliance with the HIPAA Privacy Rule. Chapter 5 discusses marketing issues in more detail.

**Healthcare Provider Marketing Checklist\*.** Generally, except as discussed later, any communication that meets the definition of marketing is not permitted unless the CE obtains an authorization. If you receive direct or indirect payment for the marketing from a third party, you must state that such remuneration is involved. See 45 CFR 164.508(a)(3).

- A communication is not "marketing" if it is made to describe your health-related product or service (or payment for such product or service) that is provided in communications about participants in a healthcare provider network or health plan network. This permits communications by a provider about its own products or services.
- It is not marketing when a hospital uses its patients list to announce the arrival of a new specialty group (e.g., orthopedic) or the acquisition of new equipment (e.g., x-ray or magnetic resonance image machine) through a general mailing or publication.
- A communication is not marketing if it is made for treatment of the individual. For example, it is not marketing when:
  - A pharmacy or other healthcare provider mails prescription refill reminders to patients, or contracts with a mail house to do so.
  - A primary care physician refers an individual to a specialist for a follow-up test or provides free samples of a prescription drug to a patient.
- A communication is not marketing if it is made for case management or care coordination for the individual, or to direct or recommend alternative treatments, therapies, healthcare providers, or settings of care to the individual. For example, under this exception, it is not marketing when an endocrinologist shares a patient's medical record with several behavior management programs to determine which program best suits the ongoing needs of the individual patient.

*Modified and paraphrased from the list provided by HHS.

- – A hospital social worker shares medical record information with various nursing homes in the course of recommending that the patient be transferred from a hospital bed to a nursing home.
- Marketing in the form of a face-to-face communication does not need authorization.
- Providing a promotional gift of nominal value for marketing purposes does not require authorization. For example, no prior authorization is necessary when a hospital provides a free package of formula and other baby products to new mothers as they leave the maternity ward.
- You must obtain patients' authorization for the following types of uses or disclosures of PHI for marketing:
  - – Selling protected health information to third parties for their use and reuse. Thus, under the rule, a hospital or other provider may not sell names of pregnant women to baby formula manufacturers or magazines without an authorization.
  - – Disclosing protected health information to outsiders for their independent marketing use. Under the rule, doctors may not provide patients lists to pharmaceutical companies for those companies' drug promotions without an authorization.
- You may not give PHI to a telemarketer, door-to-door salesperson, or other third party you hired to make permitted communications (for example, about your own goods and services) unless that third party has agreed by contract to use the information only for communicating on your behalf.
- You may not sell PHI to third parties for the third party's own marketing activities without authorization. For example, a pharmacist cannot sell, without patient authorization, a list of patients to a pharmaceutical company, for the pharmaceutical company to market its own products to the individuals on the list.
- You can share PHI with a telemarketer only if you have either obtained the individual's prior written authorization to do so, or have entered into a BA relationship with the telemarketer for the purpose of making a communication that is not marketing, such as to inform individuals about the covered entity's own goods or services.
- Disease management health promotion, preventive care, and wellness programs generally do not fall under the HIPAA Privacy Rule's definition of "marketing." To the extent the disease management or wellness program is operated by you or by a BA, communications about these programs are not marketing because they are about the CE's own health-related services. So, for example, a hospital's Wellness Department could start a weight-loss program and send a flyer to all patients seen in the hospital over the past year who meet the

definition of obese, even if those individuals were not specifically seen for obesity when they were in the hospital.

- A communication that promotes health in a general manner and does not promote a specific product or service from a particular provider does not meet the definition of marketing. Such communications may include population-based activities in the areas of health education or disease prevention. Examples of general health promotional material include mailings reminding women to get an annual mammogram; mailings providing information about how to lower cholesterol, new developments in healthcare (e.g., new diagnostic tools), support groups, organ donation, cancer prevention, and health fairs.

- Communications made to describe your health-related products or services (or payment for such product or service) are not marketing. It is not marketing for a physician who has developed a new "anti-snore" device to send a flyer describing it to all of her patients (whether or not each patient has actually sought treatment for snoring). It is not marketing for an ophthalmologist to send existing patients discounts for eye exams or eyeglasses available only to the patients.

- Communications describing the entities participating in your health-care provider network is not marketing. So, it is not marketing for an independent physicians' association to send its patients a preferred provider list.

- It is not marketing for you to make a prescription refill reminder even if a third party pays for the communication. The prescription refill reminder is considered treatment. The communication is therefore excluded from the definition of marketing and does not require a prior authorization. Similarly, it is not marketing when a doctor or pharmacy is paid by a pharmaceutical company to recommend an alternative medication to patients. Communications about alternative treatments are excluded from the definition of marketing and do not require a prior authorization. The simple receipt of remuneration does not transform a treatment communication into a commercial promotion of a product or service.

- You may use a legitimate BA to assist in making permissible communications. For instance, if a pharmacist that has been paid by a third party contracts with a mail house to send out prescription refill reminders to the pharmacist's patients, neither the mail house nor the pharmacist needs a prior authorization. However, a CE would require an authorization if it sold PHI to a third party for the third party's marketing purposes.

- Appointment reminders are considered part of treatment of an individual and can be made without an authorization.

221

- Alternative treatments are treatments that are within the range of treatment options available to an individual and do not need authorization. For example, it would be an alternative treatment communication if a doctor, in response to an inquiry from a patient with skin rash about the range of treatment options, mails the patient a letter recommending that the patient purchase various ointments and medications described in brochures enclosed with the letter. Alternative treatment could also include alternative medicine. Alternative treatments include communications by a nurse-midwife who recommends or sells vitamins and herbal preparations, dietary and exercise programs, massage services, music, or other alternative types of therapy to her pregnant patients. Authorizations are not necessary for alternative treatment communications.

- Prior authorizations are not required when a doctor distributes promotional gifts of nominal value. You may distribute items commonly known as promotional gifts of nominal value without prior authorization, even if such items are distributed with the intent of encouraging the receiver to buy the products or services. This authorization exception generally applies to items and services of a third party, whether or not they are health-related, or items and services of the covered entity that are not health-related. A covered doctor, for instance, may send patients items such as pens, note pads, and cups embossed with a health plan's logo without prior authorization. Similarly, dentists may give patients free toothbrushes, floss, and toothpaste.

- You may give or discuss products or services, even when not health-related, with patients without a prior authorization in face-to-face encounters. This prevents unnecessary intrusion into the doctor–patient relationship. Physicians may give out free pharmaceutical samples, regardless of their value. Similarly, hospitals may give infant supplies to new mothers. Moreover, the face-to-face exception allows providers to leave general circulation materials in their offices for patients to pick up during office visits.

- You may use information regarding specific clinical conditions of individuals in order to communicate about products or services for these conditions without a prior authorization. If the communication is for the individual's treatment or for case management, care coordination, or the recommendation of alternative therapies, the Privacy Rule permits the use of clinical information to the extent it is reasonably necessary for these communications. Similarly, population-based activities in the areas of health education or disease prevention are not considered marketing when they promote health in a general manner. Again, clinical information may be used for such communications, such as in a public education campaign.

**Fundraising.** It is common practice within many healthcare providers to hold fundraisers to help purchase new equipment, facilities, etc. Fundraising for a provider's own benefit is defined to be part of healthcare operations. HIPAA provides restrictions on how PHI may be used for such fundraising purposes. The Privacy Rule expressly limits the PHI that can be used for fundraising to "demographic information relating to the individual" and "dates of health care provided to an individual" (45 CFR § 164.514(f)(1)). The regulations do not define "demographic information relating to the individual." However, the Preamble to the Final Privacy Rule provides explanation.

- PHI that can be utilized for fundraising purposes without obtaining a patient's authorization includes:
  - Date of service (45 CFR § 164.514(f)(1))
  - Demographic information (45 CFR § 164.514(f)(1) (as discussed in the Preamble to the 2000 Final Rule))
  - Name
  - Address
  - Other contact information (phone numbers, e-mail, etc.)
  - Age
  - Gender
  - Insurance status
- PHI that cannot be used without a patient first signing an authorization includes:
  - Diagnosis
  - Nature of services
  - Treatment
  - Location within the healthcare provider where patient receives treatment that identifies the treatment, such as:
    - Department of Psychiatry
    - Department of Obstetrics
    - Department of Radiation Oncology

Chapter 5 discusses fundraising in more detail.

## Chapter 16: Practical Checklist

- Post your complete NPP in a conspicuous location within your facilities.
- Establish procedures for making best effort attempts to obtain individuals' receipts of the notices.
- Establish safeguards to limit incidental disclosure of PHI within your facilities.
- Include appropriate safeguard requirements within BA contracts.
- Review your marketing and fundraising plans and determine what is allowed with and without authorization.

# Chapter 17
# Healthcare Clearinghouse Issues

**Background**

The issue of whether or not an entity is a healthcare clearinghouse has been the center of interesting debate. HIPAA defines a healthcare clearinghouse as:

> *a public or private entity... that does either of the following functions:*
>
> *(1) Processes or facilitates the processing of health information ... in a nonstandard format or containing nonstandard data content into standard data elements or a standard transaction.*
>
> *(2) Receives a standard transaction ... and processes or facilitates the processing of health information [in the standard transaction] into nonstandard format or nonstandard data content for the receiving entity.*

See 45 CFR 160.103 for the complete definition.

If your organization processes or facilitates the processing of health information from nonstandard format or content into standard format or content, or from standard format or content into nonstandard format or content, then you are likely a healthcare clearinghouse, and also a covered entity (CE) subject to HIPAA requirements. Unlike healthcare providers and plans, though, healthcare clearinghouses do not have to develop a Notice of Privacy Practices (NPP) if the only protected health information (PHI) they create or receive is as a business associate (BA) of another covered entity.

**Requirements**

First review the regulatory text that applies to healthcare clearinghouses to get a good feel for what you need to do. See 164.500(b)(1) within the HIPAA regulatory text. To summarize, healthcare clearinghouses must comply with the following HIPAA requirements:

---

The information and opinions provided in this book do not constitute or substitute for legal or other professional advice.

- *Section 164.500 relating to applicability:* When healthcare clearinghouses are business associates to another covered entity, they may use and disclose PHI only as allowed by their BA agreement. When a healthcare clearinghouse functions as a covered entity, then it must abide by all the applicable HIPAA requirements for covered entities.
- *Section 164.501 relating to definitions:* The definitions made within the HIPAA regulations apply to all healthcare clearinghouses.
- *Section 164.502 relating to uses and disclosures of PHI:* Except that a clearinghouse is prohibited from using or disclosing protected health information other than as permitted in the business associate contract under which it created or received the PHI. Chapter 3 details the uses and disclosures requirements in detail.
- *Section 164.504 relating to the organizational requirements for covered entities:* Including the designation of healthcare components of a covered entity, apply to healthcare clearinghouses. See Chapter 5 for details.
- *Section 164.512 relating to uses and disclosures for which individual authorization or an opportunity to agree or object is not required:* Except that a clearinghouse is prohibited from using or disclosing PHI other than as permitted in the business associate contract under which it created or received the PHI. This issue is discussed within Chapter 5.
- *Section 164.532 relating to transition requirements:* This will be of most significance with regard to BA agreements. Such BA agreements, if they do not meet HIPAA requirements, must generally be updated to be compliant by April 14, 2003 (or April 14, 2004, if the contract is with a small plan).
- *Section 164.534 relating to compliance dates for initial implementation of the privacy standards:* Healthcare clearinghouses must be compliant by April 14, 2003, with regard to being a covered entity. If a healthcare clearinghouse is considered a BA, it must be compliant with agreement revisions as indicated in the previous item.

Please be sure to discuss all these issues with your legal counsel. As we emphasize throughout this book, each organization has its own unique characteristics and business environment. You must determine what is applicable for your specific situation.

**Transactions**

HIPAA establishes requirements for processing financial electronic data interchange (EDI) transactions using uniform electronic standards. Although this is not the focus of this book, it is an important issue and helps demonstrate why healthcare clearinghouses are covered entities and subject to Privacy Rule and Security Rule requirements. Because healthcare clearinghouses must edit electronic transactions according to HIPAA requirements, they must edit down to the data element level, which will involve accessing PHI, and also ensure all the medical codes are current and correct.

Clearinghouses and EDI translators may sometimes encounter transactions with missing information. Most of this missing information will need to be supplied by the underlying business applications that are generating the transaction information. This type of access and manipulation of information is another driver for making clearinghouses HIPAA-covered entities. These issues must be addressed within the BA agreements.

Network security requirements will also vary between a clearinghouse's information-trading partners, and also between the various communications systems used. The Security Rule does not specify technology platforms, but focuses on the security issues and requirements for the exchange of PHI. The resulting disadvantage to clearinghouses is that each information-trading partner may be using a different system or technology. Healthcare clearinghouses may need to ensure Security Rule compliance for multiple systems and security solutions and technologies. This will likely require clearinghouses to invest money, knowledge, and people to achieve and maintain compliance.

If possible, you can minimize your healthcare clearinghouse's associated compliance resources and costs by using only one network security solution for your EDI network regardless of your business associate relationship technologies. The key will be to ensure your systems are as compatible as possible with your EDI trading partners, and also have your trading partners make changes in their systems as well. Because they are also impacted by the HIPAA requirements, chances are they are going to be making changes within their systems anyway.

## Financial Institutions

A critical consideration for banks is determining what payment-processing activities qualify as covered entity and business associate activities under HIPAA. If you look at the literal interpretation of the HIPAA definition of a healthcare clearinghouse, then it would seem it does cover financial institutions. In the normal course of business, many financial institutions may receive:

- Payment instruction from a HIPAA-covered entity, such as a healthcare provider or insurance company, and will need to send ACH transactions with addenda in a HIPAA-compliant format
- ACH transactions with addenda in a HIPAA-compliant format and will pass this information on to a covered entity after editing to a human-readable or other useable form

Banks and other financial institutions processing payments need to examine their payment processing activities closely to determine if they are, in fact, covered entities. Many financial institutions may originate or receive HIPAA standard transactions (such as the Healthcare Claim Payment (835) and Premium Payment (820)), but they often will pass on the data without doing any conversions or reformatting. Even though these messages may be HIPAA transactions, the financial institution would not necessarily be considered a business associate. There are some financial institutions, however, that provide value-added services for their healthcare customers that would then qualify them as a healthcare clearinghouse. For example, some health plans and providers may use financial institutions for support services to translate or edit files to meet the HIPAA criteria for electronic transactions. Some financial institutions may also translate specific transactions or addenda from nonstandard to HIPAA-compliant formats when requested by customers. In these situations, they will likely need to comply with the HIPAA Privacy Rule and Security Rule in addition to the other HIPAA rules.

If they are not covered entities, financial institutions may very well be business associates to covered entities if they process PHI for their customers. In this scenario they will be subject to the security and privacy provisions of HIPAA as they relate to business associate agreements. To complicate matters, these HIPAA requirements may conflict with federal banking laws. The American Banking Association (ABA) and the Electronic Payments Association, NACHA, are working to clarify these issues with the Department of Health and Human Services (HHS). To obtain further information about this issue, a good site to visit is www.hipaabanking.org. Accreditation by the Electronic Healthcare Network Accreditation Commission (EHNAC) is recommended.

**Conclusion**

Healthcare clearinghouses will be either covered entities, business associates, or both. As such, all healthcare clearinghouses must understand and take actions to comply with HIPAA requirements. Financial institutions that qualify as healthcare clearinghouses will generally be well positioned to meet the confidentiality requirements of HIPAA as a result of already taking actions to comply with the privacy and information security requirements imposed by the Gramm–Leach–Bliley Act (GLBA). Privacy practices notices for organizations that are covered by both HIPAA and GLBA will likely need to be revised to incorporate:

- Standard language for confidentiality assurances that is acceptable to financial institutions as well as the HIPAA requirements
- Definitions of the financial institution's HIPAA responsibilities to maintain records of and log access to the PHI using procedures that will likely be new within their organizations

## Chapter 17: Practical Checklist

- Determine if you are considered a healthcare clearinghouse.
- Determine if you are considered a business associate.
- Designate security and privacy officers and document your security and privacy responsibilities.
- Perform a security risk assessment to determine your baseline security condition.
- Ensure that Internet and external network connections are protected.
- Review, revise as necessary, and periodically update security and privacy policies to meet HIPAA requirements.
- Review and update as necessary existing business associate agreements.
- Inventory your PHI use and disclosure.
- Provide privacy and security training for your personnel.
- Ensure that you only disclose PHI as required in BA agreements as they apply to the healthcare clearinghouse components of your organization.

# Chapter 18
# Health Plan Issues

**What Is a Health Plan?**

The term "health plan" refers to an individual or group plan that provides or pays the cost of medical care. These include amounts paid for:

1. Diagnosis, cure, mitigation, treatment, or prevention of disease, or amounts paid for the purpose of affecting any structure or function of the body
2. Amounts paid for transportation primarily for and essential to medical care referred to in item 1
3. Amounts paid for insurance covering medical care referred to in items 1 and 2

See Title 42 U.S.C. 300gg-91(a)(2) for full details of health plan medical care costs.

A health plan, as defined in the Public Health Service Act, includes any combination of the following:

- A group health plan (as defined in Section 2791(a) of the Public Health Service Act), if the plan:
  - Has 50 or more participants (as defined in Section 3(7) of the Employee Retirement Income Security Act of 1974); or
  - Is administered by an entity other than the employer who established and maintains the plan
- A health insurance issuer (as defined in Section 2791(b) of the Public Health Service Act)
- A health maintenance organization (as defined in Section 2791(b) of the Public Health Service Act)
- Part A or part B of the Medicare program under Title XVIII
- The Medicaid program under Title XIX
- A Medicare supplemental policy (as defined in Section 1882(g)(1))
- A long-term care policy, including a nursing home fixed indemnity policy (unless the Secretary of the Department of Health and Human Services (HHS) determines that such a policy does not provide

sufficiently comprehensive coverage of a benefit so that the policy should be treated as a health plan)

- An employee welfare benefit plan or any other arrangement that is established or maintained for the purpose of offering or providing health benefits to the employees of two or more employers
- The healthcare program for active military personnel under Title 10, United States Code
- The veterans' healthcare program under Chapter 17 of Title 38, United States Code
- The Civilian Health and Medical Program of the Uniformed Services (CHAMPUS), as defined in Section 1072(4) of Title 10, United States Code
- The Indian Health Service Program under the Indian Healthcare Improvement Act (25 U.S.C. 1601 et seq.)
- The Federal Employees Health Benefit Plan under Chapter 89 of Title 5, United States Code

45 CFR 144.103 defines a "group health plan" as the following:

*Group health plan means an employee welfare benefit plan (as defined in Section 3(1) of ERISA) to the extent that the plan provides medical care (as defined in Section 2791(a)(2) of the PHS Act and including items and services paid for as medical care) to employees or their dependents (as defined under the terms of the plan) directly or through insurance, reimbursement, or otherwise. For more information on what constitutes a group health plan, see our November 2000 Bulletin No. 00-06, Circumstances Under Which Health Insurance Regulated as Individual Coverage Under State Law is Subject to the Group Market Requirements of the Health Insurance Portability and Accountability Act of 1996.*

Government-funded health plans include:

- Medicare program under Title XVIII of the Social Security Act (Parts A, B, and C) (42 U.S.C. 1395, et seq.)
- Medicaid program under Title XIX of the Social Security Act (42 U.S.C. 1396, et seq.)
- Healthcare program for active military personnel (10 U.S.C. 1074, et seq.)
- Veterans' healthcare program (38 U.S.C. Chapter 17)
- Civilian Health and Medical Program of the Uniformed Services (CHAMPUS) (10 U.S.C. 1061, et seq.)
- Indian Health Service program under the Indian Healthcare Improvement Act (25 U.S.C. 1601)
- Federal Employees Health Benefit Program (5 U.S.C. Ch. 89)
- Approved state child health programs under Title XXI of the Social Security Act (42 U.S.C. 1397, et seq.) (SCHIP)

A third-party administrator (TPA) to a group health plan is not a covered entity (CE) based on TPA activities. A TPA of a group health plan is a business associate (BA) of the group health plan. It is possible that a TPA may meet the definition of a CE based on its other activities; for example, if it also provides group health insurance.

## What Is a Small Health Plan?

HIPAA defines a small health plan as one that has annual receipts of $5 million or less. Health plans should use the guidance provided by the Small Business Administration at 13 CFR 121.104 to calculate their annual receipts. Health plans that do not report receipts to the IRS (for example, ERISA group health plans that are exempt from filing income tax returns) should use proxy measures to determine their annual receipts. Small health plans have an additional year to comply with the Privacy Rule. This deadline is April 14, 2004. For additional information about the provisions of 13 CFR 121.104 and proxy measures related to "small health plans," see http://cms.hhs.gov/hipaa/hipaa2/default.asp.

## Health Plan Requirements

The Privacy Rule regulatory text has some very specific requirements for health plans as indicated in the following excerpts.

### § 164.504(f)(1)(i)

(1) Standard: requirements for group health plans.

   (i) Except as provided under paragraph (f)(1)(ii) or (iii) of this section or as otherwise authorized under Sec. 164.508, a group health plan, in order to disclose PHI to the plan sponsor or to provide for or permit the disclosure of PHI to the plan sponsor by a health insurance issuer or HMO with respect to the group health plan, must ensure that the plan documents restrict uses and disclosures of such information by the plan sponsor consistent with the requirements of this sub-part.

   (ii) The group health plan, or a health insurance issuer or HMO with respect to the group health plan, may disclose summary health information to the plan sponsor, if the plan sponsor requests the summary health information for the purpose of:

      (A) Obtaining premium bids from health plans for providing health insurance coverage under the group health plan; or

      (B) Modifying, amending, or terminating the group health plan.

   (iii) The group health plan, or a health insurance issuer or HMO with respect to the group health plan, may disclose to the plan sponsor information on whether the individual is participating in the group health plan, or is enrolled in or has disenrolled from a health insurance issuer or HMO offered by the plan.

*§ 164.504(f)(2)*

(2) *Implementation specifications: requirements for plan documents.* The plan documents of the group health plan must be amended to incorporate provisions to:

(i) Establish the permitted and required uses and disclosures of such information by the plan sponsor, provided that such permitted and required uses and disclosures may not be inconsistent with this sub-part.

(ii) Provide that the group health plan will disclose PHI to the plan sponsor only upon receipt of a certification by the plan sponsor that the plan documents have been amended to incorporate the following provisions and that the plan sponsor agrees to:

(A) Not use or further disclose the information other than as permitted or required by the plan documents or as required by law;

(B) Ensure that any agents, including a subcontractor, to whom it provides PHI received from the group health plan agree to the same restrictions and conditions that apply to the plan sponsor with respect to such information;

(C) Not use or disclose the information for employment-related actions and decisions or in connection with any other benefit or employee benefit plan of the plan sponsor;

(D) Report to the group health plan any use or disclosure of the information that is inconsistent with the uses or disclosures provided for of which it becomes aware;

(E) Make available PHI in accordance with § 164.524;

(F) Make available PHI for amendment and incorporate any amendments to PHI in accordance with § 164.526;

(G) Make available the information required to provide an accounting of disclosures in accordance with § 164.528;

(H) Make its internal practices, books, and records relating to the use and disclosure of PHI received from the group health plan available to the Secretary for purposes of determining compliance by the group health plan with this sub-part;

(I) If feasible, return or destroy all PHI received from the group health plan that the sponsor still maintains in any form and retain no copies of such information when no longer needed for the purpose for which disclosure was made, except that, if such return or destruction is not feasible, limit further uses and disclosures to those purposes that make the return or destruction of the information infeasible; and

(J) Ensure that the adequate separation required in paragraph (f)(2)(iii) of this section (§ 164.504(f)(2)) is established.

**§ 164.504(f)(3)(iii)**

(3) *Implementation specifications: uses and disclosures.* A group health plan may:

    (i) Disclose protected health information to a plan sponsor to carry out plan administration functions that the plan sponsor performs only consistent with the provisions of paragraph (f)(2) of this section;

    (ii) Not permit a health insurance issuer or HMO with respect to the group health plan to disclose protected health information to the plan sponsor except as permitted by this paragraph;

    (iii) Not disclose and may not permit a health insurance issuer or HMO to disclose protected health information to a plan sponsor as otherwise permitted by this paragraph unless a statement required by § 164.520(b)(1)(iii)(C) is included in the appropriate notice; and

    (iv) Not disclose protected health information to the plan sponsor for the purpose of employment-related actions or decisions or in connection with any other benefit or employee benefit plan of the plan sponsor.

## Marketing Issues

Health plans depend heavily on their marketing activities to create revenue. So for most if not all health plans, the HIPAA Privacy Rule marketing requirements will have a huge impact on their organizations. It is important for health plans to thoroughly review and follow the HIPAA requirements for marketing. CEs generally cannot market health-related products and services without authorization from the patient. Health plans need to review and assess their marketing plans to determine if current marketing activities or plans are in compliance with the HIPAA Privacy Rule. Chapter 5 discusses marketing issues in more detail.

### A Health Plan Marketing Checklist

- A CE can share PHI with a telemarketer only if the CE has either obtained the individual's prior written authorization to do so, or has entered into a BA relationship with the telemarketer for the purpose of making a communication that is not marketing, such as to inform individuals about the CE's own goods or services.

- The HIPAA Privacy Rule expressly requires an authorization for uses or disclosures of PHI for *all* marketing communications, except in two circumstances: (1) when the communication occurs in a face-to-face encounter between the CE and the individual, and (2) when the communication involves a promotional gift of nominal value.

- Generally, disease management, health promotion, preventive care, and wellness programs do not fall under the HIPAA Privacy Rule definition of marketing.

- It is not marketing for a CE to describe products or services that are provided by the CE to its patients, or to describe products or services that are included in the health plan's plan of benefits to members of the health plan.

- It is not marketing for a CE to describe the entities participating in a healthcare provider network or a health plan network.

- It is not marketing for an insurance plan or health plan to send enrollees notices about changes, replacements, or improvements to existing plans.

- Health plans can communicate about health-related products or services to enrollees that add value to, but are not part of, a plan of benefits.

- Prior authorizations are not required when a doctor or health plan distributes promotional gifts of nominal value.

- Insurance agents who are BAs of a health plan do not need to seek a prior authorization before talking to a customer in a face-to-face encounter about the insurance company's other lines of business.

- Nothing in the marketing provisions of the Privacy Rule can be considered as amending, modifying, or changing any rule or require-ment related to any other Federal or State statutes or regulations, including specifically antikickback, fraud, and abuse, or self-referral statutes or regulations, or to authorize or permit any activity or transaction currently proscribed by such statutes and regulations.

**Notice of Privacy Practices**

Health plans needed to provide a Notice of Privacy Practices (NPP) to individuals covered by the plan no later than April 14, 2003 (April 14, 2004, for small health plans), and must provide an NPP to new enrollees at the time of enrollment. Health plans must also provide a revised notice to indi-viduals then covered by the plan within 60 days of a material revision, and they must notify individuals then covered by the plan of the availability of the privacy practices notice, and how to obtain the notice at least once every 3 years.

The Privacy Rule does not require a group health plan to provide an NPP if it provides benefits only through one or more contracts of insurance with health insurance issuers or HMOs, and if it does not create or receive PHI other than summary health information or enrollment or disenrollment information.

### *A Health Plan Notice of Privacy Practices Checklist*

- A health plan may e-mail the notice to an individual if the individual agrees to receive an electronic notice (see 45 CFR 164.520(c) for the specific requirements for providing the notice).
- A health plan may develop more than one notice, such as when an entity performs different types of covered functions (i.e., the functions that make it a health plan, a healthcare provider, or a healthcare clearinghouse) and there are variations in its privacy practices among these covered functions.
- A health plan must have provided the NPP to individuals covered by the plan no later than April 14, 2003 (April 14, 2004, for small health plans), and must give the NPP to new enrollees at the time of enrollment.
- A health plan must provide a revised notice to individuals then covered by the plan within 60 days of a material revision.
- A health plan must notify individuals covered by the plan of the availability of the NPP and information about how to obtain the notice at least once every 3 years.
- Health plans are not required to make a good-faith effort to obtain a written acknowledgment of the receipt of the notice from their enrollees.
- A health plan does not have to provide a copy of its notice to each dependent receiving coverage under a policy.
- A health plan must send its notice to each individual covered by the plan. A health plan can send the notice to the administrator of the group product or the plan sponsor for them to distribute to employees enrolled in the plan. However, if the other person or entity fails to distribute the notice to the plan's enrollees, the health plan may be in violation of the Privacy Rule.

### Types of Insurance Plans Excluded from HIPAA

The following types of insurance generally are not considered health plans covered under HIPAA regulations:

- Long-term disability
- Short-term disability
- Workers' compensation
- Automobile liability that includes coverage for medical payments

HIPAA specifically excludes from the definition of a "health plan" any policy, plan, or program to the extent that it provides, or pays for the cost of excepted benefits, which are listed in Section 2791(c)(1) of the Public Health Service Act, 42 U.S.C. 300gg-91(c)(1). See 45 CFR 160.103 for more details and direction about the type of insurance covered by HIPAA.

## Communications

A healthcare provider may disclose PHI to a health plan for the plan's Health Plan Employer Data and Information Set (HEDIS). The Privacy Rule allows a provider to disclose PHI to a health plan for the quality-related healthcare operations of the health plan, provided the health plan has or had a relationship with the individual who is the subject of the information, and the PHI requested pertains to the relationship.

## Government and Law Enforcement

### Government Departments

State, county, and local health departments are required to comply with the Privacy Rule if the applicable department performs functions that make it a CE. For example, under the Privacy Rule a state Medicaid program is a CE (a health plan). Health departments that operate healthcare clinics are healthcare providers. If these healthcare providers transmit health information electronically in connection with a transaction covered in the HIPAA Transactions Rule, they are CEs. For more information, see the definitions of CE, healthcare provider, health plan, and healthcare clearinghouse in 45 CFR 160.103. There are also helpful "CE Decision Tools" at http://www.cms.gov/hipaa/hipaa2/support/tools/decisionsupport/default.asp to help determine whether a person, business, or agency is a covered healthcare provider, healthcare clearinghouse, or health plan. If the health department performs some covered functions and other non-covered functions, it should designate those components that perform covered functions as the healthcare component(s) of the organization. They will then be considered a hybrid entity.

### Government Enforcement

HHS is responsible for investigating complaints that the Privacy Rule has been violated and to look into other information related to noncompliance. This will sometimes require reviewing PHI, such as situations in which individuals report that they believe a CE has handled their medical records improperly. The information to which they will need access will depend on the circumstances and associated allegations. The Privacy Rule limits the Office for Civil Rights' (OCR) access to only the information necessary to determine compliance. There may be situations where no PHI is needed. Examples of investigations where the OCR may need access to PHI include:

- Accusations that a CE did not appropriately respond to a request to correct a patient's medical record
- Accusations that a CE inappropriately used health information for marketing without first obtaining authorization as required by the Privacy Rule

### Debt Collection Agencies

The Privacy Rule allows CEs to use the services of debt collection agencies. Debt collection is recognized as a payment activity within the HIPAA definition of "payment" at 45 CFR 164.501. A CE may use a debt collection agency through a BA arrangement. Disclosures to collection agencies must occur as directed by the other Privacy Rule requirements, including the BA and minimum necessary requirements.

### Law Enforcement

The Privacy Rule does not expand current law enforcement access to PHI. HHS had stated that in its opinion the Privacy Rule limits access to law enforcement to a greater degree than currently exists with the establishment of new procedures and safeguards that limit the situation under which a CE may give such information to law enforcement officers. The Privacy Rule limits the type of information that CEs may disclose to law enforcement without a warrant or similar document. For example, it specifically prohibits disclosure of DNA information without a warrant or similar approval. The Privacy Rule requires CEs to obtain permission from persons who have been the victim of domestic violence or abuse in most circumstances before disclosing the information to law enforcement. Most state laws do not currently require this type of permission. When state laws impose additional restrictions on the disclosure of health information to law enforcement, those state laws continue to apply. Even when the Privacy Rule allows disclosure to law enforcement, the rule does not require the CEs to disclose any information. Other federal or state laws may require such a disclosure, and in these cases the Privacy Rule does not take precedence over these other laws. CEs should use their best professional and ethical judgment to determine whether to disclose information. Their decisions should mirror their organization's policies and ethical principles.

### Multi-State Issues

A large number of health insurance and managed care organizations have members in more than one state. Chapter 8 explores the state preemption issues in detail. There are also implementation considerations for such organizations. If you are such an organization, following your state preemption analysis, you need to create or update your policies and procedures to comply with HIPAA and state laws based on the analysis results.

This sounds easy, right? Well, it can really be quite a complicated activity, especially for health plans that sell multiple products in multiple markets across multiple states. Some actions you should take include:

- Identify the situations within the course of your business in which you are considered a CE. You may actually be a BA in some situations; identify these situations as well.

- Identify the federal and state agencies regulating your services and products in all your jurisdictions. A preemptive analysis will be necessary for some regulatory agencies, but may not be necessary for others.

- Determine how to combine all applicable state and federal requirements into your policies, procedures, and other relevant documents.

The most common definition applicable for health insurers and managed care companies within the regulatory text is "covered entity, health plan." There are situations when a health insurer or managed care organization is not a "covered entity, health plan." If your organization is acting with a self-insured group health plan, you are not considered a CE; you are a BA of the group health plan.

However, if you sell an insured product to the employer, you may then become a "covered entity, health plan." So, in this case you would be both a CE and a noncovered entity to the same customer, depending on whether you assume insurance on some product lines. You must identify your customers and your products for which you must meet all HIPAA requirements as a CE health plan in addition to identifying when you have BA relationships to know how to comply with the laws.

Probably the most difficult activity for a multi-state CE health plan is incorporating state requirements into your policies and procedures. It is not always feasible to create policies and procedures that will be applicable across all states. In these situations you will likely need to create not only multiple policies and procedures, but also multiple forms and letters to cover the same issues.

For instance, right of access to PHI can vary greatly between states and agencies, starting with the definition of health information. The HIPAA definition of PHI usually allows individuals access to more types of information than state definitions of health information. However, some states use the definition found in the National Association of Insurance Commissioners' Insurance Information and Privacy Protection Model Act (http://www.naic.org/privacy/naic_privacy_publications.htm). This model act also requires an accounting of disclosures along with information in response to information access requests.

Attention to privacy issues is increasing. It is likely health plans will receive more questions from consumers related to privacy, and could very well experience increased regulatory reviews, fines, and litigation. Because of the huge penalties and consequences, health plans must perform rigorous analysis, provide sufficient training, and create comprehensive policies and procedures.

## Chapter 18: Practical Checklist

- Determine if you are considered a health plan.
- See the HHS Web site (http://www.hhs.gov/ocr/hipaa/guidelines/marketing.pdf) for detailed information about marketing and HIPAA.
- Generally, disease management, health promotion, preventive care, and wellness programs are not considered marketing.
- Determine if you should create more than one NPP.
- Health plans do not need to obtain a written acknowledgment of NPP receipt.
- Identify all state and federal PHI related requirements and incorporate them into your policies and procedures.

# Chapter 19
# Employer Issues

## Background

HIPAA requirements are applicable to group health plans and issuers. In most cases, if you offer a group health plan to your employees, the health plan must comply with all HIPAA requirements. Eligibility for health plan enrollment is determined according to the terms of the health plan and the rules of the issuer, but not according to an individual's health status or that of an individual's dependent. These rules and terms must comply with all applicable state laws. This chapter examines some of the common issues related to employers and HIPAA, focusing on the security and privacy issues. Because each organization is unique, you should consult with your organization's legal counsel to determine exactly how the regulations will apply to you. However, the information here can provide a good background for your meeting with legal counsel, in addition to helping you identify topics to discuss and address prior to the meeting.

A large percentage of employers believe that HIPAA does not apply to them if they do not sell health insurance or do not provide medical care and treatment. Many employers would be surprised or alarmed to learn how HIPAA can and likely will impact their operations. Employers must determine the nature of their relationship with their employee benefit plans, their use of protected health information (PHI), and how their activities must be modified to comply with HIPAA.

The Privacy Rule will apply to you indirectly as an employer or welfare benefit sponsor. The Privacy Rule will apply directly to you as a group health plan (as defined in the Employee Retirement Income Security Act, ERISA) or a health plan (as defined in HIPAA). The only ERISA plans that are exempt are those self-administered with fewer than 50 participants. Most ERISA plans and multi-employer plans are covered entities (CEs) under the rule. The regulation also makes it applicable to "any other individual or group plan or combination of individual or group plans that provides or pays for the cost of medical care."

Most employers researching their health information uses and disclosures will discover they receive health information in ways other than

---

through the health plan. For instance, health information is received through:

- Workers' compensation
- Short-term disability/Long-term disability (STD/LTD)
- Americans with Disabilities Act (ADA)
- Family Medical Leave Act (FMLA)
- Life insurance
- Long-term care
- Retiree coverage (for example, Medigap, M+C)
- Group health plan or preemployment physicals
- Federal and state drug testing

Because health information in these situations was not created or received by the group health plan, its use is not a HIPAA issue for the employer. However, there may be other applicable federal or state laws covering the information, in addition to established company policies. With specific regard to HIPAA, this health information is not considered individually identifiable health information (IIHI) or PHI for the employer. However, the provider may still need an authorization to release it. These other laws typically restrict distribution of employee health information as well as limit how employers can use such information to make employment decisions. HIPAA imposes additional requirements on all employers who sponsor employee health plans. Employers who are also CEs will be impacted in basically three major areas:

1. Organizational
2. Notice Requirements
3. Use and Disclosure Requirements

Laws that also impact the use of health information include, but are not necessarily limited to:

- Employee Retirement Income Security Act (ERISA)
- Americans with Disabilities Act (ADA)
- Federal Substance Abuse Confidentiality Requirements
- Gramm–Leach–Bliley Act (GLBA)
- Freedom of Information Act (FOIA)
- Family Educational Rights and Privacy Act
- Family Medical Leave Act (FMLA)
- European Union (EU) Data Protection Directive
- Canada's Personal Information Protection and Electronic Documents Act (PIPEDA)

### "Small" and "Large" Employers

HIPAA defines a small employer as a company (or a nonfederal government employer) that has at least two but no more than 50 employees. Be aware that some states consider a business with only one employee a small employer. A large employer is defined as an organization (or a nonfederal governmental employer) that has at least 51 employees. Some HIPAA requirements apply only to large employers.

### Small Employer Issues

HIPAA marketing rules apply to every employer group health plan that has at least two participants. HIPAA also guarantees access to health coverage for small employers. And for the most part, no insurer can exclude a worker or family member from employer-sponsored coverage based on health status. Effective July 1, 1997, insurers were required to renew coverage to all groups, regardless of the health status of any member.

Your insurer should handle the HIPAA information collection activities for you when you purchase group health insurance coverage. Be sure to discuss this with your insurer to work out the HIPAA process-related issues together. If you are self-insured, you are already performing a significant amount of insurance management and should have the systems in place for executing your self-insurance. Incorporating the HIPAA requirements will be an addition to the processes you are already doing.

### Health Benefits

Most employers now offer their employees wellness programs, on-site clinics, employee assistance programs, and similar health-related benefits. Employers are generally not considered CEs under HIPAA definitions. However, employers qualify as CEs when they sponsor healthcare components such as self-insured health plans, wellness programs, on-site clinics, or employee assistance programs. The Privacy Rule impacts the use and disclosure of PHI by the healthcare component of the employer and the applicable personnel, and requires the establishment of "firewalls," or procedural and operational separations, to keep health-related functions separate from general, employment-related functions and personnel.

### Enforcement and Penalties

States have the primary enforcement responsibility for the group and individual requirements imposed on health insurance issuers using sanctions available under the applicable state laws. If states do not take appropriate actions for their areas of responsibility, the Secretary of the Department of Health and Human Services (HHS) may determine they have failed to enforce the law, and then apply federal enforcement authority. This can result in sanctions on insurers as specified in HIPAA, as well as civil monetary penalties.

The Secretary of HHS is responsible for enforcing nonfederal governmental plans, self-funded, and insured plans. HHS can impose sanctions on plans or plan sponsors as outlined within HIPAA, including civil monetary penalties. Additionally, the Secretary of Labor enforces requirements on employment-based group health plans, including self-insured arrangements under ERISA. Individual employees can file suit to enforce ERISA.

Besides the indicated penalties and sanctions possible from HHS, the Secretary of Labor, and the states, the Secretary of the Treasury can impose tax penalties on employers or plans that are not compliant with HIPAA. The tax code obligates the employer or plan to pay the excise tax whether or not the Secretary of the Treasury has taken any enforcement action.

## Organizational Requirements

### *Employer Obligations as CEs*

As plan sponsors or plan fiduciaries, most employers need to implement the HIPAA requirements on behalf of their covered benefit plans, or ensure that the insurance provider implements the HIPAA requirements. These covered plans were required to comply with the HIPAA standard transactions by October 16, 2002 (October 16, 2003, for small health plans). If the large health plans could not make this date, they needed to file a request and a compliance plan with HHS before October 16, 2002, to obtain a 1-year extension. Small plans did not have an extension option. For the Privacy Rule, plans must develop policies, procedures, and systems to address appropriate uses and disclosures of PHI. Plans must develop procedures to ensure that only those personnel with a need to know, use, or access PHI can to comply with the minimum necessary requirements. The Privacy Rule does not apply to uses and disclosures of PHI made in accordance with individual authorizations.

Hybrid entities have components that fall under HIPAA. In general, a hybrid entity (such as a corporation) is one that qualifies as a CE, but whose covered functions are not the primary functions of the organization. For example, an employer in a nonhealth-related industry that self-administers a sponsored health plan is a hybrid entity, as is an employer that has an on-site medical clinic. (See Chapter 1 for more information about hybrid entities.) The Privacy Rule impacts hybrid entities as it applies only to the covered activities. Within hybrid entities there must be operational and procedural "firewall" separations between the healthcare components and the other components. The transfer of PHI from the healthcare component to another area of the organization is considered a disclosure under the Privacy Rule.

See the full details of CE obligations in the other applicable chapters of this book. At a high level, HIPAA requires employers acting as CEs to:

- Amend health plan documents, such as ERISA-mandated summary plan descriptions, to include many specific privacy provisions when the employer, as a health plan sponsor, receives health information beyond that needed to enroll and disenroll participants.

- Negotiate or revise written contracts with third-party administrators, insurers, HMOs, case managers, disease managers, utilization review and other managed care vendors, and other business associates (BAs). These contracts must include many specific privacy provisions.
- Appoint a privacy officer responsible for enterprise privacy issues, employee HIPAA and PHI training and awareness, and ensuring the implementation of privacy policies, practices, and procedures.
- Establish procedures for participants to inspect and copy their PHI, amend their records, and receive an accounting of all covered disclosures of their PHI.
- Implement procedures to resolve PHI-related complaints and grievances.
- Obtain authorization from each participant whose PHI will be used for any purpose other than treatment, payment, and operations (TPO).
- Separate health plan administration where PHI is used or disclosed from another organizational function, including the administration of other ERISA benefit plans.

### Employer Obligations as Plan Sponsors

Plan sponsors must comply with several HIPAA requirements related to how PHI is handled and how health plan documents must be amended. Employers who are plan sponsors must assess how their organization handles employee healthcare information, determine who needs access to this information, and determine if the information gathered by the employer qualifies as PHI according to HIPAA. Plan sponsors typically do not need to sign BA agreements.

Most employers need access to the PHI in their plans, particularly for settlement purposes. HHS has indicated that it believes most employers are probably holding or gathering PHI, which in turn likely makes them subject to the HIPAA plan sponsor requirements. As a result, most employers that act as plan sponsors need to comply with the HIPAA plan sponsor requirements. Employers that are plan sponsors, with plans that qualify as group health plans, and employers that acquire PHI from the covered plans need to address HIPAA requirements. These employers need to amend group health plan documents, agree to comply with these documents, and implement necessary safeguards. A group health plan must include provisions within the plan documents to establish the allowed and required PHI uses and disclosures before PHI can be disclosed to the sponsor.

### Employer Organizational Requirements

Employers falling under one or both of the aforementioned descriptions will need to do the following to address these HIPAA requirements:

- Amend employee sanctions and disciplinary policies
- Communicate the employee HIPAA obligations
- Apply disciplinary actions for improper use and disclosure of PHI
- Confirm employee awareness and understanding of HIPAA policy
- Appoint a privacy official
- Develop complaint processes and sanctions
- Implement personnel training and awareness programs
- Establish a plan to comply with the minimum necessary requirement
- Implement physical, administrative, and technical safeguards for PHI
- Establish a minimum 6-year records retention policy
- Implement procedures to ensure beneficiary rights
- Ensure the covered plan participants receive the Notice of Privacy Practices (NPP)
- Obtain authorizations as applicable to HIPAA requirements

HIPAA requirements exemption may be available to group health plans that provide benefits only through insurance or HMO coverage, or who do not create or receive PHI except in summary form, and for premium and plan settlement purposes. Be sure to discuss this issue thoroughly with your organization's legal counsel; each situation is unique to the organization.

### Health Information

Employer health plan sponsors are typically allowed to have access under HIPAA to summary health information. Summary health information:

- Summarizes the claims history, claims expenses, or type of claims experienced by individuals for whom a plan sponsor has provided health benefits under a group health plan
- De-identifies information by removing the following elements:
  - Names
  - All geographic subdivisions smaller than a state, including street address, city, county, precinct, zip code, and their equivalent geocodes (an exception is geographic information that can be aggregated to the level of a five-digit zip code)
  - All elements of dates (except year) directly related to an individual, including birth date, admission date, discharge date, and date of death, and all ages over 89 and all elements of dates (including year) indicative of such age, except that such ages and elements may be aggregated into a single category of age 90 or older

- Telephone numbers
- Fax numbers
- E-mail addresses
- Social Security numbers
- Medical records numbers
- Health plan beneficiary numbers
- Account numbers
- Certificate/license numbers
- Vehicle identifiers and serial numbers, including license plate numbers
- Device identifiers and serial numbers
- Web Universal Resource Locators (URLs)
- Internet Protocol (IP) address numbers
- Biometric identifiers, including finger and voice prints
- Full-face photographic images and any comparable images
- Any other unique identifying number, characteristic, or code

## Medical Surveillance

A covered healthcare provider who provides healthcare to an individual at the request of the individual's employer, or provides the service in the capacity of a member of the employer's workforce, may disclose the individual's PHI to the employer:

- For the purposes of workplace medical surveillance
- For the evaluation of work-related illness and injuries when needed by the employer to comply with OSHA, the Mine Safety and Health Administration (MSHA), or the requirements of state laws having a similar purpose

The PHI given to the employer must be limited to the provider's findings regarding the medical surveillance or work-related illness or injury. The provider must give the individual written notice that the information will be disclosed to his or her employer, or the notice may be posted at the worksite if that is where the service is provided. See 45 CFR 164.512(b)(1)(v) for regulatory text.

## Workers' Compensation

The HIPAA Privacy Rule does not apply to entities that are workers' compensation insurers, workers' compensation administrative agencies, or employers, except if they are otherwise CEs. Nonetheless, these entities need access to the health information of individuals who are injured on the job or who have a work-related illness to process or settle claims, and to coordinate care under the workers' compensation systems. This PHI is typically obtained from healthcare providers who treat these individuals and whom the Privacy Rule may cover. Because of the significant number of state and other applicable laws relating to this topic, the Privacy Rule permits PHI disclosures for workers' compensation purposes in a number of different ways. Disclosures that do not require individual authorization by HIPAA generally include the following:

- As necessary to comply with laws relating to workers' compensation or similar programs established by law that provide benefits for work-related injuries or illness without regard to fault
- To the extent state and other applicable laws require the disclosure
- To obtain payment for any healthcare provided to the injured or ill worker

Covered entities must limit the amount of PHI they disclose to the minimum that is necessary to accomplish the workers' compensation purpose. Protected health information may be shared for such purposes to the full extent authorized by applicable state or other law. Additionally, CEs must limit the amount of PHI disclosed for payment purposes to the minimum necessary. Covered entities are permitted to disclose PHI necessary to obtain payment for healthcare provided to an injured or ill worker. When a CE routinely makes disclosures for workers' compensation purposes or for payment purposes, the CE should develop procedures as part of its minimum necessary policies that detail the type and amount of PHI to be disclosed for these purposes. When PHI is requested by a state workers' compensation or other public official, CEs may rely on the official's representations that the information requested is the minimum necessary for the intended purpose.

Covered entities are not required to make a minimum necessary determination when disclosing PHI required by state or other applicable law, or when having the individual's authorization.

### HIPAA and Workers' Compensation Checklist

- For disclosures of PHI made for workers' compensation purposes, the minimum necessary standard permits CEs to disclose information to the full extent authorized by state or other law.
- For disclosures of PHI for payment purposes, CEs may disclose the type and amount of information necessary to receive payment for any healthcare provided to an injured or ill worker.
- Individuals do not have a right under the Privacy Rule to request that a CE restrict a disclosure of PHI about them for workers' compensation purposes when the disclosure is required by law or authorized by and necessary to comply with a workers' compensation or similar law.
- The Privacy Rule permits a healthcare provider to disclose an injured or ill worker's PHI without his or her authorization when

requested for purposes of adjudicating the individual worker's compensation claim.

- The Privacy Rule permits a CE to disclose PHI as necessary to comply with state law. No minimum necessary determination is required in this situation.
- A CE may disclose PHI regarding an injured worker's previous condition, not directly related to the compensation claim, to an employer or insurer when the individual's written authorization has been obtained.

## Training

Employers must provide training to their personnel regarding the safeguards necessary for PHI when the employer is insured or self-funded. Training appropriate to the job responsibilities related to PHI was required by the compliance date of April 14, 2003, and on an ongoing regular basis. Employers must also train their privacy officers and add privacy to their corporate compliance and orientation training programs. Employers should consider extending their training to BAs as well. See Chapter 24 for more information on training, education, and awareness.

## Resources

There are virtually as many unique HIPAA situations as there are employers. Some employers face especially interesting HIPAA issues because of their industries or size. Here is a short list of resources employers may find useful for their unique situations:

- *General HIPAA resources.* See the HHS Web site, called HIPAA OnLine, at http://cms.hhs.gov/hipaa/online/default.asp. It has an interactive tool to help answer HIPAA questions, including those for employer responsibilities.
- *Employer HIPAA responsibilities for church plans.* Contact the Internal Revenue Service at (202) 622-6080; or online at http://www.irs.gov/.
- *Employer HIPAA responsibilities for plans with only one employee.* Your group health plan might not be subject to HIPAA requirements. Contact the Department of Labor at http://cms.hhs.gov/hipaa/online/000022.asp to help you with this issue. Additionally, your health plan may not be eligible for HIPAA protections, but applicable state laws may protect it. Contact your State Insurance Department at http://cms.hhs.gov/hipaa/online/modules/state.asp?view=SID for more information.
- *Private employer HIPAA responsibilities.* If you are a private employer and offer a group health plan to your employees, most of the information in HIPAA OnLine at http://cms.hhs.gov/hipaa/online/default. asp will likely apply to your organization. For more specific information,

contact the Department of Labor at http://cms.hhs.gov/hipaa/online/000022.asp.

## Conclusion

The Privacy Rule helps address multiple fears that have been expressed by employees over the past several years. Multiple news reports and research reveals common employee fears with regard to their employers and health information. Employees fear:

- Employers will use health information to make employment decisions
- Prospective employers will have access to job applicants' health information and make hiring decisions based on the information
- An inappropriate person, such as an ex-spouse, will get access to health information to use against employee, such as in a custody battle
- They will be found ineligible for loans or life and disability insurance
- Privacy policies for their organizations do not provide them adequate protection
- Requesting leave or accommodations because of the access their employers will have to their health information

The requirements listed should demonstrate that employers must actively pursue compliance efforts, and that they will likely be focused on revising the policies and procedures, implementing training and education, and updating the plan documents, contracts, and other administrative forms. HIPAA likely will have a major impact on employers who provide or arrange for healthcare benefits for their workforce.

## Chapter 19: Practical Checklist

- Determine to what extent HIPAA impacts your organization.
- Conduct a CE analysis to determine if you are a CE under HIPAA.
- If you are considered a CE, conduct a CE analysis of benefit plans to determine the applicable HIPAA obligations.
- Determine if your employee benefit plan is a CE.
- If you offer covered benefit plans, identify the specific HIPAA requirements, then develop and implement a compliance plan.
- Take into account your own specific identified exceptions, and take steps to comply with the Privacy Rule with respect to use and disclosure of PHI between the group health plan and the plan sponsor.

# Chapter 20
# Business Associate Issues

**Is Your Organization a Business Associate?**

As we discussed in Chapter 1, a business associate (BA) is basically any individual or organization that performs an activity involving the use or disclosure of protected health information (PHI) on behalf of a covered entity (CE). If you are a BA, this means that you or your organization must receive PHI from a CE or on behalf of a CE, and perform a function or activity for the CE using the PHI. In addition, this means that you are not part of the CE's workforce or in their control. Not sure if you are a BA? Odds are, you are considered a BA if you meet the above criteria and are one of the following:

- Medical billing company
- Attorney
- Accountant
- Financial auditor
- Collection agency
- Bank
- HIPAA consultant
- Information technology consultant
- Software vendor
- Management consultant
- Shredding company
- Covered entity working on behalf of another covered entity
- Accreditation body such as the Joint Commission on Accreditation of Healthcare Organizations (JCAHO)
- Billing and printing service company
- Outsourced radiology and other medical service
- Durable medical supplies provider
- Ambulance service company
- Data aggregator

The information and opinions provided in this book do not constitute or substitute for legal or other professional advice.

Keep in mind that HIPAA states that any activities performed as a CE employee or contractor (if a substantial amount of work is performed at the CE's facilities) do not fall into the BA classification.

## Business Associate Requirements

HIPAA is designed to protect the communication and handling of PHI between CEs and their BAs. As stated in the Security Rule, the overall responsibility of a BA is:

> ...to implement administrative, physical, and technical safeguards that reasonably and appropriately protect the confidentiality, integrity, and availability of the electronic protected health information that it creates, receives, maintains, or transmits on behalf of the covered entity as required by this sub-part.

BA relationships with CEs are usually long term, and thus need to be established and managed carefully. Unfortunately, the days of a friendly handshake agreement are gone. Contracts must be in place before any business is transacted to protect both parties from certain liabilities and to ensure the confidentiality and privacy of PHI. These contracts should be reasonable and beneficial to both parties — not one-sided. They need to be kept as simple as possible so that there is no frustration or confusion over what is involved. There are, however, certain minimum requirements of a BA contract. The following is a list of obligations and requirements adapted from the OCR's Obligations and Activities of Business Associate:*

- BA agrees to not use or disclose PHI other than as permitted or required by the BA contract or as required by law.
- BA agrees to use appropriate safeguards to prevent use or disclosure of the PHI other than as provided for by the BA contract.
- BA agrees to mitigate, to the extent practicable, any harmful effect that is known to BA of a use or disclosure of PHI by BA in violation of the requirements of the BA contract.
- BA agrees to report to CE any use or disclosure of the PHI not provided for by the BA contract of which it becomes aware.
- BA agrees to ensure that any agent, including a subcontractor to whom it provides PHI, agrees to the same restrictions and conditions that apply through the BA contract.
- BA agrees to provide access to PHI in a designated record set to an individual; not required if BA does not have PHI in a designated record set.

*The Department of Health and Human Services (HHS) Office of Civil Rights' (OCR) Obligations and Activities of Business Associate, Sample Business Associate Contract Provisions, available at http://www.hhs.gov/ocr/hipaa/contractprov.html. Refer to this link for specific verbiage and definitions.

**Exhibit 1. Compliance Deadlines for Business Associate Contracts**

| Business Associate Scenario | HIPAA Compliance Deadline |
|---|---|
| New BA contracts | At the time the contract is executed |
| BA contracts in place on October 15, 2002, renewed or modified by April 14, 2003 | April 14, 2003 |
| BA contracts in place on October 15, 2002, renewed or modified between April 15, 2003, and April 14, 2004 | Effective date of the contract renewal or modification |
| BA contracts not renewed or modified prior to April 14, 2004 | April 14, 2004 |

*Note:* Agreements containing automatic renewal provisions are not considered agreements that must be renewed for purposes of HIPAA, and will not require a compliance deadline unless and until they are amended or modified.

- BA agrees to provide access to PHI in a designated record set to an individual for amendment as needed; not required if BA does not have PHI in a designated record set.
- BA agrees to make internal practices, books, and records, including policies and procedures and PHI relating to the use and disclosure of PHI, available to HHS for purposes of the Secretary determining CE's compliance with the Privacy Rule.
- BA agrees to document such disclosures of PHI and information related to such disclosures as would be required for CE to respond to a request by an individual for an accounting of disclosures of PHI.
- BA agrees to provide to CE or an individual, information collected to permit CE to respond to a request by an individual for an accounting of disclosures of PHI.

For a sample BA contract, refer to Appendix B. Contracts must be in place for any BA relationships that CEs have by the dates specified in Exhibit 1.

## What You Can Expect to See or Hear from Covered Entities

There are various questions and concerns that you as a BA can expect to hear from CEs, including:

- Do you know what HIPAA is?
- Can you demonstrate an understanding of it?
- What do you see as your obligations according to HIPAA?
- Do you have someone responsible for HIPAA compliance within your organization?
- Are you providing extra preventative measures to ensure PHI is protected as mandated by HIPAA? If so, what are they?
  - Privacy safeguards
  - Security safeguards

- Does your company conduct background checks on employees that have access to PHI?
- Do you have an education program in place to train your employees in the HIPAA requirements? If so, how often is it being given? May we see the training materials?
- Special letters of notification from their legal department regarding the HIPAA requirements
- Their expectations of your organization regarding HIPAA
- Certain provisions added to the BA contract including:
  - Special insurance requirements
  - Indemnification against reasonable losses, damages, costs, or other expenses
  - Ability to review your policies, procedures, and records associated with the protection of PHI
  - Greater control over BA contract termination

**Issues to Consider**

You should consider the following items when dealing with CEs and working on BA contract issues:

- CEs cannot be held liable for the actions of their BAs unless they have actual knowledge of a PHI breach and do not do one of the following:
  - Take reasonable steps to fix the breach.
  - Terminate the BA contract.
  - Report the breach to HHS if termination of the BA contract is not feasible. HIPAA allows for the continuation of the relationship as long as the breach is reported and the BA is working to address the risk that resulted in the breach.
- Regardless of who is liable, it can still be a huge public relations nightmare for both parties to deal with a PHI breach.
- If you have not already done so, identify legal counsel that can assist with BA issues.
- Determine whether or not everyone that has access to PHI in your organization actually needs that access. Minimum necessary and need to know are important rules to live by.
- CEs are not required to train or educate BAs on the HIPAA requirements.
  - If they have the ability to train and offer it, then go for it!
  - Look for the following information in any training that is offered:
    - An overview of HIPAA Administrative Simplification — the who and why
    - Explanation of terminology used in HIPAA
    - Outline of the three major rules — Privacy Rule, Security Rule, and Transaction and Code Sets Rule

- Compliance requirements (dates and penalties)
- You may also ask to hear about their HIPAA experiences and ask to see their plans
- CEs are not required to oversee how their BAs process and protect PHI, but this is why we recommend asking for and understanding their expectations of your organization.
- CEs may want only to share information that has been de-identified.
  - Both parties will have to determine whether or not that is feasible, and if so, whether or not a BA contract is even necessary at that point.
- Find out who the HIPAA compliance officer(s) are within the CEs you work with and be sure you establish a good working relationship.
- Does the CE want you to create the HIPAA-compliant BA agreement, or does the CE want you to provide the agreement? You may want to consider creating such an agreement for those CEs who ask, and advise them to modify it and have it approved by their own legal counsel based on their own organization's needs.

## Moving Forward

From trying to determine whether or not your organization is a BA to negotiating reasonable BA contracts, there are a lot of critical business decisions to be made. Be sure to obtain legal advice if there is any gray area regarding your BA status. Also, obtain legal advice before establishing new business relationships with HIPAA CEs or before revising any existing contracts. Given that there is so much at stake with regard to business liability, it is absolutely critical to get an expert involved. You can perform all the research up front and even draft your own BA contract, but always be sure to run it by your attorney before conducting business with a CE.

## Chapter 20: Practical Checklist

- Any person or organization performing work on behalf of a CE that involves PHI is considered a BA.
- CEs are not responsible for monitoring BA compliance with HIPAA.
- CEs are not responsible for educating their BAs on HIPAA.
- Take advantage of any education that is offered from CEs.
- Be prepared to tell CEs how you expect to protect PHI.
- Make sure BA contracts meet HIPAA contract requirements and are reasonable and mutually beneficial.
- Obtain legal counsel or other HIPAA consultation if you are having trouble determining whether or not you or your organization is a BA.

# Section 4: Covered Entity Issues Quiz

1. Which of the following is typically not required by HIPAA to provide a Notice of Privacy Practices to individuals?
   A. Family physician
   B. Chiropractor
   C. Health insurance company
   D. Healthcare clearinghouse

2. When must a direct healthcare treatment provider give an individual a Notice of Privacy Practices?
   A. By December 31, 2003
   B. The date of first service delivery, with exceptions
   C. The date of first service delivery, with no exceptions
   D. By April 14, 2003, and upon each office visit

3. In which of the following situations is an employer directly impacted by HIPAA requirements?
   A. When workers' compensation claims are filed
   B. When a workforce member uses the benefits allowed by FMLA
   C. When the employer sponsors an on-site clinic
   D. When the employer provides Medigap coverage to retirees

4. Many to most employers need to implement HIPAA requirements on behalf of which of the following?
   A. Their long-term care participants
   B. Their covered health insurance benefit plans
   C. Their long-term disability personnel
   D. Their casualty and fire insurance plans

5. Employer health plan sponsors are typically allowed by HIPAA to have access to what type of information?
   A. Summary health information
   B. Individually identifiable health information
   C. Protected health information
   D. Health history information

6. Which of the following is an example of a government-funded health plan?
   A. A Pacificare Plan
   B. An Indian Health Service Program
   C. An FDA Program
   D. A Voluntary Blood Bank Program

7. By what date must a qualified small health plan be in compliance with the HIPAA Privacy Rule?
   A. April 21, 2005
   B. October 17, 2003
   C. April 14, 2003
   D. April 14, 2004

8. A group health plan must require a plan sponsor to amend the plan documents to include which of the following provisions?
   A. Allow disclosures to employers for employment-related actions only after receiving a signed consent
   B. Do not allow disclosures to employers for employment-related actions
   C. Allow disclosures to employers for employment-related decisions related to any other benefit
   D. Do not allow disclosures to employers for plan-related sponsor actions

9. Which of the following is an example of marketing that requires an authorization?
   A. A face-to-face discussion with a patient where the doctor describes drugs available to treat a symptom
   B. A mailing from a health insurer promoting a mortgage product offered by the same company
   C. A mailing from a health insurer to a policyholder listing the physicians participating in the health plan network
   D. An insurer sends a mailing to subscribers nearing Medicare eligible age with information about its Medicare supplemental plan and an application form

10. How soon following a material revision of a notice of privacy practices must a health plan provide the revised notice to individuals who subscribe to the plan?
    A. Within 6 days
    B. At least once every 3 years
    C. Within 30 days
    D. Within 60 days

11. Which of the following is a distinguishing feature of a healthcare clearinghouse?
    A. Processing health information from a nonstandard format to a standard format
    B. Selling software that converts the format of health information
    C. Creating software that concerts the format of health information
    D. Electronically transferring health information from a health plan to a bank system

12. Which of the following is an example of a HIPAA-covered service provided by a healthcare provider?
    A. Body piercing
    B. Sponsoring a weight-loss plan
    C. Storing blood bank supplies
    D. Dispensing drugs for a prescription

13. Which of the following can a covered entity charge an individual for when providing a copy of their corresponding PHI?
    A. Postage, copying, preparing a summary, and the time involved with gathering all this information
    B. Postage, copying, and the costs directly involved with preparing a requested summary of PHI if applicable
    C. The total amount of time it takes to gather all information charged at the current federal minimum hourly wage
    D. Postage costs only

14. Which of the following is not allowed and is not considered an incidental disclosure under HIPAA?
    A. Calling a person's full name in a provider's waiting room
    B. A patient in a shared hospital room overhearing a doctor discuss medical treatment with the other patient in the room
    C. Placing lab test descriptions by the corresponding individual on sign-in sheets
    D. Placing a patient's file in a slot outside a hospital room with name and admission date in full view of everyone passing

15. Which of the following is most likely a Business Associate as defined by HIPAA?
    A. Temporary receptionist
    B. Collection agency
    C. Security guard for a medical clinic
    D. Trash collection service hauling shredded documents

# Section 5
# HIPAA
# Technology
# Considerations

# Chapter 21
# Building a HIPAA-Compliant Technology Infrastructure

## Overview

It specifically states in both the Privacy and Security rules that CEs must have certain administrative, physical, and technical safeguards in place to safeguard PHI. In various places throughout this book, we have stressed that HIPAA compliance is less about technology and more about business processes and culture. Having said that, you can have all the policies, procedures, and culture changes in the world, but if certain technical controls are not in place, there is no way to ensure HIPAA compliance. You cannot have one without the other. The bottom line is that a lot of policies and procedures cannot be implemented properly or enforced at all without relying on certain technologies.

Both rules touch on this but the Security Rule in particular presents a good of combination of the information technology and security standards tailored for the healthcare industry. These best practices to protect PHI are all generally well known and some of them have been around since the days of the first mainframe computer. The drawback to the HIPAA rules is that they tell you what must be done but do not tell you how to do it. This chapter picks up where the HIPAA rules leave off. In this chapter, we are going to focus on the technical safeguard requirements of HIPAA. We will not go into detail on how specific technologies work; instead we will give you ideas on certain technologies that you can use to become HIPAA compliant. We will also list some real-world experiences that we (and others) have had with these technologies, along with some practical tips that can

---

The information and opinions provided in this book do not constitute or substitute for legal or other professional advice.

save you some time, money, and effort. If you want to learn more about the specific technologies — how they work, how to best implement them, how to configure them, etc. — there are many great books and resources to which you can refer. See Appendix C for a complete listing of our favorites.

There is not a one-size-fits-all solution when it comes to information technology. For example, a firewall or VPN requirement for a large CE, such as a hospital, is not going to be the same as that for a small CE, such as a physician's office. A lot of CEs may already have the necessary technologies in place and just need them to be configured properly. Others may have to make considerable hardware and software investments in order to be compliant.

**Caution**

Do not let anyone ever tell you that a firewall, anti-virus software, or encryption alone are enough to protect your information systems and PHI. Firewalls are certainly part of the equation; however, you must layer your security to ensure that if one device fails or does not stop an attack, several more layers of protection will prevent penetration of your systems. This layered approach is referred to as defense in depth.

You should not take the technology tips we outline in this chapter as specific requirements for your organization. Please keep in mind that the HIPAA requirements are scalable and flexible, depending on your business processes, size, and associated information risks. Given the technology guidance in this chapter combined with an accurate risk analysis and a little time, money, and effort, there is no reason that you cannot be well on your way to reasonably protecting PHI within your technology infrastructure. The point we are trying to make here is that it all just depends on your organization's specific situation.

**Areas of Technology to Focus On**

HIPAA, and specifically the Security Rule, is a set of requirements that essentially provides a framework for creating and managing an effective information security infrastructure. Without the proper technical controls in place, PHI can be put at risk. There are certain technical components that HIPAA mandates such as:

- Logical access controls
- Physical access controls
- Authentication controls
- Authorization controls
- Audit controls
- Data encryption and integrity mechanisms

Although HIPAA does not specify what technology solutions are needed to meet these requirements, it can be expected that some of the following may be necessary:

- Authentication controls such as unique user names, passwords, or possibly biometric devices
- Operating system (OS), application, or even directory service access controls to permit or deny access based on user, role, or context
- Network security devices such as a firewall or an Intrusion Detection System (IDS)
- Content filtering devices such as e-mail scanning to detect vulnerable PHI going across a network and antivirus programs to detect malicious software
- Encryption software to protect PHI at rest or in transit
- Virtual private network (VPN) devices to ensure secure network-to-network or remote access communications
- Logging systems, including the built-in logging functions of OSs and applications for audit-trail purposes
- Policy management software for publishing and managing HIPAA policies and to assist in end user HIPAA awareness
- Patch management software to facilitate the ongoing management and deployment of critical software updates

### Looking Deeper into Specific Technologies

The following are specific best practices and tips on certain technologies that may be a part of your overall HIPAA technology infrastructure. These are not comprehensive solutions and every CE's needs are different. You may very well come up with some ideas on your own. Regardless, this information can help you get started on building your HIPAA-compliant technology infrastructure.

#### *Access Controls*

- Ensure that every user has a unique user ID and password. IDs that are shared by two or more people are a definite security risk and provide no accountability for the activities performed using the ID.
- Disable unused user IDs or IDs for users that are on an extended leave of absence.
- Focus on granting people access based on minimum necessary and "need to know" requirements to get a job done. Ensure that separation of duties via specific access control mechanisms is in place.
- Access controls consist of identification, authentication, and authorization — these are all integral functions of OSs, applications, and databases.
    - Identification is the process of determining who a user is.

- Authentication is the process of proving who a user is.
- Authorization defines what a user is allowed to do.
- Consider implementing role-based access controls for your OSs, applications, and databases that define the access capabilities for a particular job role or computer system.
  - User-based access is good but can be difficult to manage.
  - Group-based access is easy to manage but it can be difficult to ensure that only specific users have access to certain resources.
- Whatever your access control methods are — just have something. Never give everyone full administrative rights to computer and network resources; this is a PHI security incident waiting to happen.
- Do not log on to your OSs, applications, or databases with administrator or root privileges to perform daily job tasks that do not require those rights.
- Create standard user IDs with limited rights for everyone and encourage their use except when administrative or root privileges are needed.
- There are three ways to authenticate a person or entity: something they know (password), something they have (secure token), and something they are (biometric).
  - Implement at least one of these.
  - A combination of any two — referred to as two-factor authentication or strong authentication —offers much greater information security.
- Biometrics can be a very effective way to authenticate users — just keep cost and system administration issues in mind before rolling this technology out systemwide.
- Make sure you have policies and procedures for the creation, maintenance, and revocation of access.
- Single sign-on solutions (one password for everything) can help ease access-control administration burdens, but can be expensive and difficult to implement and administer if not done properly.
- Ensure that a system is in place to revoke accounts and passwords after termination. This is one of the most exploited vulnerabilities in a computer network.
  - Have a plan for protecting PHI in case the administrator or root account is compromised. This may include encrypted offline databases, removable storage, failover systems, etc.

### Anti-virus and Malicious Software Protection

- Anti-virus software may not be enough — look into the newer adware and "pest" software protection products.
- This software needs to be loaded on every computer that is not a mainframe/midrange system or dumb terminal.

- This software needs to be set up (if possible) to regularly and automatically download virus signature file updates.
- This software must stay installed on your computers at all times to ensure proper protection.
- This software should be centrally managed via your network if you have more than a handful of computers — otherwise, it can be too difficult to manage.
- Disable the ability for your end users to uninstall this software.
- Complete scans of your computer system are important after you first install the software and then every month or so — you should not have to do these too often if the software is never uninstalled.
  - Instead, focus on keeping your software installed to check for viruses, etc., in real-time upon file access, e-mail sending and receiving, etc.

### Applications and Databases

- Certain clinical, practice management, and other healthcare applications have built-in user accounts.
  - Use them only if necessary — use user ID and password integration with local OS or directory services if it is available.
  - Create an account/password combination for each user.
- Apply the latest vendor software updates — especially the critical security patches — on a regular basis.
- Ensure that strong passwords are used — tips on passwords are discussed later.
- Ask your software vendor(s) how accounts and passwords are stored (clear text, proprietary encryption format, etc.) and take security precautions as necessary.
- Do not display the last user ID that logged in on the log-in screen.
  - If it is displayed, a malicious user can use this against you and try to log in with that user ID.
- Use automatic log-off. There is no set time specified by HIPAA — just use common sense based on what you find in your risk analysis and what works best in your environment.
- Some applications have built-in features that allow or even force users to log off manually or after a few seconds or minutes of inactivity.
- Treat databases as one of your most critical assets — this is where the "good stuff" is — this is where your PHI spends most of its waking hours.
  - Databases are often the most highly targeted yet the most vulnerable part of your information systems.
  - Specific attention must be given to your databases during and after your risk analysis.

- Leave database maintenance and administration up to the database experts or users that have received formal training.
  - A great way to expose or otherwise damage a database and thus affect the confidentiality, integrity, and availability of PHI is for an untrained user to perform administrative functions in a haphazard fashion.

### Data Backups and Storage

- Consider backing up your data at least daily.
  - Consider real-time backups for larger systems with heavy transaction volumes.
- Back up your OS and application files as well.
  - This will help decrease system restoration times dramatically.
- Make complete backups of your system periodically — once a month or every few months — and keep them indefinitely.
- Backups can be made to tape, CD, another computer, or even a secure Internet-based data repository.
- Magnetic media including tapes and disks fail eventually so consider replacing your media every few years.
- Backups must be tested to ensure they contain valid data that you may need in an emergency.
- Backups must be stored offsite — at least some of them such as your weekly backups — in case a disaster destroys or damages them.
- Offsite backup media must be handled only by authorized and trusted personnel.
- Do not store backup tapes near a computer monitor or UPS — the electromagnetic interference coming from these devices can corrupt data on them or completely erase them.
- Ensure that backup media are adequately protected from extreme hot or cold temperatures and are readily accessible.
- Encrypt or at least password protect your backups.
- Print out hard copies of important files periodically and store them in a safe location.
- Ensure that swap file space for your OSs and applications is sufficient for daily usage and to prevent DoS attacks.

### Encryption

- Although encryption is an "addressable" Security Rule implementation specification, data must be encrypted if your risk analysis turns up specific threats and vulnerabilities to PHI at rest or in transit, and if encryption is the only viable solution to reduce the risk.
- It can be difficult and expensive to deploy and manage — but it might be a necessary evil.

- A common practice is to deploy encryption for data in transit and not for data at rest.
  - This is not good!
  - At a minimum, focus on data at rest, including e-mail attachments, because this is where the true vulnerability lies.
- Ensure that strong passphrases are used for encryption keys — otherwise encryption's value is diminished.
- Any well-known 128-bit or greater encryption method such as AES, IDEA, or Triple-DES will suffice.
- PGP is a free and excellent way to encrypt e-mails and your computer's file system if you only have a small number of computers to manage.
- Zip utilities, such as PKZip Professional and WinZip, can also encrypt files and is a cost effective way to encrypt and share confidential files.
- Consider enabling encrypted file systems if your OS supports it.
- Consider using PGP to create and validate digital signatures on files to verify their integrity.
- Use an MD5 utility to create a one-way encrypted hash for files to verify their integrity.
- Consider establishing a public key infrastructure (PKI) if you can justify the cost and support it will require.
- If you use PKI or some other form of digital signatures, keep in mind that content filtering, antivirus software, and IDSs may be rendered ineffective when data is encrypted.
- Encryption can be an inconvenience to users.
  - You must balance security with convenience based on what was discovered in your risk analysis.
- Your goal with encryption should be to keep users out of the loop.
  - Have ways to automatically encrypt PHI so that your users will not have to remember to do it.
- Implement data in transit encryption methods within your applications at the perimeter of your network instead of at the desktop level via PKI, SSL/TLS for e-mail and Web applications, or e-mail firewalls for secure messaging — see Appendix C for some specific vendors and products.
- Implement data at rest encryption methods within your applications and databases if possible.
  - If not, integrate third-party database encryption software — see Appendix C for some specific vendors and products.
- Never, ever rely on password protected files in your word processor, spreadsheet, or file compression utility to ensure the security of the file's contents.
  - There are dozens of utilities that can be downloaded for free that can crack most of these passwords in typically less than one minute.

- Always use Secure Shell (SSH) or a similar technology method instead of telnet for encrypted remote computer access.
- Understand the applicable federal laws for exporting cryptography.

### *Faxes*

- Faxes sent via computers through fax-modems are covered under the Security Rule. Regular fax machines are not considered "computers" in the context of the Security Rule.
- Faxes sent via a regular fax machine are covered by the Privacy Rule.
- If you fax PHI, make sure someone is at the other end to receive the fax by calling them while sending it or immediately thereafter. Do not let faxes sit around on fax machines.
- Make sure that fax machines are in a physically secure location away from public access.
- Immediately file or securely dispose of faxes (shred, etc.) before unauthorized people can see the fax.
- Something to keep in mind about faxes — many organizations, including clinics, hospitals, laboratories and other providers, are using e-faxes now.
  - This is a growing trend, and there is no way to tell that a given fax number goes to an e-fax unless it is specifically documented or someone tells you.
  - An e-fax number looks like any other phone number. Basically, an e-fax converts the faxed information into an electronic file that is sent to a person's computer or to an organization's mail server and is typically delivered to an e-mail account as an attachment.
  - PHI within an e-fax is electronic PHI — keep this in mind, and check with the recipient of the entity to which you are faxing information to see if their fax number is an e-fax number.

### *Firewalls*

- Use the best firewall you can afford — for a small network, you can get a really good firewall with most of the fancy bells and whistles for well under $1,000.
- Use the built-in features of your existing network firewall, router, or other Internet connection device including the following:.
  - Block all traffic by default.
    - Open only the ports required for the traffic you need leaving or entering your network.
    - If you allow all traffic by default, it will be much more difficult to secure and manage.
  - Block all outbound packets (this is called egress filtering) going to the Internet that did not originate from your network.

- Block all inbound packets (this is called ingress filtering) coming from the Internet that are addressed from the broadcast address (0.0.0.0 or 255.255.255.255) or other reserved addresses such as 10.x.x.x, 172.16.x.x–172.31.x.x, or 192.168.x.x).
  - This can help prevent IP spoofing and Denial of Service (DoS) attacks involving your network.
- Use packet filtering to only allow specific types of traffic through.
- Enable stateful packet inspection to increase packet filtering security if it is available.
- Do not rely on IP addresses or DNS information to authenticate users or hosts via your packet filters as they can be forged to look like they are coming from anyone.
- Use network address translation (NAT).
  - This is a good start for network security, but should not be the only security mechanism you use.
  - Helps conceal your internal network configuration.
  - Helps restrict incoming and outgoing traffic.
  - Do not rely on NAT for logging or traffic inspection.
- Use port forwarding if your firewall supports it.
  - This forwards specific inbound traffic on to the proper host inside your network.
- Use application proxies, if possible, to help "hide" your systems behind the firewall and let the proxy software do all the work on behalf of your computers.
- Keep in mind that most firewalls cannot block application-specific or malicious software attacks.
  - Web applications need to be protected by content filtering or IDSs.
  - All computers must be protected by antivirus software.
- Log all firewall activity.
  - Consider logging to a remote syslog server — see below for more info on logging.
- Consider outsourcing your firewall monitoring to make sure that security anomalies and attacks do not go unnoticed.
- Limit the number of applications running on your firewall device such as content filtering, antivirus, etc. — you do not want to have your "layered" approach to security on a single point of failure device.
- Disable all possible user IDs on the firewall system.
- Consider load balancing by adding a second firewall to increase firewall throughput and ensure the availability of your Internet connection in case your firewall fails.
- Change the default firewall password and assign a very strong password — see below for more info on passwords.

- Run the firewall service as an ID other than administrator or root if possible.
- Patch the firmware, OS, and application software for your firewall on a regular basis.
- Remember that a firewall might not be able to prevent security attacks originating from inside your network.
- Keep your firewall rule set as simple as possible and make sure that it stays in line with your security polices.
- There is a good National Institute of Standards and Technology document titled Guidelines on Firewalls and Firewall Policy, which provides more detailed information on firewall security, at: http://csrc.nist.gov/publications/nistpubs/800-41/sp800-41.pdf.

### Intrusion Detection Systems

- IDSs can be very effective to detect malicious use on your network, but they can also consume a lot of time and resources when monitored properly.
  - Consider outsourcing the monitoring of your IDS.
- A common mistake is to install an IDS and forget about it.
  - You (or third party) must monitor your IDS constantly to be able to effectively respond to attacks.
- There are two types of IDS — network and host; consider getting both.
  - Network-based IDSs can detect attacks across your entire network.
  - Host-based IDSs can detect attacks on specific computer systems or applications.
- Typical network IDSs may be defeated fairly easily if the attack:.
  - Is new or one the IDS does not recognize in its signature database.
  - Takes place too fast sending too much traffic that overloads the system.
  - Uses packet fragmentation.
  - Is encrypted.
  - Takes place on a switched network.
- Although there is not an ideal location for network-based IDS, a good location to consider placing it is behind a firewall on a non-switched segment so it can catch all traffic that was allowed in by the firewall.
- You may also consider placing another IDS outside the firewall, especially if you want to monitor the effectiveness of your firewall system — the returns are generally not that great for this setup though as there are other, less expensive, utilities to monitor the effectiveness of your firewall.

- Typical host IDSs can monitor system usage and detect local misuse of the system — see more below when we talk about personal firewalls/IDSs.
- Consider installing host-based IDS software that can check the integrity of files to determine whether or not they have been modified or tampered with by an unauthorized user.
- Look for IDSs that have some or all of the following beneficial features:.
  - Do not solely rely on attack signature but can also detect network protocol anomalies and behavior-based attacks.
  - Can cut off an attack immediately (referred to as intrusion detection and prevention or IDP).
  - Can monitor network bandwidth usage.
  - Can detect:
    - Trends
    - Malicious software
    - Unauthorized hardware or software
    - Specific network events
    - Network analyzers
  - Can be distributed with multiple sensors across the various segments of your network.
  - Can track the attack back to its source.
  - Can reconstruct and playback network attacks.
  - Has good alerting capabilities such as e-mail, pager, etc..
  - Has good reporting capabilities — preferably through one centralized management console.
- Patch the firmware, OS, and application software for your IDS on a regular basis.
- Do not rely on IP addresses or DNS information to authenticate users or hosts as they can be forged to look like they are coming from anyone.
- Consider supplementing your IDS with a network analyzer — especially in the case of a security incident.
- Consider outsourcing your IDS monitoring to make sure that security anomalies and attacks do not go unnoticed.

### Modems

- You can have all the security in the world — firewalls, IDSs, encryption, strong passwords, etc. — but all it takes to cancel every bit of that out is a simple unsecured modem on your network.
- Ensure that the software that controls the modem is always unloaded or disabled except when you need to send or receive information.

- Ensure that the modem cannot receive incoming calls — unless it has to — by any means.
  - Test this from the outside to confirm.
  - This may require a special call out only phone line.
- Ensure that the computer hosting the modem is very secure to prevent remote reprogramming of the modem or dialing lists.
  - Anti-virus and personal firewall/IDS software is a must here.
- Consider enabling caller ID on incoming phone lines for audit trail purposes.
- Consider using an encrypting modem if necessary.

### Operating Systems

- Use server OSs that have strong built-in security features for authentication, access control, and logging.
  - Built-in directory services are really helpful in creating user, role, and context based permissions to protect PHI.
- Use client OSs such as Windows 95/98/Me that have strong built-in security features for authentication, access control, and logging.
  - Older desktop OSs have very few security mechanisms built in and may not be sufficient for HIPAA compliance.
- Centrally manage your client OSs via group policies.
  - This will allow you have to granular control over client security features.
  - Another benefit of group policies is that you can prevent users from modifying the OS settings that could inadvertently put PHI at risk.
- If group policies are not available, configure local client OS policies at a minimum to ensure PHI protection.
- Harden your OSs by implementing well-known best practices that we provide reference to in Appendix C.
  - Disable all unnecessary services.
  - Disable all unnecessary protocols.
  - Make specific registry or configuration changes to plug known security holes.
    - These will help reduce potential vulnerabilities as well as help the computer run at its optimum performance.
- If possible, setup your OSs to clear their swap files before shutting down.
  - This can prevent someone from accessing PHI, etc. off of the drive if the system is stolen.

- Apply the latest vendor software updates — especially the critical security patches — on a regular basis.
  - Some OSs have an update feature built into them — use this at a minimum.
  - Be careful not to install software updates on production computers that your business relies on without fully testing them first or having a quick and easy backout plan in case they cause problems or fail.
  - Consider using a third party patch management product that you can use to centrally test, deploy, and manage these patches with — see Appendix C for a listing of some of these products.

    *Caution:* There has been some concern regarding recent Windows service packs and HIPAA compliance. By agreeing with the End User License Agreement during the installation of these service packs, you are granting the ability for a third party to "provide upgrades or fixes that will be automatically downloaded to your computer." As there are issues here based on your installation that could possibly take your organization out of HIPAA compliance, this should be taken into consideration during your risk analysis and ongoing HIPAA compliance audits.

  - To prevent these automatic updates from occurring without your testing and approval, you can consider turning off the auto-update functionality within the OS.
- Ensure that strong passwords are used — see below for tips on passwords.
- Turn on logging — most new, network friendly OSs support it.
  - Enable system, application, security, and any other applicable logging features.
  - This will help you create audit trails for PHI access.
- Do not display the last user ID that logged in on the log-in screen.
  - If it is displayed, a malicious user can use this against you and try to log in with that user ID
- Remove, or at least disable, any guest accounts on your systems.
- Automatic log-off — there is no set time specified by HIPAA — just use common sense based on what you find in your risk analysis and what works best in your environment.
  - Some OSs have built-in features such as screen savers that will allow or even force users to log off manually or after a few minutes of inactivity.
- Consider using radio frequency-based proximity sensors to automate this when users come and go around workstations — especially nursing stations.

### Personal Firewall/IDS Software

- Use personal firewall/IDS software on every computer possible inside your network.
  - We cannot stress enough how critical it is to have this software in addition to your regular firewall — it will help catch attacks destined for specific computers and applications that most network firewalls cannot block on their own.
- In fact, the protection that some of the more-advanced personal firewall/IDS products offer may be sufficient enough for your overall firewall and IDS needs, especially for smaller CEs, so you do not have to purchase a more-expensive network-based firewall or IDS.
- This software should be centrally managed via your network if you have more than a handful of computers — otherwise, it can be too difficult to manage.
- You may have to experiment with your software's application protection feature. It might be important to you to protect against Trojan horse programs and other applications that can send information out of your computer — but the protection may also be more of a hassle than it is worth.

### Logging

- Logging is required and an essential element to create PHI audit trails.
- Turn on logging on every possible system.
- Logging-event successes and failures may prove to be too much information to sift through and store — consider logging-event failures and access to critical PHI files only.
- There are specific logging applications that can sift through all of your logging data to search for important security events — see Appendix C for a reference to some of these products.
- Log to a remote syslog server that is running on dedicated hardware.
  - This helps to ensure security of the logs and helps prevent tampering of the logs by a malicious user trying to cover his tracks.
  - There are various free, open source, commercial syslog products — see Appendix C for a reference to some of these products.
- Place strict access controls on any remote logging servers or log files.
- Make sure your log files are backed up daily.

### Passwords

- Do not make users choose complicated passwords or have to change them so often that they are difficult to remember and end up getting written down in obvious places such as on sticky notes placed on the monitor or keyboard.

- Never write down passwords.
- Never record passwords electronically unless you are using an encrypted password database — and never send passwords via unencrypted e-mail.
- Never program shortcut keys on keyboards to store passwords.
- Enforce passwords within the OS, application, or database — most newer OSs have this ability and certain applications and databases either have this or can be customized to have it.
- Enforce password reuse and complexity such as minimum length, upper and lower case, and special characters at the OS, application, or database level — never rely on your users to create strong passwords.
- 8 characters is a good minimum length for passwords.
- Encourage users to create passwords that are easy to remember yet difficult to guess.
- It is sufficient that passwords be changed every 6 to 12 months as long as they are strong passwords that are difficult to guess — if users are required to change them more frequently, odds are they will be written down.
- Consider running password-cracking utilities against your password database to ensure that strong passwords have been selected; however, do not assume that passwords that were not cracked are secure.

## Messaging

### E-Mail

- HIPAA does not ban the use of e-mail to send PHI if no threats or vulnerabilities are found during the risk analysis.
- Having said that, as far as we are concerned, any e-mail that is sent in clear text is at risk — during transmission inside your network; across the Internet; and once it arrives at its destination, during transmission on the recipient's network; and while it is stored on the recipient's e-mail server or local computer.
  - Without specific technologies in place, there is no way to prevent those e-mails from being printed or forwarded on to another user — see Appendix C for software that can prevent these two security risks from occurring.
- Users should not be given the option to encrypt e-mails because if you give them that responsibility, it might not get done.
- Have a policy against sending PHI via e-mail.
  - If that is not possible, then you must have policies, procedures, and encryption technologies in place.

- Do not rely on an e-mail's subject line or the sender's e-mail address to verify the authenticity of the sender.
  - E-mails can be forged or spoofed to look like they are coming from anyone and can be used to trick people or contain malicious code that can compromise PHI.
- Do not put PHI in the e-mail subject line.
- One thing you might want to consider is using a perimeter-based e-mail encryption solution.
  - These products encrypt/decrypt e-mails at the network perimeter, thus taking e-mail security responsibilities away from users.
  - Some have the ability to notify users that they have messages waiting for them; after clicking a link, the user is directed to a secure Web site to read the e-mail.
- If no risks are found to exist for internal e-mail, then encryption may be optional.
  - Just make sure your e-mail server and message stores are highly secured from malicious attacks originating from inside or outside your network.
- There is a good NIST document titled "Guidelines on Electronic Mail Security," which provides more-detailed information on e-mail security at http://csrc.nist.gov/publications/nistpubs/800-45/sp800-45.pdf.

**Instant Messaging (IM)**

- Do not forget about IM — it is a great way to communicate — but it has even more threats and vulnerabilities than e-mail:
  - Weak or no encryption, allowing clear text to go across the network.
  - Potential leakage of PHI
  - Could possibly contain malicious code
  - Potential breach of firewall policies
  - Could permit unauthorized access to your network shares
  - Potential DoS attacks
- IM may log everything (including PHI) locally or on remote servers that are not in your control in clear text, which could be compromised as well.
  - This is actually a greater vulnerability than when the data is being transmitted across the network.
  - These logs are subject to review under other laws as well.
- Allow only one type of IM software.
  - Keep that software current on all computers running it.
- Enable IM encryption.

- Enforce strong passwords for the IM application.
- Consider configuring your OSs to prevent users from installing unapproved IM software.

### Remote Access/Virtual Private Networks

- Personal firewall/IDS software must be used — no ifs, ands, or buts — otherwise a malicious user can compromise the remote computer and have full access to your systems through the dial-up or virtual private network (VPN) connection.
- Only provide remote access to the systems necessary for your users to get their jobs done.
- Treat remote computers as company computers when it comes to security policies and minimum system requirements.
  - Consider supplying company-owned equipment for remote access to eliminate any policy enforcement issues.
- Consider the following minimum system requirements for remote access:
  - Anti-virus software installed
  - Personal firewall/IDS software installed
  - The latest OS and application patches
  - Strong passwords
  - Secure authentication
  - Automatic log-off
  - Secure physical location
  - Contingency plan if the computer will be storing PHI
- Any VPN system that uses 128-bit encryption or greater will suffice.
- Strong encryption pass phrases are essential for secure VPN operation.
- Strong user authentication passwords can be the weakest link in a VPN configuration.
  - Have a policy forbidding users to allow their VPN software to store, or "remember," their VPN password; for instance, if a laptop is stolen, the thief could have a direct VPN connection into your network.
  - Do not forget the physical security of remote clients — a laptop with a VPN client that has a password saved in it can be very dangerous!
- Just because VPN information is encrypted does not mean that someone with a network analyzer cannot figure out what is going on, such as the time of day transmissions occurred, the length of the transmissions, etc., to help launch an attack on your VPN.
- You can even use VPN software built into your existing OSs; for example, with some of the newer OSs, you can use standard protocols such as PPTP, L2TP, and IPSec.

## *Physical Security*

- Ensure that physical access to your critical infrastructure devices such as your firewall, IDS, router, and servers is tightly controlled, as unsecured areas can be one of the best ways for PHI to be compromised.
    - Having a locked door on the computer room where only a limited number of people have access is ideal.
    - Bottom line: If you have an option or a way to lock it up, then do it — this can eliminate a lot of vulnerabilities.
- Biometrics and magnetic-strip ID badges work well.
- Limit physical access to network infrastructure equipment, including cables and patch panels.
- Consider fiber-optic cabling, especially for dispersed campuses where physical access to the network hardware is possible.
- Limit the use of glass around computer rooms and equipment to prevent the possibility of someone gaining access.
- Place your computer systems in a safe place in the event of an earthquake or other threat that may cause structural damage to the building.
- Use physical tie-downs for computers and equipment that are susceptible to physical security risks.
- Ensure that media (CDs, diskettes, tapes, etc.) are stored in locked containers or safes away from daily office traffic.
- Install heat and smoke detectors in your computer room — both above and below raised floors and ceilings.
- Ensure that fire suppression systems are installed but do not unnecessarily put personnel or equipment at risk.
- Install humidity and temperature controls in your computer room to ensure that equipment is not damaged by too much or too little moisture or too high temperatures.
- Have a policy against eating, drinking, or smoking near any computer equipment.
- Install antiglare filters on computer monitors where there might be a chance of someone seeing what is on the screen — these not only help reduce glare, but also can prevent anyone from seeing what is on the screen unless directly in front of the computer.
- Utilize media shredders and bulk erasers to destroy media or data before disposing of them.
- Utilize paper shredders or locked bins for paper that contains PHI.

## Mobile Computing Concerns

### *Wireless Networks*

Wireless local area networks (WLANs), sometimes referred to as Wi-Fi (wireless fidelity), are inexpensive and easy to implement. Medical professionals do not have to be tied to a desktop computer or take down notes on paper and have to reenter them later. They can just walk around with a laptop computer that is connected to a WLAN and enter or retrieve data immediately. Other benefits that WLANs offer are:

- Make work more convenient
- Can increase healthcare worker productivity
- Permit greater mobility in a healthcare environment
- Can come in handy during meetings by providing remote connectivity to the network
- Can be very cost effective, perhaps even cheaper than running regular copper or fiber network cabling
- Can bring network connectivity to otherwise difficult-to-access areas

Of course, along with such a useful and beneficial technology, there are various associated technical concerns and security risks, including:

#### Technical Concerns

- Speed concerns: 802.11b runs at a theoretical speed of 11 Mbps, and 802.11a and 802.11g run at 54 Mbps; however, as with other Ethernet network standards, real-world speed is typically only 40 to 60 percent of the theoretical speed, depending on various factors such as distance, types of access point (AP) antennas used, and whether or not encryption is enabled
- Reliability concerns: Coverage and signal strength are not always optimal; this also depends on distance, antenna, and other factors
- WLAN networks only support a limited number of hosts
- In-depth technical skills are needed for large WLAN design and deployment
- Network troubleshooting can be difficult
- Cross-vendor equipment compatibility problems

#### Security Concerns

- Practically anyone can purchase a WLAN AP from an electronics department store, bring it into the office, and immediately connect it to your network.
  - Difficult to know when these rogue APs are being used.
- Sensitive information (PHI) may go across WLANs — both inbound and outbound.

- PHI is also at risk while at rest if a malicious user gains access to the network via an insecure AP.
- The wired equivalent privacy encryption scheme (WEP) can be cracked.
- Telecommuters use WLANs and thus the associated threats and vulnerabilities now include remote computers.
  - Policy enforcement and system requirements must extend out to users' homes.
- The risk of lost data may outweigh any benefits — a risk analysis will help determine this.

### *What Can Be Done to Secure Wireless Networks?*

The WLAN standards bodies, along with the various WLAN vendors, have realized that for WLANs to be viable network connectivity alternatives in the future, these security issues must be addressed. Certain protocol standards as well as proprietary solutions are being developed and integrated into existing WLAN technologies as well as being built into emerging technologies. In addition, there are various well-known WLAN security best practices that, if followed, can help justify their use in a healthcare environment without worrying about major PHI threats and vulnerabilities. The following is a list of practical ways you can secure your WLANs to help ensure PHI is not at risk:

- Change default AP passwords.
- As with any other perimeter security device or critical host, use strong passwords on your APs.
- Use WEP — 40- or 128-bit will work the same because the WEP flaw is not related to encryption key length.
- Change the default WEP encryption keys (if any), and keep changing them on a regular basis.
- If your equipment supports it, use a unique WEP key for each session or at least for a limited number of frames.
- Use a VPN over your WLAN to eliminate WEP concerns.
- Use the newer WEP replacements found in the Wi-Fi Protected Access (WPA) standard and IEEE 802.11i security standard that utilize TKIP (Temporal Key Integrity Protocol) and EAP (Extensible Authentication Protocol) that address WEP's well-known vulnerabilities.
- Turn on MAC address access controls so you can specify which WLAN network cards can connect to your APs, if possible.
  - Just remember that MAC addresses can be forged or spoofed to allow unauthorized users on your network.
- Enable user authentication, if possible.
- Disable or at least change the default community string for SNMP.

- Change the default network numbers known as service set identifiers (SSIDs).
- Physical security of your APs is a must — like other network infrastructure devices, if they are compromised, your entire system can be compromised.
- Consider adjusting AP signal strength to prevent stray signals that others could tap into.
- Install firmware and WLAN network driver updates on a regular basis.
- Consider adding a WLAN firewall device — see Appendix C for references to some of these products.
- Test to see what happens when your APs lose power.
  - Can they be easily tapped into if physical access is available?
- Do not forget to turn on logging and monitor your APs.
  - Back up your log files or log to a remote syslog server.
- Save your AP configurations after any changes are made and store them somewhere safe and secure.
- Perform ongoing vulnerability assessments of your WLAN.
  - Assess your WLAN from the inside and outside.
- Ensure that client systems connecting to your WLAN meet these minimum requirements:
  - Anti-virus software installed
  - Personal firewall/IDS software installed
  - The latest OS and application patches
  - Strong passwords
  - Secure authentication
  - Automatic log-off
  - Secure physical location
  - Contingency plan if the computer will be storing PHI

Do not let the security issues associated with WLANs keep you from using them. If properly secured, WLAN benefits can definitely outweigh the risks. As Chuck Yeager has said, "You do not concentrate on risks. You concentrate on results. No risk is too great to prevent the necessary job from getting done." Some WLAN security best practices and a little common sense will enable you to securely use WLANs in your healthcare setting. WLAN convenience and ease of use, when managed properly, can help to increase the overall efficiency and quality of patient care.

### *Personal Digital Assistants*

It is increasingly common to see handheld computing devices, more commonly called PDAs (personal digital assistants), being used within healthcare facilities by care providers, as well as within organizations that are health plans and healthcare clearinghouses. If you are using PDAs to store or process PHI, or in some other way to provide patient care, then you must follow the HIPAA Privacy Rule and Security Rule requirements. PDAs can easily become the source of inadvertent disclosure of PHI.

PDAs are used for a wide range of activities, such as storing scheduling and contact information, accessing the Internet, executing clinical reference applications, among many other activities including the storage of patient information. Healthcare workers like the efficiency and ease with which this information may be downloaded into a network system to include within patient records. News releases and professional journals detail the growing trend of technology-savvy physicians who are increasingly using PDAs for patient care for such activities as a portable device to store patient treatment information.

It is likely that most of the PDAs used today within the healthcare industry were not formally issued by the organization, but instead were brought into the facility by workers as their own personal devices. Such use of technology and organizational information does not include the implementation of associated safeguards, such as standardized software and hardware, policies, procedures, and centralized support and maintenance, which are typically deployed within organizational supported solutions. These differences highlight risks related to protecting PHI associated with PDAs.

**How Are the PDAs Used?** If you decide to allow PDA use within your organization, you must consider specifically how they will be used. The HIPAA Privacy Rule and Security Rule regulate securing PHI on PDAs, and so the PDA must have safeguards implemented to guard against unauthorized use. In general, PHI may only be accessed and used within covered entities for appropriate treatment, payment, or healthcare operations purposes. So, physician-to-physician consultation for treating patients and sharing PHI stored on their PDAs is an acceptable use of PHI. However, the size and portability of a PDA make it extremely easy to lose or misplace, or to be stolen. Additionally, the information stored on the PHI must be secured so that others physically obtaining the device cannot get access to the PHI. Another consideration is the transmission of data from a PDA to the computer network. Information may be intercepted while the PDAs are transferring information to the network. The risks increase dramatically when the transmissions are wireless. Sending PHI from a PDA to another individual outside of the organization is most certainly covered by the Security Rule requirements. Encryption and other access controls requirements may be established, and the transmissions must be planned and appropriately coordinated with the business associates.

**PDA Risks.** Used correctly, PDAs and other mobile computing devices such as laptops can increase efficiency and potentially decrease the rate of medical and insurance errors. However, PDAs are inherently less secure than traditional desktop and mainframe computers. Their size and portability creates many risks, including but not limited to the following:

- Theft or loss
- Lack of passwords or bad password management
- Lack of file access controls
- Viruses infecting PDAs and subsequently networks
- Unauthorized network access using stolen PDAs
- Wireless transmission concerns
- Network bandwidth issues can negatively impact networks to which PDAs connect
- Device retrieval from terminated employees can be very difficult

PDA users must be responsible for knowing the information stored and processed on their PDAs. Although it may be impractical for each person to know exactly the files that are on their PDAs, they must know the types of information, especially as it relates to PHI, that they have on their PDAs. This is necessary to determine the information that has potentially been compromised in case of loss, theft, or inappropriate use, and to activate the appropriate mitigation procedures.

**Securing Health Information on PDAs.** HIPAA does not specifically state requirements for the use of PDAs. However, their security and safeguard requirements apply to PDAs. If you are using PDAs within your organization, or plan to use them, you need to establish policies, procedures, and training covering their use to ensure the security of the information processed and stored on them.

Consider establishing the following directives within your PDA policies and procedures to ensure the security and privacy of PHI on PDAs. Determine the feasibility of each of these suggestions based on your business and environment.

- Management must approve the installation and use of synchronization software from corporate systems to and from PDAs prior to use.
- PDA users must participate in PDA security and use training prior to using the PDA.
- Each PDA user must sign a PDA use contract or agreement.
- PDAs containing PHI must be physically secured when left unattended.
- Corporate-approved access controls and encryption must be used on PDAs containing PHI.
- A central inventory of all information stored, or allowed to be stored, on PDAs must be maintained.
- Employees must back up data, using an approved corporate method, on a regular basis to avoid loss of valuable PHI.

- PDAs used for job responsibilities are subject to audits just like any other electronic device, even if employee owned.
- PDAs must use centralized synchronization on the corporate network. Local synchronization is not allowed.
- All PDAs owned by the organization must display ownership information and log-in banner on start up. Information to be displayed includes the following:
  - User name
  - Organization name
  - Business address
  - Business phone
  - Approved log-in notice regarding ownership and monitoring
- Power-on passwords must be used on all PDAs containing PHI.
- Passwords must be used to enable data transfers to and from the corporate network and the PDA.
- PDA passwords must comply with corporate password policies.
- Network system passwords are not allowed to be stored on PDAs.
- PDAs must be configured to automatically power off following a maximum of 10 minutes of inactivity (less time is recommended). A password must be required to reestablish access with the PDA.
- Individuals are not allowed to share PDAs or PDA passwords.
- PDA passwords must be different than other passwords used on the corporate network.
- PDAs are not allowed to connect to noncorporate networks (such as the Internet) simultaneously while connected to the corporate network.
- Files loaded onto PDAs must be in PDF format.
- Only corporate-approved applications can be used on PDAs.
- PDAs that are lost or stolen, or belong to terminated personnel, must be immediately locked out from network access.
- Only certain classification(s) of data are allowed to be accessible by PDAs (this requires that you have a data classification process in place).
- Dynamic (single-use) passwords must be used on all PDAs (e.g., via tokens, etc.).
- Anti-virus software must be used on all PDAs.
- PDAs may not be used in wireless modes.
- Wireless transmission from PDAs must be encrypted.
- Only PDAs provided and configured by the organization can be used to process and access corporate information and PHI.
- All PDAs used must be approved by the Security Officer or other IT administrator or manager.
- Information about all PDAs used must be maintained in a central inventory. This inventory info must include person's name, title,

department, phone number, manager, and handheld model and serial number.

- All PDAs must be covered by the corporate-approved PDA insurance.
- Each PDA must have a corporate security tracking tag attached.
- Software must be implemented on PDAs to create an audit trail of system activity, including log-in attempts, security incidents, and attempts to access files containing PHI.
- PDAs that will no longer be used must be wiped using disk-wiping software to clear out or overwrite the PHI. If this is not possible, the PDA must be physically destroyed, or the storage removed and destroyed.

## Summary

The tips we have provided in this chapter are not comprehensive, but we believe we have touched on some of the more important elements. What we have provided here is a lot of information to take in at once. Do not let this intimidate you. If you build your HIPAA-compliant technology infrastructure a little at a time and show reasonable effort, you will do fine.

Ultimately, there is no such thing as a 100-percent secure technology infrastructure, so do not strive for absolute perfection; strive for the most possible within your organization. Also, keep in mind that you cannot buy a complete, prepackaged HIPAA-compliance solution, no matter what vendors tell you. All of these technology considerations must be integrated with solid policies, procedures, and daily business practices to ensure HIPAA compliance.

Keep in mind that security cannot effectively be added onto a system after it has been installed. We are not saying it is impossible — it is just very difficult. Instead, strive to design security into your technology systems and infrastructure from the beginning wherever possible. It will be cheaper and much easier to manage in the long run. Also, we cannot stress enough how important it is to keep in mind the scalable and flexible characteristics of HIPAA. As long as reasonable efforts are being made to protect PHI, you should have no problems attaining and maintaining HIPAA compliance.

## Chapter 21: Practical Checklist

- Perform a risk analysis to determine what PHI threats and vulnerabilities exist, which policies and procedures will have to be developed, and which technologies will have to be used to enforce your policies and facilitate your procedures.
- Remember that firewalls are not enough — you must have a layered security architecture to ensure "defense in depth" in the event one or more security controls fails.

- Encrypt all e-mails if there is a chance they will contain PHI — e-mails sent and stored in clear text may present too many vulnerabilities.
- Harden your OSs to ensure they are not vulnerable to attack.
- WLANs are fine if they are secured properly.
- The Security Rule requirements cover computer-based faxes and the Privacy Rule requirements cover hard-copy faxes.
- Do a walk-through of your facility and assess your physical security.
- All other security mechanisms can be defeated by lax physical security — make sure all electronic devices are under secure control.
- Determine if and how PDAs are being used within your organization.
- Establish PDA usage policies and procedures.
- Specify acceptable PDA hardware and software to use for processing and storing PHI.
- Determine how to reclaim PDAs from terminated personnel.

# Chapter 22
# Crafting Security Incident Procedures and Contingency Plans

## Background

The Security Rule sets forth very high-level standards and implementation specifications for dealing with information security incidents and unexpected information systems emergencies. Security incident procedures and contingency plans, as the Security Rule refers to these, are two different yet closely related areas of information security that are absolutely critical to the confidentiality, integrity, and availability of protected health information (PHI). They both define who, what, when, where, why, and how in planning for and responding to critical incidents involving your healthcare information systems. You certainly cannot expect to defend against all security incidents and disasters, but you do need to plan for the ones that could likely occur. In this chapter, we will explain the differences between security incident procedures and contingency plans, expand upon what is required for these two standards by the Security Rule, and provide some practical advice and checklists so you can ensure that your healthcare information systems are well protected from events such as hacker attacks, virus outbreaks, and natural disasters.

## Handling Security Incidents

Computer security incidents are rarely thought of until they occur. In most situations, information security threats are not taken seriously until an organization suffers damage or loss. Security incidents can be caused by anything from malicious users inside or outside your network to a rogue virus or worm outbreak that disables a system or deletes critical healthcare information. There are massive amounts of serious computer security incidents that occur on a daily basis. Most of these either go unnoticed, unreported, or simply do not gain a spot in the media headlines.

Security incident occurrences are becoming more frequent due to the ease of performing computer attacks and not getting caught, the increasing

---

The information and opinions provided in this book do not constitute or substitute for legal or other professional advice.

number of vulnerabilities found in the software we use, and the widespread use of the Internet. A majority of organizations do not take information security seriously, and the bad guys know that. Do not fret. Short of unplugging your computers or not using them at all, there is no way to completely secure PHI. You can, however, put a set of procedures in place, which, combined with your other information security initiatives, will allow you to be assured that your systems are reasonably secured and you are well prepared to respond to an incident when that time does come.

An incident response program basically requires forming a team, developing incident handling and reporting procedures, testing those procedures, and being able to formally respond to security incidents when they occur. You may recall from Chapter 11 that a security incident is defined in the Security Rule as "the attempted or successful unauthorized access, use, disclosure, modification, destruction, or interference with system operations in an information system." Given this, we provide guidance on developing procedures that will allow you to effectively respond if a security incident occurs. These security incident program building blocks are not application or operating system dependent. We have kept them at a high enough level so they can be applied within any organization yet detailed enough to match up with the Security Rule requirements. For other security incident resources, please refer to Appendix C.

### Security Incident Procedure Essentials

When the time comes to respond to a computer security incident, an expert team and a solid set of procedures must be in place to successfully maintain the confidentiality, integrity, and availability of your PHI and business operations. The following sections outline the Security Rule implementation specifications for security incidents along with some things you can do to meet these requirements.

### *Response and Reporting (Required)*

The Security Rule lists security incident response and reporting as a required implementation specification. Response and reporting is defined in the Security Rule as:

- Identify and respond to suspected or known security incidents
- To the extent practicable, mitigate harmful effects of security incidents that are known to the covered entity
- Document security incidents and their outcomes

Now consider the individual implementation specifications in Exhibit 1 for this standard and define what can be done to meet them.

Once you completely document your security incident procedures, you should securely store them in a safe place that will be accessible to every

## Exhibit 1.  Individual Implementation Specifications

**Identify and respond to suspected or known security incidents**

- Security incident team
  - First and foremost, you must have a team in place that can help plan for and formally respond to security incidents. This team, sometimes referred to as a Computer Emergency Response Team (CERT), or Computer Security Incident Response Team (CSIRT), should consist of key internal employees who will formally respond to security incidents. Keep in mind that responding to security incidents is not just an IT issue. Anyone that plays a key role in your information systems and healthcare operations should be included. The following is a list of people you need to consider having on your team:
    - HIPAA Security Officer
    - HIPAA Privacy Officer
    - Network or Security Administrator
    - Security Manager or Executive
    - Risk Management Executive
    - Chief Information Officer (CIO)
    - Legal Counsel
    - Public relations representative
    - Local, state, or federal law enforcement cyber crime investigator
  - Be sure to document in detail what each team member's roles and responsibilities are. If you choose to outsource your incident response to a consultant or other firm, be sure that someone in your organization still has ownership and responsibility for coordinating security incident response (most likely the HIPAA Security Officer).
  - Document each team member's full contact information, including:
    - Home phone number
    - Friend, relative, or spouse home or work number, if possible
    - Mobile phone number
    - Pager number
    - Personal e-mail address, if possible
    - Instant messaging address, if possible
  - Determine which methods the team members will use to communicate in the event of a security incident.
- Security incident detection system. This could include one or more of the following items, some of which were discussed in detail in Chapter 21:
  - IDS
  - Network analyzer
  - Anti-virus software
  - Log file monitoring system
  - Manual (human) monitoring of log files
    - Only use this as a last resort. This might not be what you want a full-time employee doing all day! Besides, it is extremely tedious, boring, and attacks are easy to miss.
- Formal response procedures. These procedures clearly define what steps your CSIRT will take when a security incident is detected. They should include the following at a minimum:

**Exhibit 1. Individual Implementation Specifications (Continued)**

- What criteria will be used to determine if a security incident has occurred
  - IDS alerts, system unavailability, data loss, etc.
- The order in which CSIRT members will be contacted
  - This should also include every member's detailed contact information
- How the security incident will be analyzed
  - What methods (IDS, log analysis, network analyzer, etc.)
  - Which tools will be used in the analysis
- Documentation on how you are currently collecting and storing your log files before the security incident occurred
  - The word "before" is critical here. If you intend to pursue a formal investigation and prosecution of the perpetrator(s), you must ensure that logging is enabled before an incident occurs. If you start logging after you suspect a security incident has occurred, your logs may not be considered business records maintained in the course of normal business activities and thus may not be admissible in court.
- How you will communicate with the media, your customers, and the general public
  - You should prepare a communications plan in advance of a security incident so that everyone is not scrambling to figure what to do and what to say.
  - Be sure to include who will communicate the message of a security incident (internal or external PR, HIPAA Security Officer, etc.), when it will be communicated, what will be said, and what is being done to resolve the issue and prevent further damage.
- How your team will handle potential evidence
  - How log files will be saved and stored
  - Who has primary responsibility for preserving evidence and leading the forensics collection?
  - Will an image be made of the drives?
  - Will an expert cyber crime investigator be involved?
  - What will be the chain of custody if a formal investigation is deemed necessary due to major losses or criminal activity?
- What steps will be taken to restore or rebuild systems
  - How backups will be used
  - What other systems may be put in place of the victim systems?
  - How OSs, applications, and configurations will be reinstalled and reset
  - Estimated timeline to operate at a minimal level
  - Estimated timeline to be back to business as usual
  - Who will help with your recovery efforts?

**Mitigate, to the extent practicable, harmful effects of security incidents that are known to the covered entity**

- How you will protect your healthcare information systems from further intrusion or damage:
  - Disconnect affected systems
  - Reboot affected systems
  - Place affected systems on different network segments
  - Patching or somehow fixing the vulnerability

**Exhibit 1. Individual Implementation Specifications (Continued)**

**Document security incidents and their outcomes**
- Document in as much detail as possible:
  - — What happened
  - — When it happened
  - — The symptoms of the incident
  - — Systems or information that were damaged, lost, or stolen
  - — Outcomes of the investigation
- Follow-up actions with all members of the CSIRT and any others involved to discuss lessons learned and how to prevent this incident in the future

---

member of your Computer Security Incident Response Team (CSIRT) when a security incident occurs. Because your business operations may change from time to time, remember to test these procedures and manage them on an ongoing basis as you would any other information security documentation.

## Basics of Contingency Planning

Contingency planning involves preparing for the worst — anything from a system outage to outright loss of an entire database or data center. Although it is extremely difficult to protect against something that has not happened, certain fundamental steps can be taken to mitigate risks to information systems and critical business functions. Being unprepared for an information systems disaster can mean severe business interruption or even failure.

Although the terms "disaster recovery" and "business continuity" are often used interchangeably, technically there is a difference. Disaster recovery concerns the retrieval or recreation of information systems and business functionality to the state they were in before a disaster occurred. Business continuity refers to maintaining a minimum level of business operations in order to fulfill critical operating requirements in the midst of a disaster or other type of operational or systems disruption. Despite the differences in terminology, the concepts for implementing and managing successful disaster recovery and business continuity plans are basically the same.

As covered in Chapter 11, the Security Rule contains a contingency plan standard that requires establishing "policies and procedures for responding to an emergency or other occurrence (for example, fire, vandalism, system failure, and natural disaster) that damages systems that contain electronic protected health information." The specific implementation specifications for this standard include:

- Data backup plan
- Disaster recovery plan
- Emergency mode operation plan
- Testing and revision procedures
- Applications and data criticality analysis

Now consider the individual implementation specifications for this standard along with what can be done to meet them.

### Data Backup Plan (Required)

The Security Rule defines the data backup plan requirement as "establish and implement procedures to create and maintain retrievable exact copies of electronic protected health information." Keep in mind that this rule (like all of the security rules) is flexible and scalable, depending on your organization's size. The following suggestions, although certainly not comprehensive for all situations, should be a good starting point for your data backup plan procedures.

- Specific backup technologies used
  - Floppy disks (Don't laugh — this is better than nothing!)
  - Tape backups
  - Optical disks (CDs and DVDs)
  - Mirrored hard disks in servers and workstations
  - Redundant Network Attached Storage (NAS) devices
  - Redundant Storage Area Network (SAN) devices
  - Internet-based backups (where data is transmitted to a storage facility via your Internet connection)
  - Software or other methods used to create the backups
- Specific backup methodologies used
  - When data is backed up
    - In real-time (constantly)
    - Hourly
    - Daily
    - Weekly
    - Monthly
  - Backup media (tape, disk, etc.) rotation schedule
    - Use the same media every day
    - Use different media every day
    - Have media labeled for each day, such as Monday–Thursday
    - Have other media labeled for Fridays, such as Friday1 through Friday4
  - Type(s) of backups performed
    - *Full:* All data is backed up

- *Incremental:* Backs up only the files that have changed since the last full or incremental backup and marks the files as being backed up (clears the archive file attribute)
- *Differential:* Backs up only the files that have changed since the last full or incremental backup and does not mark the files as being backed up (does not clear the archive file attribute)
  - Consider backing up your applications and database schemas, especially if any customization has been performed
- Backup management and media storage
  - Assigned backup responsibility
    - Who will manage your backups on an ongoing basis?
  - Backup testing methodology; this is very critical to ensure that your backup media actually contain valid data and will be reliable when you need them
  - Where the backup media will be stored, which is very critical to ensure that backups are not destroyed in the event of a disaster
    - In-house vault
    - Offsite backup storage facility
    - Someone's home (not preferred but better than nothing)

### Disaster Recovery Plan (Required)

Disaster recovery concerns the restoration or recreation of information systems and business functionality to the state they were in before a disaster occurred. Disaster recovery plans should address who is responsible for the information systems and various business operations; what information systems, PHI, and business functions are involved; and when the plan should be invoked. Keep in mind that there are parallels between disaster recovery and security incident response. If a security incident is bad enough, it could be considered a disaster. For example, if a malicious user deleted an entire patient database, this could lead to some, if not most, services coming to an abrupt halt. This might be considered a state of disaster for your organization.

All of the implementation specifications required for your contingency plan can help with your overall disaster recovery plan. The following is a set of minimum requirements needed to establish a disaster recovery plan to define the who, what, and when of disaster management.

- Disaster recovery team
  - Similar to your security incident team, you must have people in place that can help plan for and respond to information systems disasters. In the same fashion, anyone that plays a key role in your information systems and healthcare operations should be included. The following is a list of people you need to consider having on your team:

- • HIPAA Security Officer
- • HIPAA Privacy Officer
- • Network or Security Administrator (or both)
- • Security Manager or Executive
- • Risk Management Executive
- • Operations Manager
- • Legal Counsel
- • Public Relations Representative
- − Be sure to document in detail each team member's roles and responsibilities. If you choose to outsource your disaster recovery to a specialty firm, be sure that someone in your organization still has ownership and responsibility for coordinating disaster recovery (most likely your HIPAA Security Officer).
- − Document each team member's full contact information, including:
  - • Home phone number
  - • Friend, relative, or spouse home or work number, if possible
  - • Mobile phone number
  - • Pager number
  - • Personal e-mail address, if possible
  - • Instant messaging address, if possible
- − Determine which methods the team members will use to communicate in the event of a disaster.
- • Anticipate that a disaster will occur eventually and plan for it.
  - − The disaster recovery team should consider beforehand:
    - • What could go wrong
    - • What it would do in the event of a disaster
    - • What is the worst that can happen
    - • What is likely to happen
  - − Ensure that critical applications, systems, and data are distributed among facilities that are reasonably easy to get to but not so close that they could be affected by the same disaster.
- • Determine which information systems and business functions are involved.
  - − Most of the systems and business functions involved along with the specific PHI that must be considered will have been determined during your information risk assessment.
  - − More specifically, you can perform a business impact analysis that is outlined in the Applications and Data Criticality Analysis section; this will help you obtain a detailed inventory of specific information, business processes, and other assets that must be protected and thus made part of this plan.
  - − Ensure that your system and data inventories and network diagrams are kept current.

- When the disaster recovery plan should be invoked
  - Your organization might categorize different levels of disasters such as:
    - A hacker or disgruntled employee attack that causes system outages or severe data losses
    - A computer virus, worm, or other malicious code that infects critical information systems and renders them unusable
    - A hardware failure on a critical computer system
    - An environmental catastrophe such as a tornado or fire
    - A building that is physically damaged or destroyed
  - It should be top priority to ensure that people are protected and it is safe to implement your plan.
  - When a disaster occurs, do not react impulsively and immediately; stop and think before acting.
  - Get the facts first and find out:
    - What has occurred
    - When it occurred
    - How it occurred
    - Who and what was involved
- How you will communicate with the media, your customers, and the general public
  - You should prepare a communications plan in advance of a disaster so that public relations decisions do not have to be made during a crisis and your organization will know what to say.
  - Be sure to include:
    - Who will communicate the message of the disaster (internal or external PR)
    - When it will be communicated
    - What will be said
    - What is being done to resolve the crisis and get the business back on track
- Confirm that emergency shelter and other staple items are considered in your overall plan.
  - Must consider the following items:
    - Shelter
    - Food
    - Water
    - Clothing
    - Backup communications devices such as mobile phones
  - Determine who will facilitate all of this.
- What is the process of restoring data
  - Who will do it?
  - What systems will the data be restored to?
  - What data is most critical and will be needed first?
  - How will data be tested for proper restoration and integrity?

- A major objective of your disaster recovery planning should be to develop a plan that can be implemented by practically anyone in case the disaster recovery team becomes incapacitated and the organization's leadership becomes unreachable.
- Distribute copies of the written plans to everyone involved and also store extra copies in an offsite, fireproof vault to which each team member has access.

### Emergency Mode Operation Plan (Required)

Emergency mode operation is essentially business continuity. As stated in the Security Rule, the goal here is to "establish procedures to enable continuation of critical business processes for protection of the security of electronic health information while operating in emergency mode."

There is a great amount of overlap between disaster recovery and business continuity, including forming a team, and determining which systems and business processes are involved and when the plan should be invoked. These may be identical for both of these implementation specifications or perhaps combined into one document. The following items are specific to business continuity planning and should be considered in developing your overall emergency mode operation plan:

- Based on the results of your risk analysis, document the systems that are absolutely mission critical to keep your business running.
- Establish written policies, contracts, and service level agreements with third-party hosting, collocation, telecommunications, and Internet service providers that facilitate business continuity.
  - You will want to ensure that your service providers (if any) have the ability to provide redundant systems, Internet, or WAN connections, phone systems, and even technical expertise to assist in a crisis; this may involve:
    - *Hot sites:* Facilities that have fully redundant systems that can take over within minutes
    - *Warm sites:* Facilities that have partially ready computer systems such as hardware and network connections but no data or applications installed
    - *Cold sites:* Facilities that have no equipment, applications, or data but are ready to be moved into
- Confirm that not only an emergency shelter is available, but also that an offsite work facility is free to move into.
  - Must consider the following items:
    - Offsite office space
    - Backup communications devices such as mobile phones
    - Computers
    - Business supplies

### *Testing and Revision Procedure (Addressable)*

The Security Rule states that testing and revision procedures must be in place for periodic testing and revision of contingency plans. This is an addressable implementation specification. Considering the criticality of contingency plans, we cannot imagine a scenario where they should not be tested and updated on an ongoing basis. Your information systems and business operations will change over time thus requiring future testing and updating as necessary. Otherwise, you might not know that your plans are not going to work until the worst possible time. Here are a few tips on developing your contingency plan testing and revision procedures:

- Develop testing standards
  - What will be tested
    - Team communication plans
    - Data center failover plans
    - Data backup plans
    - Data restoration plans
  - If your information systems and business processes change regularly, consider performing a business impact analysis on a regular basis
  - How often testing will occur
- Test plans at least annually and when major systems changes occur
  - Document and review your test results
  - Update the plans as needed
  - Analyze plans on an ongoing basis to ensure alignment with current business objectives and requirements

### *Applications and Data Criticality Analysis (Addressable)*

The Security Rule requires CEs to "assess the relative criticality of specific applications and data in support of other contingency plan components." This analysis is also known as a business impact analysis. This will help you to document and understand the interdependencies among business processes and determine how the business would be affected by an information systems outage. The Security Rule states that this is only a required implementation specification, but just like with the testing and revision procedure, we highly recommend integrating this step into your overall plan and your initial and ongoing risk analyses. In fact, we cannot imagine being able to effectively develop contingency plans without the information discovered in this analysis. Here are a few key steps to keep in mind when performing an applications and data criticality analysis:

- Take an inventory of information systems assets such as computer hardware, software, applications, and data (including PHI).

- Identify single points of failure within the information systems infrastructure.
  - For example, this could include the following:
    - A single computer or server that all employees rely on that only has a single hard drive as opposed to mirrored drives or a redundant array of inexpensive disks (RAID), or a single power supply as opposed to dual power supplies
    - A single Internet connection
    - A single administrator-equivalent user ID
    - Only one network administrator or manager that knows all of the system passwords
- Identify critical applications, systems, and data.
  - What systems are must-haves
  - What systems are needed but not critical
  - What systems are not absolutely necessary until your team can restore business as usual
- Prioritize key business functions.
  - Business functions to consider:
    - Emergency healthcare operations
    - Healthcare claims submissions
    - Supply chains
    - Lines of communication between patients and their caregivers

**Moving Forward**

Security incident and contingency plans are not only HIPAA requirements, they are also an essential component of an overall information risk management program that makes good business sense. When developed and implemented properly, they are key to information systems and business survival. Moving forward, covered entities can leverage the technological benefits inherent in the Internet's distributed computing environment for offsite data backups and redundant standby equipment to reduce the impact of a disaster.

Long term, it is much less expensive to implement proper security incident and contingency plans than it is to restore business operations and customer confidence. Computer intrusions and disasters cannot be stopped completely; however, if something does happen and the proper plans are in place, covered entities will know they have a contingency plan to follow to return to business as usual as quickly and efficiently as possible.

## Chapter 22: Practical Checklist

- Have you formed your security incident team?
- Have you formed your contingency plan teams?
- Have you documented everyone's full contact information?
- Do you have systems in place to detect security incidents?
- Have you thought about all the different disaster scenarios that could occur?
- Have you performed a business impact analysis to determine what information and business processes are must-haves and which ones are optional during a crisis?
- Are offsite office facilities and emergency shelters available to move into in the event of a crisis?
- Do you have plans in place to test and update your security incident and contingency plans on an ongoing basis?

# Chapter 23
# Outsourcing Information Technology Services

## Background

Outsourcing is certainly nothing new to the healthcare industry. Healthcare executives and HIPAA officers are constantly facing new projects and technological changes, including compliance initiatives, that force them to rethink their information technology (IT) strategies. Healthcare in particular is faced not only with having to embrace the information technologies of the twenty-first century but also to perform overall healthcare operations more efficiently. As mentioned previously in this book, this is the backbone of HIPAA Administrative Simplification. With the growing HIPAA compliance pressures, there simply is not enough manpower and expertise in-house to get everything done, especially when it comes to information security. According to the Spring 2003 U.S. Healthcare Industry Quarterly HIPAA Compliance Survey published by HIMSS and Phoenix Health Systems, 44 percent of respondents are currently outsourcing various HIPAA initiatives. Most of these outsourced services are in the areas of HIPAA assessments, project planning, and user awareness. Even if your organization has never outsourced IT or information security services, you might be able to replicate the proven outsourcing methodologies used in other functions in your organization to make outsourcing work for you here as well.

## Reasons to Consider Outsourcing

The "make or buy" decision on IT services is one that every covered entity (CE) must consider. For many CEs, there are simply too many complex HIPAA and information security issues to handle them all alone. Information technology and security are critical functions of all CEs, regardless of size. If your organization is like most, your protected health information

---

The information and opinions provided in this book do not constitute or substitute for legal or other professional advice.

(PHI) is continuously vulnerable. You can put the policies, procedures, and technologies in place that we discuss in this book; however, they will still need constant nurturing and management. Sooner or later, one or more people will have to get involved in managing your security infrastructure. You will have to ask yourself if it makes good business sense to tie up your internal resources on managing these ongoing initiatives. Also, you will need to think long and hard about whether or not you and your team should be or want to be on call 24/7 to respond to those inevitable late-night security incidents.

Outsourcing can help your organization focus on what it does best — providing healthcare services. You must have a clear understanding of your organization's abilities in the IT and information security departments before moving forward. Here are some reasons to consider outsourcing your IT and information security work:

- Information technology, and specifically information security, is not a core competency of your business.
- Your current staff does not have the proper skill sets.
- Attracting and retaining employees with the proper skills is difficult.
- Outsourcing can make it easier to manage ongoing costs by allowing you to convert otherwise variable costs into fixed costs.
- It can be cheaper than hiring full-time staff to do it.
- If done properly, it can help reduce the overall cost of the IT function.
- Ongoing staff training costs are skyrocketing.
- Outside expertise is available and willing to help.
- Outside experts have less exposure to internal politics.
- Outside experts can provide fresh and unbiased insight into what really needs to be done to secure your information and help you toward compliance.
- Gives access to the latest information technologies and aggregated expertise.
- It can allow you to obtain network trending intelligence that otherwise would be impossible to acquire.

**What Functions to Outsource**

Before outsourcing, you must first determine your specific needs and what makes the most business sense. You can outsource some or all of your IT and information security work. Just keep in mind that HIPAA requires information security responsibility to be assigned to one individual within the organization. This person can manage and oversee HIPAA security initiatives but certainly has the flexibility to outsource the needed services.

Do not outsource for the sake of outsourcing. You must look at this important decision from both a strategic and a tactical perspective. Do you really need to outsource? If so, then why? Is it because of lack of internal expertise? Time? Money? You must then determine: (1) what areas you need to outsource and in what capacity, (2) how long the outsourcing will need to last, and (3) guidelines to which your outsourcing vendors must adhere. All of this should be documented in Service Level Agreements (SLAs), which need to be mutually beneficial, must clearly articulate the opportunity and issues, and show the benefits to both parties. They should be flexible but at the same time outline specific deliverables, target dates, and expectations on responsiveness. They must be reasonable for both parties, with penalties clearly outlined for breach of contract or sub-par service. Also, be sure to outline specific incentives to encourage the highest levels of performance.

The following is a list of areas that can be outsourced to help you with your HIPAA compliance:

- HIPAA Security Rule gap analysis
- Risk analyses
  - Penetration testing
  - Vulnerability assessments
  - Initial audits
- Security policy and procedure development
- Network infrastructure design, installation, and maintenance
- Server and workstation security
- Web and application security
- Software development, quality assurance, and maintenance
- Security awareness and training
- Security planning and strategy development
- Security incident plan creation and documentation
- Contingency plan creation and documentation
- Data center operations
- Network security monitoring
- Physical security design, installation, and maintenance
- Security incident response and forensics
- Ongoing security audits

## What to Look for in Outsourcing Firms

Given that IT and information security is one of the most critical functions of your business, you will need to make sure you find quality vendors with which to partner. Expertise can vary widely, so you must ask questions and check references from several potential vendors. Look at their credentials and focus more on experience than certifications. Consider the following certifications as a baseline requirement:

- CISSP® (Certified Information Systems Security Professional, sponsored by ISC²)
- CISA® (Certified Information Systems Auditor, sponsored by ISACA)

- CISM™ (Certified Information Security Manager, sponsored by ISACA)
- CHS (Certified in Healthcare Security, sponsored by HIMSS)
- GIAC (Global Information Assurance Certification, sponsored by SANS)
- Security+™ (sponsored by the Computing Technology Industry Association)
- IAM (Infosec Assessment Methodologies, sponsored by the National Security Agency)
- Various vendor-specific certifications

Whatever you do, do not let certifications lead you to believe you are getting top-notch experts every time. There are other factors to consider such as technical and business experience, communication skills, and documentation skills. Besides, nothing can ever substitute for real-world experience.

The more important the outsourced function, the more control you will want to maintain. Given the criticality of IT and information security not only regarding HIPAA compliance, but also the fact that PHI needs to remain confidential, intact, and available at all times, you will certain want to maintain input and control over what is done by your outsourcing vendors. Look for the following characteristics in your potential outsourcing vendors:

- Trustworthy, reliable people you can work with every day
- Long track record of integrity — check several references
- Proven expertise — again, check several references
- Flexible people that can change project direction and scope (within reason) when necessary
- Avoid know-it-alls — it is practically impossible to know everything about all aspects of IT and information security; they need to know their limits and must be willing to pull in other subject matter experts when necessary
- Team of resources (either internal or subcontract) they can pull in almost immediately and rely on when more resources are needed
- Specialized expertise in information security and preferably business management and healthcare as well
- Solid and proven methodologies for all the services they perform
- Open to recommending and implementing open-source, commercial off-the-shelf (COTS), and proprietary or in-house solutions
- Vendor neutrality so there is no conflict of interest in them selling you products that are a better fit for them than they are for you
- Reasonable and competitive rates for the particular service and expertise being provided

### Questions to Ask Outsourcing Firms

- How will you bill for projects — hourly or by the project? (Both may be fine — you just need to know up front.)
- What is your regular maintenance schedule to apply patches on our systems? (This needs to be done frequently — very soon following patch release.)
- Do you have an incident response plan in place to handle intrusions or disasters related to your own information systems that could affect our organization? (Their systems could be housing critical data that your organization is dependent on — make sure they have a "Plan B.")
- Will you sign a HIPAA BA contract? (If the answer is no, you will be forced to look elsewhere.)
- How will you determine and evaluate the technologies and products we need? Is it based on our specific requirements, or certain vendor relationships you have? (Look for any signs of vendor bias and sales opportunities that you do not consider in your organization's best interest that take from your bottom line and add to theirs.)
- Are your solutions typically open-source, commercial off-the-shelf (COTS), or proprietary? (They should be open to all three, depending on what is the best fit for your organization.)
- How do you plan to keep me informed regarding project status, milestones, reviews, and overall documentation? (They must have a formal, documented methodology that will keep you in the loop at all times.)
- How does your staff keep up with new security threats and vulnerabilities? (Look for answers such as subscribing to security bulletins, attending security conferences, reading information security trade publications, collaborating with colleagues and other companies, etc.)
- Does your organization have both general liability and professional liability insurance? What other services do you offer? Do you try to offer everything to everyone, or are you focused on information security? Are general IT services your core competency? Do you focus solely on information security? Are you healthcare-industry specific? (Keep in mind that greater specialization can result in a better fit for your organization's HIPAA needs.)
- If you will be monitoring my network, how and what will you monitor?
  - Do you simply monitor devices, or can you monitor my entire network? (Look for an organization that can monitor anything you have or may add in the future, including applications and database systems. You do not want to limit your network growth to their technical constraints and abilities.)

- Do you only monitor one technology (firewall, intrusion-detection systems, etc.) or one vendor's products? (A direct tie-in to your specific products can be a plus, but you do not want to be limited to just one vendor. They must be flexible and willing to work with virtually all products that your needs require.)
- Will you also monitor for network performance, etc., that can help me assess our future growth and needs? (This can be a nice value-added service.)
- How do you keep abreast of and monitor for newly discovered threats and vulnerabilities? (Look for partnerships with other public (e.g., CERT) and private (partner company) security alert systems.)
- Do you monitor for unknown threats and vulnerabilities? If so, what techniques are used? (Look for behavior-based analysis that can search out anomalies in specific protocols and applications that would not otherwise be detected.)
- How do you assess logs, etc., for attacks? Is it all automated? Is any of it done manually? (There should be a combination of both automated and manual assessments, because neither is method perfect or foolproof.)
- If a security anomaly or breach is detected, how will you respond? (There should be a formal security incident plan that you can review. This plan needs to be integrated with your security incident plan.)
- Is this service scalable regardless of how large my network grows? (If their systems cannot scale, then yours may be limited as well.)
- How is data correlated and analyzed to pick up specific anomalies? Do you look for specific trends across various systems?
- How will the data be presented to me? (They need to have formal procedures for presenting you with their ongoing reports; hard copy and Web-based are preferable.)
- What expertise will my team need to have to read and interpret your monitoring data? (The reports should be presented in a nontechnical fashion that anyone can read and understand. If this is not done, it somewhat defeats the purpose of outsourcing your security monitoring altogether.)
- What requirements will you have of our network? (You need to know if your network will have to be reconfigured or adapted to fit their monitoring technologies.)

**Common Outsourcing Mistakes**

Be sure not to do any of the following common actions and activities:

- Outsourcing solely to save money — remember that outsourcing costs can be greater, especially up front
- Outsourcing to fix a management or operations problem that should be addressed internally
- Viewing outsourcing with short time perspective without thinking about long-term goals, benefits, and relationships
- Believing that your internal team has the time, energy, and wherewithal to handle everything
- Not running background checks on the people that will have access to PHI
- Failure to look at the context in which outsourcing will be done — outsourcing must be fit into the bigger picture of your organization's overall mission
- Not requiring your outsourcing firms to keep logs of what they do
- Not ensuring that solid SLAs are put in place that can facilitate quick problem resolution
- Not monitoring the performance and stability of outsourcing vendors to stay ahead of any organization problems they may have
- Not having a fall-back plan in case the outsourcing vendors have trouble
- Relying on one vendor, which may amplify any problems that occur
- Failure to communicate the decision to outsource to current employees
- Not keeping upper management up to date on outsourcing initiatives
- Not thinking through possible negative scenarios that could occur when outsourcing; it could be that outsourcing is really not worth the risks or the best option for your organization after all

## Chapter 23: Practical Checklist

- Determine whether or not IT and information security is your organization's core competency — if not, consider outsourcing.
- Do not outsource for the sake of outsourcing — make a good business case for it based on skill sets, time, and money.
- Determine what areas of information security need to be outsourced.
- Consider hiring an outside firm at least to help you get started on your HIPAA compliance efforts.
- Perform your due diligence in interviewing and selecting your outsourcing partners — you will want to make sure you do this right the first time.
- Ensure a mutually beneficial SLA is in place to ensure outsourcing success.

# Section 5: HIPAA Technology Considerations Quiz

1. Which of the items below is *not* a technical component that HIPAA mandates based upon the risk analysis results?
   A. Physical access controls
   B. Authentication controls
   C. Barcode scanner methodologies
   D. Data encryption mechanisms

2. Why should you use network address translation (NAT) on your network firewall?
   A. This is a guaranteed measure to stop spam
   B. Helps to conceal your internal network configuration
   C. Because it forwards inbound traffic to the proper host
   D. It can help prevent IP spoofing

3. You should look for Intrusion Detection Systems (IDSs) that have which of the following beneficial features?
   A. Can cut off an attack immediately
   B. Can monitor network bandwidth usage
   C. Can detect specific network events
   D. All of the above

4. Where should you use personal firewall/IDS software?
   A. On management's computers
   B. On those computers that receive the most e-mail
   C. On every computer possible inside the network
   D. You do not need a personal firewall

5. Access controls consist of what?
   A. Identification, authentication, and authorization
   B. Modification, cancellation, and hyper scripting
   C. Messaging, alerts, and random checks
   D. All of the above

6. Which of the following is NOT an acceptable technical way to authenticate a person or entity?
   A. Password
   B. Secure token
   C. Biometric
   D. Recognize

7. What are often the most highly targeted yet the most vulnerable part of your information systems?
   A. Databases
   B. Firewalls
   C. Servers
   D. E-mail accounts

8. Although encryption is an "addressable" Security Rule implementation specification, when must your data be encrypted?
   A. After two or more security breeches
   B. If you have a wireless network
   C. If your risk analysis turns up specific threats and vulnerabilities to PHI at rest or in transit
   D. If your organization decides to transmit PHI electronically

9. Which of the following is NOT a reason security incident occurrences are becoming more frequent?
   A. The simplicity of performing computer attacks and not getting caught
   B. The increasing number of vulnerabilities found in the software we use
   C. New government regulations that require computer accessibility for all U.S. citizens
   D. The widespread use of the Internet

10. What should you be sure to include in your communications plan?
    A. Who will communicate the message of a security incident
    B. When it will be communicated
    C. What will be said
    D. All of the above

11. The Security Rule defines the data backup plan requirement as what?
    A. A set of standards for how you save files on your computers
    B. The ability to save hard copies of all PHI
    C. A plan for how you will back up your files if a security incident occurs
    D. Procedures to create and maintain retrievable exact copies of electronic protected health information

12. Who of the following does NOT need to be part of your security incident team?
    A. CIO
    B. Legal Counsel
    C. HIPAA Security Officer
    D. ER Nurse

13. An Intrusion Detection System (IDS) is used to do what?
    A. Monitor for well-known and suspected attacks on your network
    B. Keep strangers out of your office
    C. Stop spam e-mail
    D. Alert you when you sent out PHI

14. According to the Spring 2003 U.S. Healthcare Industry Quarterly HIPAA Compliance Survey, what percentage of respondents were currently outsourcing various HIPAA initiatives?
    A. 2
    B. 25
    C. All
    D. 44

15. Which of the following certifications should NOT be considered as a baseline requirement for an outsourcing firm?
    A. GIAC
    B. CHS
    C. PA
    D. CISSP

# Section 6
# Managing Ongoing HIPAA Compliance

# Chapter 24
# HIPAA Training, Education, and Awareness

**Creating an Effective Awareness Program**

Ensuring organizational awareness of privacy and security policies and practices is a requirement of the HIPAA regulations. It is also a good idea, and has been for many years. Your staff members are the foundation of ensuring your policy compliance. If they do not know and understand what is expected of them with regard to meeting HIPAA and other privacy and security requirements, then they will probably unwittingly do things that could very well put your organization at risk.

Healthcare organizations must develop and implement an awareness program that meets the following goals:

- Ensures compliance with HIPAA privacy and security regulations
- Establishes an executive owner or sponsor to champion, maintain, and ensure senior level involvement; this will be necessary to get the message across and secure support of the HIPAA compliance activities throughout the organization
- Instills the privacy and security requirements and concerns into the organizational culture
- Clearly communicates the HIPAA privacy and security issues and challenges
- Supports your strategic and tactical HIPAA implementation strategies

Your awareness strategy should include the following:

- An awareness budget that accounts for the communications, planning, and implementation activities that will be proportionate to this piece of the total amount of the HIPAA compliance budget
- A timeline indicating target dates for all phases of the awareness and training program

---

- A procedure or tool (or both) for measuring the overall effectiveness of the awareness program
- Identification of integration points and windows to effectively coordinate the privacy and security awareness and education practices within the overall HIPAA compliance plan
- A strategy to integrate the awareness processes throughout all departments and teams of the organization to help ensure a successful awareness program
- Execution of an awareness risk assessment to identify awareness compliance gaps and form the baseline to use for measuring future awareness compliance success
- A description of the tactical objectives of the awareness and education program
- The development, implementation, communication, and enforcement of policies and procedures to mitigate risk and ensure ongoing compliance with HIPAA privacy and security regulations

The privacy and security awareness and education program you create must address your organization's interpretation of HIPAA and support the activities your organization will take to mitigate risk and ensure patient privacy based on the results of the baseline assessment. Creation and delivery of a common message, interpretation of the regulations, and a process for addressing and communicating issues will speed the implementation and reduce the overall cost in complying with HIPAA.

Follow a structured process for the development and maintenance of your awareness program:

- Clearly define your HIPAA privacy message (why, value, strategic approach, policies, procedures, contacts, etc.)
- Clearly document the desired tactical outcomes
- Clearly document the details of what will be done (awareness activities and tasks)
- Provide examples of case studies and suggestions

Continue to assess, refine, and update the awareness program throughout all the phases of developing and maintaining your organization's HIPAA compliance.

Does your organization have the resources necessary to develop and deliver a privacy and security awareness and education program? If not, you will need to allocate or contract resources necessary to develop an awareness program. In the event you must obtain external resources, or an outsourced arrangement is desired, be sure to establish guidelines for qualifying an experienced consultant to develop your privacy and security awareness program, in addition to any other help you outsource for HIPAA compliance activities.

**Exhibit 1. Privacy and Security Training Groups and Timing**

| Times | A | B | C | D | E | F | G | H | I | J |
|:-----:|:-:|:-:|:-:|:-:|:-:|:-:|:-:|:-:|:-:|:-:|
| a |   | X | X | X | X | X |   | X |   | X |
| b | X | X | X | X | X | X | X |   |   | X |
| c | X | X | X | X | X | X |   |   |   | X |
| d |   |   |   | X |   |   |   |   | X |   |
| e | X | X | X | X | X | X | X |   | X | X |
| f | X | X | X | X | X | X | X |   |   | X |

## Identify Awareness and Training Groups

The following groups should be targeted for specialized privacy and security training and awareness. These will vary, depending on the type of covered entity (CE) and other business organization factors.

A. HIPAA implementation sponsors
B. Executive team and legal counsel
C. Department managers and supervisors
D. Information technology staff
E. Office managers
F. Medical practitioners
G. All employees, including newly hired
H. Business associates impacted by HIPAA requirements
I. Call center and customer service staff
J. Human Resources Staff

Generally, there are six times when training should be given to one or more of these identified groups:

1. New employee orientation soon after employment start
2. Initial general training to all employees
3. Initial in-depth training to target groups
4. Business associate training following contract updates or when initiating new contracts
5. Specialized training when HIPAA policies or procedures change
6. Ongoing training for all groups; recommend at least once a year

Exhibit 1 visually represents training times and the associated groups, based on the groupings and descriptions previously discussed.

## Training

Training is more formal and interactive than an awareness program. The goal of training should be to build specialized skills and knowledge in the topic, and to facilitate job responsibility, performance, and capabilities.

Training should also motivate the participants. The importance of training to help ensure information security has been recognized in recent years as being one of the most effective ways to help secure information and protect privacy. In fact, the realization of this led to the National Institute of Standards and Technology (NIST) release of document SP800-16 in 1998. "IT Security Training Requirements: A Role- and Performance-Based Model" provides guidelines for federal agencies to develop their own IT security training programs. It provides a nice structure for nongovernment organizations to use as well, and will be helpful in building your privacy and security training program to meet HIPAA compliance requirements. If you use this as a guide, remember that you will need to modify the curriculum to match your own organization's unique training needs.

Keep in mind that it is job function and associated responsibilities that should determine what information security and privacy courses each target group needs. An employee may have multiple job responsibilities, and thus may need to attend more than one training session. This approach to training, although effective, may be a challenge to implement within some organizations because of time constraints or unwillingness to acknowledge that training is of such importance.

### Specialized HIPAA Topics

Training content should be specialized for target groups based on specific issues that they must understand and with which they must comply. Match the course content to job responsibilities and roles as much as possible to be most effective. For instance, assume you have the following defined roles:

R1: Healthcare Delivery Personnel (for example, physicians, nurses, etc.)
R2: Clinic and Provider Facility Managers
R3: Health Plan Claims Examiners
R4: Information Technology Personnel
R5: Privacy and Security Officers
R6: Plan Member Service Representatives
R7: Billing Personnel
R8: Health Plan Enrollment Personnel
R9: Legal Counsel and Human Resources
R10: Marketing and Sales
R11: Customer Services and Call Centers

You want the people filling these roles to know and understand their job responsibilities related to HIPAA compliance. Based on this, and taking into account your own unique business environment, you may determine the course content that should be given to the associated indicated roles. Exhibit 2 shows an example of how to do this.

**Exhibit 2. HIPAA Training Matrix**

| Course Topic | R1 | R2 | R3 | R4 | R5 | R6 | R7 | R8 | R9 | R10 | R11 |
|---|---|---|---|---|---|---|---|---|---|---|---|
| Complete HIPAA Privacy Rule | | X | X | | X | | | | X | | |
| Complete HIPAA Security Rule | | X | | X | X | | | | X | | |
| Notice of Privacy Practices | | X | | | X | X | | X | X | X | X |
| Authorizations | | X | X | | X | X | X | X | | X | |
| Business Associates | | X | X | X | X | X | X | | X | X | |
| Accounting of Disclosures | X | X | X | | X | X | X | | | | |
| Marketing | | X | | | X | | | X | X | X | |
| Identity Verification | | X | X | X | X | X | | X | X | | X |
| Technical Security Mechanisms | | X | | X | X | | | | | | |
| Penalties and Preemption | | X | | | X | | | X | X | | |
| Exceptions for Authorizations | | X | | | X | X | | | X | | |
| Access to Information | X | X | X | X | X | X | X | | X | | X |
| Uses and Disclosures | X | X | | | X | | X | | | | X |

## *Training Delivery Methods*

The size of your training groups may vary greatly. Large organizations may have as many as 50 in a classroom-setting training session. However, for the most effective training, we recommend you keep the number to 25 or less in this type of face-to-face training, to promote the most interaction, and also to help reduce side discussions and maintain attention. Another good option for training, especially for the initial all-employee sessions, is via a computer-based training (CBT) method, an online interactive method (such as a "Webinar"), or via a conference-call training session. The most effective delivery method will largely depend on your target audience. Methods for you to consider include:

- General classroom lectures to small- to medium-size groups
- Classroom training with group activities and tests to small- to medium-size groups
- Auditorium presentations to large groups
- Web-based interactive training
- CBTs with progress and achievement measures
- Audio instruction
- Video instruction
- Satellite or fiber-optic live distance training
- Outsourced training with professional education services
- Education provided by professional societies
- Government-sponsored training provided by regulatory agencies

## Training Design and Development

Design the training curriculum based on the learning objectives for the associated target groups. The training delivery method should be based on the best way to achieve your objectives. In choosing a delivery method, select the best method for the learning objectives, the number of students, and your organization's ability to efficiently deliver the material.

### Design and Development

During the design and development phase, keep these things in mind:

- Outline your class content.
- Divide into instructional units or lessons.
- Determine time requirements for each unit and lesson.
- Create content based on the things personnel need to know to perform their job responsibilities.
- Include interactive activities that can be taken back to their job and used right away.
- Be clear about the behaviors, actions, and activities expected of the students when performing their jobs.
- Describe the actions personnel should exhibit to demonstrate successfully meeting objectives being taught.
- Build on existing capabilities and experiences within the group.
- Sequence topics to build new or complex skills onto existing ones, and to encourage and enhance the students' motivation for learning the material.
- Use multiple learning methods.

When determining the best instructional method for your target groups, keep the following in mind:

- *Consider the people within your target group audience.* Consider the audience size and location. Consider experience levels. Consider time constraints. If the audience is large and geographically dispersed, a technology-based solution such as Web-based, CD, satellite learning, or something similar may work best.
- *Consider the business needs.* If you have a limited budget, then a technology-based delivery may be applicable, or you may want to bring in an outside instructor with already-prepared materials.
- *Consider the course content.* Some topics are better suited for instructor-led, video, Web-based, or CBT delivery. There are many opinions about what type of method is best. Much depends on your organization. It will be helpful if you can get the advice of training professionals who can assess material and make recommendations.
- *Consider what kind of student/teacher interaction is necessary.* Is the course content best presented as self-paced individual instruction

or as group instruction? Some topics are best covered with face-to-face and group interaction, others are best suited for individualized instruction. For example, if the goal is just to communicate policies and procedures, a technology-based solution may be most appropriate. However, if students need to perform problem-solving activities in a group to reinforce understanding or demonstrate appropriate actions, then a classroom setting would be better.

- *Consider the type of presentations and activities necessary.* If the course content requires students to fill out forms, use a specialized software program, or do role-playing, a classroom setting is best.
- *Consider the stability of the class content.* The stability of content is a cost issue. If content will change frequently (for instance, if procedures are expected to change as a result of mergers, acquisitions, or divestitures), or if new software systems are planned, the expense of changing the material needs to be estimated by considering difficulty, time, and money. Some instructional methods can be changed more easily and cost efficiently than others.
- *Consider the technology available for training delivery.* This is a critical factor in deciding the instructional strategy. Will all students have access to the technologies you will require? If doing Web-based training, will all students have access to the intranet or Internet? Do students have the necessary bandwidth for certain types of multimedia?

There are many instructional elements that will be consistent from course to course regardless of the instructional methods used. Most courses will involve delivery with voice, text, and graphics. To make instruction more effective you should also incorporate the use of pictures or graphics, video, demonstrations, role-playing, simulations, case studies, and interactive exercises. Several of these presentation methods will be used in most courses. Remember that it is generally considered most effective for student understanding to deliver the same message and information multiple times using multiple methods. Your students have their own unique learning styles, and what works well for one person will not necessarily be effective for the others. Develop your instructional methods based on instructional objectives, course content, delivery options, implementation options, technological capabilities, and available resources.

Web-based training is often a good alternative for large audiences, to provide an overview of the topic, and communicate policies and facts. However, this type of instruction method is often not appropriate for audiences that are learning procedures or need to know how to act in specific types of situations in which role-playing is necessary.

If you decide you need to get outside help for your training, research the organizations you are considering and determine the following:

- Do they use trained and experienced instructors?
- Do they have healthcare (with providers, health plans, or clearing-houses) experience?
- Do they have metrics to support their training?
- Do they offer multiple training methods?
- Are their training offerings comprehensive for the HIPAA requirements?
- Do they have local training facilities or staff? Travel expenses can impact costs.
- Do they belong to an association with existing or proposed HIPAA certification authorities? Beware of vendor-created HIPAA certifications! These were not endorsed, or even recognized, by HHS at the time we wrote this book.

Effective privacy and security training is necessary to help you achieve HIPAA compliance. There are many resources freely available on the Internet. Keep in mind that these can be helpful, but that any training needs to be tailored to the organization's own unique environment and needs. To be effective, organizations must take advantage of different types of training methods. Training must support making HIPAA privacy and security policies and procedures a learned and consistently practiced behavior.

### Awareness Options

Awareness activities are different from training activities. The objectives for delivering HIPAA privacy and security awareness are similar to training options. However, there are some very important differences between training and awareness activities. The options and methods for awareness activities are typically much different than the more-formal and structured training. Awareness activities should:

- Occur on an ongoing basis
- Use a wide range of delivery methods
- Catch the attention of the target audience
- Be less formal than training
- Take less time than training
- Be creative and fun
- Reinforce the lessons learned during formal training

Think of positive, fun, exciting, and motivating methods that will give employees the message and keep the HIPAA privacy and security issues in their mind as they perform their daily job responsibilities. The success of an awareness program is the ability to reach all personnel using a variety of techniques. Examples of awareness materials and methods include:

- Guest speakers
- Newsletters

- Intranet Web sites
- Posters
- Computer screen savers
- Lunch and "coffee break" presentations
- Departmental presentations
- Posting motivational or catchy slogans on screen savers, browser marquees, etc.
- Videotapes
- Computer-based awareness quizzes, games, etc.
- Brochures and flyers
- Pens, pencils, key chains, note pads, Post-It notes, and other types of promotional items with short privacy and security messages
- Stickers for doors and bulletin boards
- Cartoons and articles published monthly or quarterly in in-house newsletter or department-specific notices
- Daily privacy or security thought or advice of the day
- Special topical bulletins
- Monthly e-mail notices related to privacy and security issues
- Privacy and security banners or messages that appear on the monitor at log on
- Distribution of food items as an incentive; for example, packages of gummy-bugs with an attached label that reads something similar to "Real Computer Viruses Are Not This Sweet"
- Travel first-aid kit with privacy or security slogan printed on the package such as "Help Ensure Customer Privacy Health"
- Badge holders with a privacy or security slogan such as "Protect Privacy" or "Think Security"
- Flashlight with a label such as "Spotlight Privacy"

It is critical to remember that an awareness program never ends. An effective awareness program must repeat your message many times in many ways. The more important the message, the more often it should be repeated using multiple methods. Because it is an ongoing activity, it requires creativity and enthusiasm to maintain the interest of all audience members. The awareness messages must demonstrate that privacy and security are important not only to your organization, but also to each employee and each customer and patient.

An awareness program must remain current. As HIPAA regulations change, and subsequently privacy and security policies and procedures, personnel must be notified. We recommend establishing a method to deliver immediate information and updates when necessary. Perhaps new information is sent as the first alert item personnel see when logging onto the network for the day. The awareness messages and methods must also be simple. The purpose is to get messages and ideas out to personnel quickly and easily. They cannot be confusing or convoluted so as to dissuade personnel from reading them, and eventually not paying attention at all to the messages. Make it easy for personnel to get privacy and security information, and make the information easy to understand.

Depending on your available personnel, resources, and budget, you may need to consider outsourcing the design and development of your awareness program. Be sure to qualify any vendor you consider as being experienced and qualified for the topic of healthcare privacy and security. You can review literally thousands of such vendors on the Internet. When you have narrowed the field, ask for references from the vendors to discuss their experiences and satisfaction. Asking your peers within professional organizations or on healthcare privacy or security mailing lists can also be revealing and help you with your decision.

### Document Training and Awareness Activities

HIPAA regulations require privacy and security training for all members of your organization workforce, and all contractors who handle protected health information (PHI). Training must include coverage of privacy and security policies and procedures. All existing personnel must have been trained by the Privacy Rule compliance date of April 14, 2003. All new employees must be trained within a reasonably short period of time after starting work for your organization. You must log the people who have been trained and you must provide follow-up training when your policies and procedures change. Although it is not specifically required, it is a good idea to measure the understanding of the people who have participated in training and have received the awareness messages.

There are some automated systems that log the people who have taken training and received awareness messages. If you do not have the budget or resources for such a system, you need to log the people who have taken training and maintain this information for future reference, and to provide to HIPAA regulators when they request to see who has taken training. Use a log similar to Exhibit 3 to keep track of training and understanding. Add rows and columns as appropriate for your training program. Make an entry only after the training has been completed. If you utilize a testing process you can add a column to indicate that the test was administered and results of the testing.

### Get Support

To be successful, senior management must support your HIPAA privacy and security training and awareness efforts. Not only must they provide financial support to effectively develop the program, but they must also provide visible support to demonstrate to the workforce the importance and necessity of your efforts. Create a project plan that includes your objective for HIPAA privacy and security awareness and training, and

**Exhibit 3. HIPAA Training Log**

| Name | Department | Phone | Date | HIPAA Training Topic | Test Results (percent) |
|------|-----------|-------|------|---------------------|------------------------|
| Sue Smith | Plan Administration | X89356 | 04-02-03 | Notice and acknowledgment | 94 |
| Dr. Herold | Family Practice | X00000 | 05-03-03 | Confidential channel requests | 92 |
| Dr. Beaver | Obstetrics | X99999 | 03-12-03 | Minimum necessary | 92 |
| Joe Black | IT Manager | X77777 | 05-13-03 | Technology safeguards | 71 |

include estimates for necessary personnel, materials, time schedules, and any other associated costs (such as videos, manuals, etc.). Ask management to provide funds to support the organization's HIPAA privacy and security training and awareness compliance requirements. If you do not have perceived support from senior management, it is likely you will encounter passive resistance from a significant percentage of the workforce; they may not attend training for which they were scheduled, may ignore your requests to read and acknowledge policies and procedures, or may blatantly violate your policies and procedures. It is important to prevent this by having senior management clearly communicate the importance of everyone's participation prior to your training and awareness rollout.

### Measure Effectiveness

All management programs must be periodically reviewed and evaluated for effectiveness. This holds true for your HIPAA privacy and security training and awareness program. The methods you use for quantitative and qualitative measurement to determine the effectiveness of your program will depend in large part on the size and composition of your organization. In small clinics it may be sufficient to discuss the issues and determine understanding with your workforce members. In large health plans you may need a sophisticated automated system to help determine effectiveness. Consider using one or more of the following for determining effectiveness within your organization.

- Give quizzes immediately following training.
- Distribute a privacy and security awareness survey to all personnel or to a representative sample.
- Send follow-up questionnaires to people who have attended formal training approximately 4 to 6 months following the training to determine how well they have retained the information presented.
- Monitor the number of compliance infractions for each issue for which you provide training.
- Measure privacy and security knowledge as part of the yearly performance evaluation.

- Place feedback and suggestion forms on the intranet Web site.
- Track the number and type of privacy and security incidents that occur before and after the training and awareness activities.
- Conduct spot checks of personnel behavior. For instance, walk through work areas and note workstations that are logged in while unattended or patient information print-outs that are not adequately protected.
- Record user IDs and completion status for Web- and network-based training. Send a targeted questionnaire to those who have completed the online training.
- Have training participants fill out evaluation forms at the end of the class.

Your evaluation of training and awareness effectiveness has four distinct purposes, to measure:

1. The extent that conditions were right for learning and the learner's subjective satisfaction
2. What the student learned from a specific course or awareness activity
3. A pattern of student outcomes following a specified course or awareness activity
4. The value of the class or activity compared to other training and awareness options

Besides obtaining these measurements, the evaluation should also help you to identify how to:

- Assist employees in determining their own performance success
- Assist managers in determining their own workforce performance
- Compile trend data to assist instructors in improving both learning and teaching
- Create return on investment statistics to support training and awareness funds

**Conclusion**

Until comparatively recently in the history of healthcare, physicians personally hand-wrote their patients' medical records, and they were typically locked in a file cabinet with very little access by anyone other than the nursing and support staff within the immediate office. Today, healthcare delivery and payment systems are some of the biggest industries within the United States, with many intermediaries touching the systems and associated data. Integrated processing systems and networks have virtually replaced the pen, paper, and locked file cabinets. There are now so many players, public and private, involved with the processing and handling of health information, it is almost impossible for all but the very smallest healthcare office to do business without some type of data processing. The HIPAA regulations are leading the industries in many ways with privacy and security mandates. Complying with the multitude of requirements within all the HIPAA regulations will be a great challenge to most, if not all, healthcare organizations. Every healthcare organization covered by HIPAA must know, understand, and address the requirements set forth by HIPAA if it wants to remain a viable healthcare entity and maintain its patients' and customers' trust. To accomplish this, effective training and awareness activities are necessary.

## Chapter 24: Practical Checklist

- Analyze your organization's training and awareness needs and define the goals and objectives for the program.
- Create a training and awareness program.
- Obtain visible senior management support of the program.
- Obtain sufficient funding.
- Provide general and specialized training to all personnel, targeting specific groups according to their organizational roles.
- Use simple and straightforward awareness methods.
- Repeat messages using multiple methods to keep HIPAA awareness at the front of everyone's mind.
- Tell personnel what the threats are and how they are expected to address those threats.
- Constantly evaluate the effectiveness of your program and make changes accordingly.

# Chapter 25
# Performing Ongoing HIPAA Compliance Reviews and Audits

## Background

HIPAA compliance is not a one-time event. Once you have achieved HIPAA compliance, you are not finished with your efforts. You must now work to ensure your organization stays compliant. This may become challenging in an environment where there are many facilities in different locations, or where the organization is large and maintains constantly changing systems and networks.

Between the increasing demands of the Department of Health and Human Services (HHS), business partners, and customers, covered entities (CEs) simply cannot afford to be in a state of noncompliance. In a recent study by Harris Interactive, 83 percent of respondents said they would stop doing business with a company if they found out the company had misused customer information. Performing ongoing reviews and audits will not only ensure HIPAA compliance, but can also help build customer and business partner confidence and ultimately lower operating costs due to streamlined operations.

The Privacy and Security Rules must be managed on an ongoing basis indefinitely. In fact, as we have covered in this book, HIPAA specifically mandates creating audit trails and ongoing compliance efforts. Your business will change, people will come and go, new processes will evolve, new technologies will be developed, new information threats and vulnerabilities will emerge, and new policies and procedures will be put in place. All of these issues will require you to continuously manage HIPAA compliance as you would any other business matter.

Keep in mind that audits compare what an entity says it is doing to what is actually taking place. Audits are not necessary evils or negative HIPAA side effects. If the business value is understood and accepted by everyone involved,

---

The information and opinions provided in this book do not constitute or substitute for legal or other professional advice.

HIPAA audits should be viewed as constructive criticism that can help provide guidance to move forward. Before starting any HIPAA compliance audits, you will need to gather as much information as possible, including:

- Privacy policies and procedures
- Security policies and procedures
- All forms of protected health information (PHI) stored or transmitted both in hard copy and electronic formats
- The methods and systems in place to protect PHI

In this chapter we outline both privacy and security areas you should focus on, questions you should ask yourself and your HIPAA compliance team, along with some steps you can take to make this all happen.

**Privacy Issues**

Analysis by HHS* determined that the average cost of ongoing Privacy Rule compliance would be approximately 0.05 percent of each small entity's annual expenditures. HHS estimates that by 2008 the Privacy Rule will cost an estimated 0.07 percent of projected national health expenditures for ongoing compliance by all CEs.**

Privacy compliance activities will become most effective on an ongoing basis when they become integrated within the business processes and functions they are intended to control. Incorporating a privacy architecture within your applications and business process development projects is the best way to ensure that privacy processes are addressed from the very beginning of planning a new process.

Certainly another recommended method of staying compliant is to perform a yearly Privacy Rule gap analysis using the method described in Chapter 5. After performing the gap analysis, always compare the results to the previous gap analysis results to see where you have improved or where you have slipped and need to address new problems and issues.

In between the full gap analyses, you need to stay aware of ongoing privacy issues and changes. Items to review to determine whether privacy compliance and issues are continuing to be adequately addressed include the following:

- Does a Privacy Officer position still exist? Is this a dedicated role, or the role someone has assumed while performing other job responsibilities?
- Is the privacy official at the proper level within the organization?
- Does the privacy official have the authority to impose policies and procedures?

* Available at http://aspe.hhs.gov/admnsimp/nprm/pvc53.htm.
**Available at http://www.hhs.gov/ocr/part4.html.

- Do communications regarding privacy and references to the privacy official regularly occur?
- Have privacy noncompliance incidents been appropriately handled, and have sanctions been enforced?
- Have a privacy compliance budget and associated resources been identified?
- Have the security implications of privacy requirements been identified and documented?
- Are privacy activities scheduled and tracked?
- Have your applicable state laws been compared with HIPAA requirements to determine preemption issues?
- Is someone responsible for keeping up with new and updated privacy regulations?
- Has a complete set of privacy requirements to meet HIPAA compliance been identified for your organizational environment?
- Has a Privacy Rule gap analysis been performed within your organization?
- Do you continue to update your PHI uses and disclosures as necessary?
- Has the privacy impact on business processes been determined?
- Do you continue to map your privacy practices to the Privacy Rule requirements as the practices change?
- Do you track privacy changes and identify where modifications within procedures must be made?
- Do you create new privacy policies, procedures, and forms as necessary?
- Are updates to your privacy policies and procedures planned as rules and business processes change?
- Does the appropriate staff receive ongoing privacy training?
- Does the privacy training get updated periodically?
- Do you perform periodic privacy reviews within business units where PHI is processed?
- Do you ensure that your business associates have up-to-date privacy plans?
- Do you require business associates to participate in regularly scheduled privacy impact assessments?
- Has your organization implemented the technology required to send and receive encrypted PHI?
- Are new business associate agreements created with privacy clauses?
- Have routers, firewalls, and intrusion-detection systems (IDS) been implemented and updated to control access to PHI on networks from outside sources?
- Are new applications created that support your privacy policies and Notice of Privacy Practices (NPP)?

- Are audit logs regularly reviewed and followed up?
- Are regular (for example, quarterly or biannual) reports created and submitted to upper management detailing privacy risk and impact, along with improvements and degradations to privacy compared to previous reports?
- Are auditors experienced and trained to do privacy impact assessments?

## Security Issues

Similar to an automobile or even the human body, once a security infrastructure has been built, proper maintenance is by far the most critical element to ensure it stays in proper working order. There is the old saying, "An apple a day keeps the doctor away." Similarly, in the context of information security, a patch a day keeps the vulnerabilities away. The saying, "An ounce of prevention is worth a pound of cure," applies equally as well. A little tune up — a little monitoring, a little training, and a little maintenance of log files and configurations — can keep your information systems' infrastructure sound and secure.

The first step of security audits and reviews is to understand the business objectives and HIPAA requirements of what is being audited. The actual Security Rule verbiage* for ongoing monitoring, referred to as evaluation, is as follows:

> *Perform a periodic technical and nontechnical evaluation, based initially upon the standards implemented under this rule and subsequently, in response to environmental or operational changes affecting the security of electronic protected health information, that establishes the extent to which an entity's security policies and procedures meet the requirements of this sub-part.*

One key area to focus on to maintain your information's security is to perform a risk analysis on a regular basis. This is essentially the same analysis we outlined in Chapter 12 that you need to perform at the beginning of your Security Rule compliance efforts. The only major differences will be that many new threats and vulnerabilities will exist and there will be new tools available for you to assess them. Speaking of new vulnerabilities, over 8600 security vulnerabilities were reported to the Carnegie Mellon CERT Coordination Center between 2000 and 2003! This number alone should help justify why security needs to be reassessed so often.

Here is another set of items to review to ensure that HIPAA security compliance is properly addressed:

- Does the Security Officer position still exist?

*U.S. Department of Health and Human Services HIPAA Security Rule, available at http://a257. g.akamaitech.net/7/257/2422/14mar20010800/edocket.access.gpo.gov/2003/pdf/03-3877.pdf

- Are security roles and responsibilities being adhered to?
- Do you suspect that business associates are reasonably handling PHI in a secure manner?
- Is there an overall auditing policy? Are there associated procedures? How often are they updated?
- Does the plan include testing a cross-section of both information systems and physical security systems?
- Are audits and reviews performed on a regular basis?
- Do budgets exist for audits and reviews?
- What specific metrics are in place for monitoring Security Rule compliance?
- Are there new methods of collecting and handling PHI since your last audit or review?
- Are your inventory and classifications of PHI current?
- Are your information flows, network hardware and software inventory, and network diagrams current?
- Is PHI being backed up and stored adequately?
- Are personnel security issues such as authorizations, access controls, and terminations being considered?
- Do you update all of your security policies and procedures as needed?
- Are new policies and procedures being created as needed?
- Is security awareness training occurring?
- How is training comprehension measured?
- Are you or your security team members subscribing to and reading security bulletins that come out practically every day?
- Are network and application vulnerability assessments being performed on a regular basis (monthly, quarterly, biannually, etc., depending on needs) or after any major system changes?
- Is your software (applications, operating systems, etc.), especially the software on critical computers or servers, tested for updates and patches on a weekly if not a daily basis?
- Are the software updates and patches that are found properly tested before they are applied?
- Are new security standards and best practices from NIST, SANS, etc., being kept up with and integrated into your security infrastructure?
- Do the incident and contingency plans cover the most critical information systems and reflect key business processes?
- Do the plans get tested at least annually?
- Do the resources required to test these plans still exist?
- Is there a contingency plan that addresses partial or complete lost or access to PHI?
- Do you document who is making changes to your systems (applying patches, configuration changes, etc.), along with the changes being made, why they are being made, and the back-out procedures?

- Are you logging all system activity that is related to the access, storage, or transmission of PHI to create sufficient audit trails?
- Do you monitor your system (firewall, IDS, server, workstation, etc.) log files to ensure that signs of impending system failure are addressed and malicious activity is not occurring?
- Do you back up your log files in case you need to go back and determine what PHI was accessed at a specific time by a specific entity?

## Making Audits Work

The results of your audits will, and probably should, vary from year to year. If everything turns up clean, perhaps the audit is not detailed enough. If your results get progressively worse over time, perhaps there is an internal process or management issue. Either way, any gaps or discrepancies found in your HIPAA privacy and security audits need to be addressed as soon as possible.

If the audits are performed by outside entities, make sure that they have your organization's best interests in mind. See Chapter 23 for more information on outsourcing. You will want to keep an eye out for auditors recommending that you fix all problems regardless of their significance or impact to your organization or the privacy and security of PHI. You will have to consider the cost of remediation for each issue vs. the benefits remediation will provide. You cannot be expected to remediate every single issue that turns up. If you cannot justify fixing certain problems that are uncovered, just make sure that you document the business reasons behind your decisions.

Ongoing HIPAA compliance is similar to any other compliance program. There needs to be a designated person in charge, the proper policies and procedures need to be maintained, and risk management techniques need to be applied in a common sense and business-oriented (not technical) fashion. The bottom line is to make sure your auditing practices can provide a critical view of the protective measures in place for PHI to help your organization reasonably comply with the HIPAA regulations into the future.

## Chapter 25: Practical Checklist

- Is someone still in charge of HIPAA privacy and security compliance?
- Are privacy and security audits and system reviews being performed at least annually?
- Are privacy and security policies and procedures being updated and added as needed?
- Make sure that whoever is performing your HIPAA audits has your organization's best interests in mind.
- Clearly document the results of your ongoing HIPAA audits.
- Treat privacy and security compliance just as you would any other compliance program.

# Section 6: Managing Ongoing HIPAA Compliance Quiz

1. Which of the following should be a goal of your HIPAA awareness and training program?
   A. Instill privacy and security requirements and concerns into the organizational culture
   B. Describe the history and background of HIPAA
   C. Identify those within your organization who have been in non-compliance with the HIPAA regulations
   D. Describe how to coerce individuals into waiving their rights under HIPAA

2. Which of the following should be included within your training and awareness strategy?
   A. A strategy to use marketing techniques to raise training budget
   B. Identify states to create preemption procedures
   C. A procedure for measuring the overall effectiveness of the awareness and education program
   D. A procedure for answering complaints related to HIPAA compliance

3. Which of the following most accurately describes the difference between training and awareness?
   A. Training is less formal and interactive than an awareness program
   B. Training is more formal and interactive than an awareness program
   C. A training program is more expensive than an awareness program
   D. An awareness program is more expensive than a training program

4. Which of the following is the most likely group to target for HIPAA privacy and security training?
   A. Customer services and call centers
   B. Personnel who have received recent promotions

---

The information and opinions provided in this book do not constitute or substitute for legal or other professional advice.

    C. Third parties

    D. Trash removal contractors

5. Training delivery should best be created based upon which of the following?

    A. The preferences of your upper management

    B. The time of year

    C. The number of personnel

    D. The best way to achieve your objectives

6. Which of the following most accurately describes a characteristic of awareness activities?

    A. Should only occur during new-employee orientation

    B. Should be detailed within business associate contracts

    C. Should occur on an ongoing basis

    D. Should be very formal and structured

7. Your evaluation of training and awareness effectiveness has four distinct purposes, including which one of the following?

    A. Determine the total budget for HIPAA compliance efforts

    B. Identify privacy and security officers

    C. Compare your organization with other healthcare organizations

    D. Determine what the student learned from a specific course

8. According to research by HHS, ongoing Privacy Rule compliance efforts will cost CEs how much of their projected national health expenditures by 2008?

    A. 0.007 percent

    B. 0.07 percent

    C. 0.7 percent

    D. 7 percent

9. Which of the following is the best way to ensure that privacy processes are addressed during process planning?

    A. Incorporating a privacy architecture within your applications and business process development process

    B. Performing a periodic risk analysis

    C. Hiring a third-party reviewer

    D. Implement a privacy software implementation package

10. In a recent study by Harris Interactive, what percentage of respondents said they would stop doing business with a company if they found out the company has misused customer information?

    A. 83 percent

    B. 100 percent

    C. 2 percent

    D. None of the above

11. What sort of information should you gather before starting any HIPAA compliance audits?
    A. Privacy policies and procedures
    B. Security policies and procedures
    C. The methods and systems in place to protect PHI
    D. All of the above

12. What is the first step of security audits and reviews?
    A. Hire a consultant with a strong security background
    B. Gather your HIPAA compliance team and brainstorm how to protect PHI
    C. Understand the business objectives and HIPAA requirements for what is being audited
    D. Isolate known vulnerabilities on your network

13. How many new vulnerabilities have been have been reported to the Carnegie Mellon CERT Coordination Center between the years 2000 and 2003?
    A. Over 8600
    B. 1+ million
    C. 25,000
    D. 42

14. What should you do if your audit turns up clean?
    A. Relax until next year
    B. Consider that perhaps the audit is not detailed enough
    C. Hire an outside consultant to do the audit again
    D. None of the above

15. What are some things you should consider if the audits are performed by outside entities?
    A. Make sure that they have your organization's best interests in mind
    B. Keep an eye out for auditors recommending that you fix all problems regardless of their significance or impact to your organization or the privacy and security of PHI
    C. Both A and B
    D. None of the above

# Section 7
# Appendices

# Appendix A
# Case Studies

## Case 1: Healthcare Clearinghouse

We could not find a clearinghouse willing to share their HIPAA compliance experiences. Many of them feared that by discussing their experiences they would either draw attention to themselves and face an HHS compliance audit, or that their competitors would learn too much from the information and they would lose a competitive advantage. Additionally, it seems by the published reports that the HIPAA requirements may in some ways threaten the existence of clearinghouses, and the counter points state that the Transactions and Code Sets requirements will make clearinghouses more desirable. Clearinghouses may be able to help many CEs meet the electronic data interchange security requirements in a cost effective way and reduce the CE's risks. Time will tell what in fact will come to fruition.

We were able to glean information about clearinghouse HIPAA compliance from multiple news reports and articles covering healthcare clearinghouse experiences. The Transactions and Code Sets Rule apparently is the biggest challenge for clearinghouses and has been written about the most. However, we were able to find some information about how the Privacy Rule and the Security Rule affected clearinghouses as well.

Nearly all clearinghouses use payer patient information. However, often no individual at a clearinghouse ever directly accesses the patient information. But, because the information passes from the payer to the clearinghouse, the clearinghouse must assure the payer that the information is secure. Thus, a BA Agreement is often created.

Administrative requirements now imposed by HIPAA have historically been absent from clearinghouses. Clearinghouses usually focus on technical controls primarily, and physical controls secondarily. Often, from what we could determine, no privacy or security policies already exist within clearinghouses. Therefore, most clearinghouses are now scrambling to create a full set of policies to address the HIPAA privacy and security requirements.

HIPAA requires security controls as well as audit capability on the network. Although many clearinghouses have at least some functions meeting

---

The information and opinions provided in this book do not constitute or substitute for legal or other professional advice.

these requirements, there are still many more clearinghouses that have not yet invested in intrusion detection systems or similar security alarms, and also do not have any formal audit logging or audit procedures in place. Of the clearinghouses indicated in various reports that have taken steps to address these requirements, tools such as Snort are being installed in the hosting center, at least as a short-term solution until a more-comprehensive solution can be planned and integrated into the network.

Another HIPAA security requirement that many clearinghouses have apparently indicated they have not previously had is a formal incident response policy and procedure. To help them meet this requirement, many have reported going to public Internet sites, such as the government NIST site, and using the example documents as an interim solution. Some are planning to develop intrusion detection system architecture in the coming year or two by implementing a commercial system.

### Background on a Typical Clearinghouse
- Transaction processing for 30 to 50 plans, 6 to 10 million members
- 80 to 100 million claims per year
- Involves many IT vendors
- Maintains multiple data and application centers
- Tests applications and provides Customer Plan training

### Clearinghouse HIPAA Compliance Challenges
- Complex organization
- Relationships and contracts with dozens of health plans
- Involves many BAs, vendors, and other third parties
- There are many E-business initiatives to address, such as providing healthcare benefits on the Internet Web site
- Typically no in-house legal department
- Lack of centralized responsibility to track contracts, BA relationships, permission letters
- Lack of formalized process for releasing PHI
- Use of PHI in training materials
- Many BAs have access to PHI that is not necessary to perform their jobs
- Lack of formal, written privacy policies and procedures for protecting PHI (fax, e-mail, training manuals, etc.)
- Informal policies and procedures exist surrounding the uses and disclosures of PHI
- Lack of process in place to track disclosures of PHI
- Existing confidentiality statements do not meet HIPAA BA agreement requirements
- Informal authorization procedures
- Lack of tracking procedures to document disclosures

### Clearinghouse Lessons Learned

- The cost of implementing user authentication can be "huge." Unfortunately, we could not find any actual numbers.
- Confirm what you are under the HIPAA regulations; for example, a CE, a BA, etc.
- Understand and document PHI business process flows.
- Take a coordinated, organized, and structured approach.
- Identify your use of data collection tools.
- Identify BAs and communicate with them.
- Understand HIPAA impacts on your future business initiatives.
- Obtain assistance from your HR department for policies and procedures, training, etc.
- Involve legal counsel as appropriate.
- All HIPAA security requirements should be addressed in parallel.
- Getting multiple business partners to agree to the clearinghouse's single security policy can be quite challenging and can take a very long time to accomplish. Be prepared to create multiple policies for multiple business partners.
- The more closely you inspect some of the HIPAA requirements, such as auditing, the more complex and intimidating they can seem. Do not put off a close review of the requirements!
- Identify and address version control issues between your business partners.
- Your networking solutions will vary with each business partner. Not all business partners need to exchange transactions over the Internet. You will likely need multiple network types (such as SNA, asynchronous, TCP/IP, etc.) to deal with all situations.
- Document, document, document.

### Typical Clearinghouse Implementation Plan

1. Coordinate identifying and updating contracts with BAs and trading partners.
2. Develop strategy for training materials.
3. Develop privacy policies and procedures.
4. Develop standard authorization forms and procedures for outside disclosures.
5. Coordinate a privacy and security workgroup to facilitate discussion of HIPAA related to ongoing business initiatives.
6. Develop an ongoing privacy and security awareness education program.
7. Determine preemption issues.
8. Assign a point of contact for privacy and HIPAA questions.
9. Develop procedures for documentation storage requirements.

10. Create methods to support individual rights of confidential communications.

11. Create methods to support revocation of authorizations as required.

## Case 2: Metropolitan Area Healthcare System Case Study

A large, Southeastern healthcare system that has a network of hospitals, urgent care centers, physicians' groups, and hospice and home care facilities shared its experiences with HIPAA compliance preparation. These questions were answered by a member of the organization's HIPAA compliance team. For privacy purposes, we have kept this team member's name and organization anonymous. Although other healthcare systems will have different needs and be affected by HIPAA in different ways, these organizations should still find the experiences and information contained in this study very useful.

1. **Approximately how many employees are in your organization?** We currently have about 9,000 employees.

2. **When did you start your HIPAA compliance efforts?** March 2000.

3. **Has your organization's size affected your compliance efforts? If so, in what ways?** Because we are so large and geographically spread out, our compliance efforts are complex. We have to constantly be aware of how we are going to get the same, consistent information and awareness education to all the staff across all shifts. We also have to work out and coordinate the logistics of posting the notices of privacy practices and delivering the first batch of HIPAA-related forms to all the departments at each facility.

4. **Do you have one person or team devoted to HIPAA privacy and security compliance efforts, or do you have different people or teams for each?** We have one team responsible for the overall HIPAA strategy of the organization. Responsibilities on the team are divided, with some team members focusing primarily on privacy and others focusing primarily on security. However, we often cross over and back each other up and coordinate efforts on items where it makes sense.

5. **How many people were on your HIPAA compliance team at the beginning of your compliance efforts? How many are there now?** Our HIPAA compliance team has five members — a director and four employees. The team has been this size since May 2000. The director of the team reports to the Vice President of Compliance and Insurance Services.

6. **What area is responsible for HIPAA compliance?** HIPAA compliance is everyone's responsibility. However, the Compliance and Insurance Services Division is responsible for setting the overall HIPAA strategy for the organization.

7. **Have you hired a Privacy Officer to specifically address the HIPAA directive to appoint such an official? Or, are these required responsibilities given to an existing staff member who is also performing other job duties?** This responsibility has been assigned to an existing staff member who was/is also performing other duties.
8. **Have you identified a separate contact person to handle HIPAA compliance complaints and questions? If so, did you hire someone specifically for this role, or is it being filled by an existing staff member who has other job responsibilities?** This responsibility has been assigned to an existing staff member who was/is also performing other duties. This person is also the Chief Privacy and Security Officer.
9. **If applicable, did you meet October 2002 Transactions and Code Sets compliance deadline, or did you have to file for an extension?** We filed for an extension.
10. **What was the first thing you did as part of your HIPAA compliance effort?** After establishing a budget and getting the team in place, we had a consulting firm do a HIPAA gap analysis for us. They reviewed our policies, procedures, processes, as well as our applications.
11. **Did you meet full Privacy Rule compliance by April 14, 2003?** Based on our interpretation of the HIPAA regulations and state law, we were compliant with privacy on April 14, 2003.
12. **In how many states do you provide services?** 1
13. **Do you have any international offices?** No.
14. **How are you reconciling your HIPAA Privacy Rule activities with other privacy regulations with which you must comply (for example, GLB, EU Data Protection Directive, Canada's PIPEDA, etc.)?** We researched the various privacy regulations that we must comply with and developed our policies and procedures to comply with the most restrictive regulations.
15. **How have you addressed state preemption issues?** We researched the various privacy regulations at both the State and Federal level, and developed our policies and procedures to comply with the most restrictive regulations.
16. **What have been the most difficult challenges for you with regard to HIPAA compliance?** Systemwide communications and training; getting a consistent message about what HIPAA is and how it affects our staff's day to day duties out to staff on all shifts at all facilities.
17. **Have you hired any consultants or contractors specifically to work on HIPAA compliance activities? How have you integrated external help with your internal efforts?** We are doing most of the HIPAA compliance activities in-house. We have used some outside firms to help perform gap analysis and to implement some of the solutions we have decided to use.

18. **Have you started addressing the business associate HIPAA requirements? Have all your business associates been coopera- tive? What have been your biggest challenges?** We have been working with our business associates to add HIPAA language to their contracts. Most business associates have been easy to work with on this. Getting mutual agreement on language in the contract has been the biggest challenge.

19. **What training initiatives, if any, have you implemented so far?** HIPAA awareness training has been accomplished through a variety of methods. We have used general orientation, manager orientation, town hall meetings, department meetings, HIPAA booklets, and online HIPAA training software to make all staff members aware of HIPAA and their day to day responsibilities for compliance with it.

20. **Are you integrating security efforts with your privacy efforts or are you tackling them one at a time?** Some of our security and privacy efforts are combined (like awareness training), but most of them are handled separately. However, both projects are being implemented at the same time (running parallel to each other).

21. **What have been your biggest surprises with regard to achieving compliance within your organization?** The level of detail to which we have had to implement in order to address privacy rights in accordance with the HIPAA regulations has been very surprising.

22. **What are five tips you would give to other organizations that are getting started with HIPAA compliance that perhaps they have not thought about yet?**

    1. Develop a communications plan for how HIPAA initiatives will be communicated to all staff.
    2. Create a security plan and a privacy plan and implement common project activities at the same time.
    3. Create an incident response plan and team (for both privacy and security incidents).
    4. Project growth rates for audit logs and ensure you have enough disk space to hold the logs.
    5. Set up a committee that is a cross section of clinical and financial folks to review policies and procedures before they are approved and implemented.

23. **How are other applicable regulatory requirements (for example, GLBA, state and local privacy requirements, etc.) impacting your HIPAA compliance work?** It extends the amount of research that has to be done because we must compare state laws to HIPAA and determine which is more restrictive. We then must architect our overall HIPAA strategy to ensure compliance with the most restric- tive of the laws.

24. **Approximately how much has your organization spent, or budgeted to spend, on HIPAA compliance?** Around $3 million dollars has been budgeted for HIPAA compliance.

25. **Did you purchase any computer/network systems for your HIPAA compliance requirements? If so, what kind (for example, audit, logging, encryption, etc.)?** So far we have purchased content scanning, vulnerability assessment, configuration management, auditing, and encryption software. We will be buying other items over the next 2 years.

26. **Does your Compliance and Insurance Services area consist of lawyers? Privacy experts? Security experts? Some other specialty?** The Compliance and Insurance Services division does not directly employ a lawyer, but does utilize outside legal services. There are privacy and security experts in the division whose job it is to decide strategy and provide answers to any privacy or security related issues.

27. **Around how many BA contracts did you have to modify?** There have been too many to count at this point.

28. **What is the highest level of executive (CEO, Sr. VP IT, etc.) who is visibly supporting your HIPAA compliance efforts (for example, used his/her name on organizationwide memos, newsletters, etc.)?** President and CEO (same individual). The Board has also been supportive of HIPAA compliance activities.

29. **How do you track the personnel who have received training? Do you give these people any type of quiz or test to determine comprehension and understanding?** There is a computerized training and tracking system that employees log into, read the material, and take quizzes about the material.

## Case 3: Small Physician's Office

A small, Southeastern physician's office that offers obstetrics and gynecological healthcare services shared its experiences with HIPAA compliance preparation. These questions were answered by this organization's Office Manager and HIPAA Officer. For privacy purposes, we chose to keep the Office Manager's name and organization anonymous. Although other physicians' offices will have different needs and be affected by HIPAA in different ways, these organizations should still find the experiences and information contained in this study very useful.

1. **Approximately how many employees are in your organization?** We have 3 physicians and 15 staff members.

2. **When did you start your HIPAA compliance efforts?** In early 2002, I went to my first HIPAA workshop and started seriously collecting information. In early 2003, I started implementing the HIPAA require-

ments including creating updated manuals and changing our training programs.

3. **Has your organization's size affected your compliance efforts? If so, in what ways?** Being a small practice, everyone needs access to patients' PHI. Nothing other than making sure everyone gets the same training.

4. **Do you have one person or team devoted to HIPAA privacy and security compliance efforts, or do you have different people or teams for each?** We currently do not have anyone that focuses solely on HIPAA compliance. Our office manager (myself) and our HIPAA compliance team are responsible for HIPAA among other things.

5. **How many people were on your HIPAA compliance team at the beginning of your compliance efforts? How many are there now?** There has always been one HIPAA officer and three committee members.

6. **What area is responsible for HIPAA compliance?** Office Manager/HIPAA Officer. I have set up a committee, one staff member from each of our office areas (business office, front desk, and back office) but I'm responsible for training physicians and staff.

7. **If applicable, did you meet October 2002 Transactions and Code Sets compliance deadline, or did you have to file for an extension?** We filed for the extension.

8. **What was the first thing you did as part of your HIPAA compliance efforts?** I changed my sign-in sheets and had "HIPAA Privacy Cover Sheets" made for our entire office to cover the charts and paper containing PHI to use on desk, at island, front desk, etc.

9. **Did you meet full Privacy Rule compliance by April 14, 2003?** Yes, to the best of my knowledge.

10. **What have been the most difficult challenges for you with regard to HIPAA compliance?**
    1. Putting together my office HIPAA manual for each staff and physician
    2. Front desk area — it is so open that the staff has to be very careful when on telephone checking patients in and out and when appointments need to be made for another office, etc.
    3. Making sure the physicians keep the charts covered in a back office area where patients, visitors walk by.

11. **Approximately how much has your organization spent, or have budgeted to spend on HIPAA compliance activities? Has the budget changed since the original amount?** $1,000 — This amount has not changed.

12. **Have you hired any consultants or contractors specifically to work on HIPAA compliance activities? How have you integrated external help with your internal efforts?** No, we are doing it all ourselves. Our printing company is doing our copies of forms, etc. for us.

13. **Have you started addressing the business associate HIPAA requirements? Have all your business associates been cooperative? What have been your biggest challenges?** Yes, all of my business associates have signed agreements that we keep on file. They have all been completely fine with doing these for us.

14. **What privacy technologies, if any, have you implemented, or plan to implement, to address the security-related requirements of the Privacy Rule?** We have currently implemented computer backup tapes which are kept in a fireproof, locked safe.

15. **What tips can you give to other physicians offices regarding their HIPAA compliance activities?** Don't panic — using common sense is the key. We have been doing most of the HIPAA compliance requirements anyway.

16. **What training initiatives, if any, have you implemented so far?** I put together HIPAA manuals for each doctor and staff person. We had training sessions to go over HIPAA after they had read the manuals. They also have them to refer back to.

17. **Are you integrating security efforts with your privacy efforts or are you tackling them one at a time?** A lot overlap — like backup tapes for computer, stored away in a fireproof, locked safe. I have not totally read the security rule yet.

18. **What have been your biggest surprises with regard to achieving compliance within your organization?** How easily the staff has been trained. We are doing a lot of the compliant things normally. We have always stressed and respected patient confidentiality.

19. **What are five tips you would give to other organizations that are getting started with HIPAA compliance that perhaps they have not thought about yet?**
    1. Divide your office into areas, and do a walk-through, looking for problems to correct.
    2. Create an authorization form showing patient has received office privacy notice. Make this a permanent item in each patient's chart and make it a colored piece of paper so it can be spotted easily.
    3. Having a committee helps in overall compliance because each office area is represented.
    4. Add HIPAA sections to your office manuals for each employee. If incidents happen, they can re-read the manual.
    5. Integrate HIPAA training with new employee orientation.

20. **How are other applicable regulatory requirements (for example, GLBA, state and local privacy requirements, etc.) impacting your HIPAA compliance work?** We know that state laws always take precedence over the HIPAA regulations if they are more stringent.

21. **Have you purchased any computer/network systems for your HIPAA compliance requirements? If so, what kind (for example, audit, logging, encryption, etc.)?** No.

22. **If you have had a state preemption analysis performed, would you recommend it to other physicians' offices? How much did it cost? Is it an online tool, or a paper document? From what company?** We did not have one done and don't plan to at this time.

23. **Around how many business associate contracts did you have to modify?** 9

24. **How do you track the personnel who have received training? Do you give these people any type of quiz or test to determine comprehension and understanding?** We used sign-in sheets at training sessions. I have not given quizzes, but I did ask questions during the training to confirm their understanding.

### Case 4: Multi-State Health Insurance Plan

A medium-sized, multi-state Midwest insurance company that offers a wide range of insurance and financial services, such as health insurance, life insurance, casualty, pension, etc., shared its experiences with HIPAA compliance preparation. Because some of the information involved may be considered as competitive information with other health plans, the company has requested to remain anonymous. However, other health plans specifically, and any covered entity generally, should find their experiences and information useful.

1. **How many employees are in your organization?** We have around 20,000, including brokers and agents and other independent sales staff.

2. **Approximately when did you start your HIPAA compliance efforts?** We started our compliance efforts for both the Transactions Code Sets and Privacy requirements about halfway through 2000. It seemed as soon as our Y2K efforts were finished, we started on this!

3. **Has your organization's size affected your HIPAA compliance efforts? If so, in what ways?** Yes, it has been a factor. Compared to many CEs, we are a large organization with many different products, departments, and geographic locations. This has created both positive situations and negative situations with respect to addressing HIPAA compliance. Fortunately, we have dedicated training, programming, and administrative staff. Unfortunately, we are also a hybrid entity, and implementing the access controls and internal administrative "firewalls" has been a challenge. We had initially planned to only concentrate on HIPAA compliance within those departments handling PHI. However, as we pursued this strategy we realized that almost every area within the organization has some opportunity to access PHI. This is especially true within our Infor-

mation Technology areas. So, we then restructured our plan to identify and target specific groups based upon job responsibility.

4. **Do you have one person or team devoted to HIPAA privacy and security compliance efforts, or do you have different people or teams for each?** We have two distinct compliance groups working on the HIPAA rules. One is addressing HIPAA privacy and security and the other is addressing HIPAA transactions and codes. We also have a subgroup within our Information Technology area looking specifically at updating systems for the transactions and codes requirements.

5. **How many people were on your HIPAA compliance team at the beginning of your compliance efforts? How many are there now?** We initially started addressing HIPAA compliance like Y2K compliance, and had 20 people on just the HIPAA privacy compliance team alone. Over the months we've found we didn't need this many, so our group was reduced to half the size. We have a corporate compliance department that is ultimately responsible for HIPAA compliance for all applicable rules.

6. **Have you hired a Privacy Officer to specifically address the HIPAA (and GLB) directives? Or, have these required responsibilities been given to an existing staff member who is also performing other job responsibilities?** We have given these responsibilities to an existing staff member. Our Privacy Officer is also the Corporate Compliance VP.

7. **Does your corporate compliance area consist of lawyers? Privacy experts? Security experts? Some other specialty?** Our corporate compliance department is comprised of lawyers. The security knowledge and expertise necessary for meeting certain compliance requirements is provided from other appropriate areas within the company. Our lawyers meet with the others areas as necessary.

8. **Have you identified a separate contact person to handle HIPAA compliance complaints and questions? If so, did you hire someone specifically for this role, or is an existing staff member who has other job responsibilities filling it?** Our health insurance area has had a customer complaint, or call center, area for several years to address questions and service issues. Our public relations department is also addressing HIPAA compliance issues and questions from the public as necessary.

9. **What is the highest level of executive (CEO? Sr. VP IT? etc.) who has visibly supported your HIPAA compliance efforts (for example, used his/her name on organizationwide memos, newsletters, etc.)?** Our Compliance VP (also the Privacy Officer).

10. **If applicable, did you meet October 2002 Transactions and Code Sets compliance deadline, or did you have to file for an extension?** We needed to file for an extension to October 2003.

11. **What was the first thing you did as part of your HIPAA compliance efforts?** We created a project plan and compliance plan. We had our management services area help the project team to identify appropriate deliverables.

12. **Did you meet full Privacy Rule compliance by April 14, 2003?** Yes! We met the deadline. Starting early was the key.

13. **In how many states do you provide services?** We provide insurance and financial services in approximately 20 U.S. states.

14. **Do you have any international offices?** No. And we have no plans to go international.

15. **How are you reconciling your HIPAA Privacy Rule activities other privacy regulations with which you must comply (for example, GLB, EU Data Protection Directive, Canada's PIPEDA, etc.)?** We are complying with all regulations that apply, with the guidance of our compliance department, and trying to reconcile all actions to the most restrictive requirements.

16. **What have been the most difficult challenges for you with regard to HIPAA compliance?** We've had difficulties trying to accurately translate and understand the finer points of the Privacy Rule. The wording was very difficult to understand, ambiguous in places, and the interpretation was very subjective, and then, creating the procedures to support the requirements.

17. **How much did you budget to HIPAA compliance activities? Has the budget changed since the original amount?** We did not have a separate budget for HIPAA compliance activities. We used our existing security and privacy budget to achieve HIPAA compliance ... from the planning, policies, and procedures, to training and resources.

18. **Approximately how much did you spend on HIPAA compliance?** Hmm ... good question!! Because we were using money from our security and privacy budget, we were not keeping close track. Plus, the various business units also spent money on compliance efforts in response to our new HIPAA-compliant policies and procedures. Here are some of the more quantifiable activities:
    1. For around 12 months 20 people were working on HIPAA compliance, followed by around 12 months of 10 people working on HIPAA compliance. Total hours used were approximately 700.
    2. We performed a gap analysis to determine where additional compliance actions were necessary. Our management services group created the project plan for this, and also did a PHI flow analysis.
    3. We had a dedicated team review the Business Partner Agreements.
    4. Our training department created a HIPAA privacy-training video course that all employees were required to view.

5. We hired a consulting company to perform some HIPAA-specific tasks for some of the very specialized requirements.

6. We physically rearranged some of our areas. For example, our health insurance department was physically moved to a separate, consolidated location with more restrictive physical access controls.

7. We did training for all employees ... around 30 minutes each for around 20,000 people.

19. **Have you hired any consultants or contractors specifically to work on HIPAA compliance activities? How have you integrated external help with your internal efforts?** The primary task for our hired consultants was for the HIPAA transactions and code sets compliance activities. We also hired another consultant do a short project to help identify group health plan compliance issues and develop flow processes.

20. **How have you addressed state preemption issues? Would you recommend your state preemption analysis to other health plan CEs? How much did it cost? Is it an online tool, or a paper document? From what company?** We purchased and used a state preemption analysis tool from a healthcare membership organization. We do not give vendor or product recommendations publicly.

21. **Have you started addressing the Business Associate HIPAA requirements?** Yes.

22. **Have all your Business Associates been cooperative?** For the most part they have.

23. **What have been your biggest challenges?** Trying to get the final details of the BA agreement contracts mutually agreed upon with each BA. And, trying to ensure we were covering all necessary BA requirements within the agreements unique to each BA.

24. **Around how many BA contracts did you have to modify?** We had a lot ... but we did not keep track; probably around one hundred or so.

25. **What privacy technologies, if any, have you implemented, or plan to implement, to address the security-related requirements of the Privacy Rule?** We did not implement any privacy-specific technologies. We already had security technologies in place that should also address all the Security Rule requirements.

26. **Did you purchase any computer/network systems for your HIPAA compliance requirements? If so, what kind (for example, audit, logging, encryption, etc.)?** No, we have not purchased any specifically for HIPAA compliance. We were planning upgrades anyway, so we ensured the systems purchased had features, such as logging, incident detection, security controls for stored and in-transit information, etc. The HIPAA requirements helped to justify the expenditures for these extra, often additional cost, features.

27. **What tips can you give to other healthcare plans (payers) regarding their HIPAA compliance activities?**
    1. Thoroughly read and review the regulatory text.
    2. Don't use purchased policies and procedures ... at least not verbatim. Always make policies and procedures specific to your organizational needs.
28. **What training initiatives, if any, have you implemented so far?** Besides the video referenced earlier, we also created information that we posted to our corporate intranet Web site, and we have created a CBT course. We are planning to create targeted, separate classroom classes for specific groups such as underwriters, sales, marketing, claims, etc.; basically the areas handling the PHI the most.
29. **How do you track the personnel who have received training? Do you give these folks any type of quiz or test to determine comprehension and understanding?** We track our CBT usage, and we quiz the people who take it. Our CBT is divided into different modules for different target audiences. We also keep track of who has viewed the training video.
30. **What have been your biggest surprises with regard to achieving compliance within your organization?** Our training efforts took substantially more effort than we expected. Our information technology changes took significantly less effort than expected.
31. **How are other applicable regulatory requirements (for example, GLBA, state and local privacy requirements, etc.) impacting your HIPAA compliance work?** We were impacted by GLBA, and the work we did for it significantly cut the amount of work necessary for HIPAA. We used many of the same compliance systems for HIPAA that we already had established for GLBA. We are combining the NPP with the GLBA privacy notices in mailings. We also have some logging and tracking in place for HIPAA now that we had implemented for GLBA. HIPAA implementation costs would probably have been much higher if we had not already done a lot for GLBA compliance.
32. **For the customers for whom GLBA and HIPAA applies, are you combining the GLB and HIPAA privacy notices into one privacy notice that covers the requirements for both, or are you sending the same customers two different versions, one for GLB and one for HIPAA?** No, we are definitely not doing this, and we would not advise anyone else to do this. Our customers receive multiple privacy notices from us, but at least we're covering all our regulatory notice requirements for GLBA and HIPAA in this manner.
33. **Are you using a layered notice of privacy practices?** No, we are not. We did not even consider doing this.
34. **What are five tips you would give to other covered entities, of any kind (health plan, healthcare provider, healthcare clearinghouse,**

**business associates, employers, etc.), that are getting started with HIPAA compliance that perhaps they have not thought about yet?**

1. Read, research, examine, and understand the HIPAA rules.
2. Know what HIPAA requires for your own specific organization.
3. Create a detailed project plan.
4. Use purchased policies and procedures if you already do not have some in place, but invest time in updating them to meet your specific organization.
5. Share your experiences with your industry peers, and in turn learn from their experiences.

# Appendix B
# Sample Documents

**HIPAA Privacy Officer Job Description**

*The Privacy Officer Role*

It will sometimes be difficult to clearly separate the roles and responsibilities of the Privacy Officer from the rest of the organizational responsibilities. Healthcare organizations often assign privacy responsibilities to the Chief Information Officer. The risk of doing this is that privacy may then be perceived as a technology-only issue. Addressing privacy truly is a business issue and must be integrated into and addressed by all areas of the organization, including each business practice, and within all processing systems.

Ideally the privacy function should be a separate function within the organization, reporting directly to the CEO, with communication and integration into all other areas of the company. But, is this a function that one person can accomplish alone? Perhaps, but it really depends upon if you can find all the skills necessary for this job within one person, and also the size of your organization. It may be impossible to find someone with all the necessary skills within a small- to medium-sized organization. In these situations the responsibilities are often included within the responsibilities of another executive role, such as CIO.

In complex and large organizations, however, the Privacy Officer is more likely to be a full-time position reporting to the CEO, possibly even with a small staff of his or her own to address all the organization's privacy issues, in addition to having the Privacy Oversight Council. If staffing does not make having dedicated personnel feasible, then you must seriously consider hiring a consultant to spend some time reviewing your privacy practices, evaluating your situation, and getting you on track with all the assorted privacy requirements applicable to your organization. Or, outsource your privacy functions to a qualified and experienced organization that provides such a service. However, if you choose to do this, you must still identify a privacy official from your workforce to be the primary point of contact with the outsourced organization.

---

The information and opinions provided in this book do not constitute or substitute for legal or other professional advice.

## Sample Chief Privacy Officer (CPO) Job Description

This position reports to: <Chief Executive Officer, President, Board of Directors>

### *Goal*

The CPO is responsible for ensuring the implementation, compliance, and ongoing activities within the company as they relate to employee and customer privacy. The CPO will promote a corporatewide privacy philosophy supporting a comprehensive and practical set of privacy policies, procedures, and technology to not only protect the organization from privacy-related liability, but also to use privacy practices as a way to create customer goodwill and market returns, and to ensure HIPAA privacy rule compliance.

### *Qualifications*

- <5, 10, X> years knowledge and experience in information privacy laws, access, security, release of information, and access control technologies.
- <5, 10, X> years knowledge and experience in the <financial, health-care, manufacturing, government, etc.> industry.
- Demonstrated organization, facilitation, communication, and presentation skills.
- Experience in creating and following a departmental budget.
- Experience and effectiveness in leading initiatives and projects.
- CISSP® or CISA® preferred, but not required.

### *Roles and Responsibilities*

- Know, understand, and ensure corporate compliance with HIPAA regulations and all other relevant privacy laws, regulations, and standards that apply to the company. This includes the laws of any jurisdiction in which the company conducts business, including state and international locations.
- Keep current with local, state, federal, and international privacy related laws and accreditation standards, and monitor privacy technologies.
- Provide leadership and oversight for all privacy-related activities of the company.
- Communicate and work with corporate senior management and corporate compliance officers to establish, maintain, and provide leadership for a corporate Privacy Oversight Committee.
- Coordinate the development, implementation, and maintenance of corporate customer and employee privacy policies and plans with the Privacy Oversight Committee.

- Create and implement procedures to help prevent loss and inappropriate distribution of corporate information.
- Work with Public Relations and Marketing to increase the public awareness of the company's privacy efforts, and address privacy-related issues and incidents.
- Analyze and assess information flows across and between business units, and address the privacy implications of the flows.
- Investigate and handle every privacy-related incident and consumer complaint.
- Ensure that privacy compliance benchmarks and regularly scheduled information privacy risk assessments and compliance monitoring activities occur.
- Coordinate and work with Law, business department leaders, and appropriate committees to ensure the organization has and maintains appropriate privacy and confidentiality consent, authorization forms, and information notices and materials reflecting current corporate and legal practices and requirements.
- Promote essential privacy policy elements organizationwide, including the following common regulatory requirements: Notice, Choice, Access, Security, Recourse, and Verification.
- Ensure procedures are implemented to allow customers to view and correct their personal data files processed by the organization.
- Oversee and ensure the development of ongoing corporate privacy orientation, training, and awareness activities and communications for personnel at all levels and business partners.
- Ensure all trading partner and business associate agreements include privacy requirements and responsibilities, and address all related concerns.
- Ensure procedures are implemented to track access to information protected by regulations.
- Oversee and work with the Privacy Oversight Committee to create, implement, and maintain procedures for receiving, documenting, tracking, investigating, and addressing complaints concerning the company's privacy policies and procedures.
- Oversee and work with Human Resources and Law to ensure compliance with corporate privacy policies and procedures and consistent application of sanctions and disciplinary actions for noncompliance throughout the organization.
- Participate in and review information security plans throughout the organization to ensure alignment between security and privacy practices, and act as a liaison to Information Security and Information Technology departments.
- Understand the organization's technical infrastructure, and promote the use of privacy enhancing technologies.

- Advise and work with corporate personnel involved with any aspect of access to personally identifiable information, or any other type of regulated information, to ensure compliance with the corporate privacy policies and procedures and applicable laws.
- Cooperate with law enforcement and regulatory groups in privacy-related compliance reviews and investigations.
- Represent the company's information privacy interests to third parties, privacy commissioners, and other officials responsible for the development, oversight, and enforcement of privacy legislation to update or adopt privacy-related legislation, regulations, and standards.

### Sample HIPAA Security Officer Job Description

**Note**

We have intentionally formatted this job description differently from the CPO job description to point out that there are many ways for CEs to write both of these positions. Keep in mind that this information can be tweaked slightly to cover a Chief Security Officer (CSO) job position if needed. Just remember that both of these job descriptions will need to be tailored for your organization's specific needs.

The HIPAA Security Officer is responsible for the ongoing management of all HIPAA-related information security policies, procedures, and technology systems in order to maintain the confidentiality, integrity, and availability of all organizational healthcare information systems and protected health information.

### *Actions and Accountabilities*

- Responsible for implementing, managing, and enforcing information security directives as mandated by HIPAA
- Ensure the ongoing integration of information security with healthcare system business operations, strategies, and requirements
- Ensure that the access control, disaster recovery, business continuity, incident response, and information risk management needs of the organization are properly addressed
- Lead information security awareness and training initiatives to educate workforce about information risks
- Perform ongoing information risk assessments and audits to ensure that information systems are adequately protected and meet HIPAA evaluation requirements
- Work with vendors, outside consultants, and other third parties to improve information security within the organization
- Lead an incident response team to contain, investigate, and prevent future computer security breaches
- Hold everyone, including self, accountable for established information security policies and procedures

## General Skills and Experience Requirements

- Minimum 10 years of experience in information technology and security positions

- Experienced in the management of both physical and logical information security systems

- Strong technical skills (application and operating system hardening, vulnerability assessments, security audits, TCP/IP, intrusion detection systems, firewalls, etc.)

- Outstanding interpersonal and communication skills

- Must possess a high degree of integrity and trust along with the ability to work independently

- Excellent documentation and presentation skills

- Ability to assess and weigh current and evolving business risks and enforce appropriate information security measures

- In-depth knowledge of the HIPAA Security Rule and other government technology laws and standards

- CISSP® or CISA® certifications preferred, but not required

### Sample HIPAA Business Associate Agreement

The following is an outstanding example of a good HIPAA Business Associate Agreement that provides a relatively easy way for covered entities to modify it to meet their own requirements. This document is just part of a very good comprehensive HIPAA compliance software tool called PrivaPlan that is used by thousands of providers.

<To customize this template document, replace all of the text that is presented in angle brackets (i.e., "<" and ">") with text that is appropriate to your organization and circumstances. After completing the customization of this document, the document should be reviewed by an attorney who is familiar with health privacy laws and regulations in the state in which this agreement is executed, and who is in a position to provide legal counsel to your organization.>*

### HIPAA Business Associate Agreement

This Business Associate Agreement ("Agreement") is entered into this ___ day of ___, ___ between <covered entity>, a <state corporation> ("Company") and <business associate>, a <state corporation> ("Contractor").

## *Recitals*

I. Company is a <type of organization> that <description of primary functions or activities> with a principal place of business at <address>.

II. Contractor is a <type of organization> that <description of primary functions or activities> with a principal place of business at <address>.

III. Company, as a Covered entity defined herein under the Health Insurance Portability and Accountability Act of 1996 ("HIPAA") is required to enter into this Agreement to obtain satisfactory assurances that Contractor, a Business Associate under HIPAA, will appropriately safeguard all Protected Health Information ("PHI") as defined herein, disclosed, created, or received by Contractor on behalf of, Company.

IV. Company desires to engage Contractor to perform certain functions for, or on behalf of, Company involving the disclosure of PHI by Company to Contractor, or the creation or use of PHI by Contractor on behalf of Company, and Contractor desires to perform such functions.

In consideration of the mutual promises below and the exchange of information pursuant to this agreement and in order to comply with all legal requirements for the protection of this information, the parties therefore agree as follows:

A. Definitions of Terms
   1. Agreement means this Business Associate Agreement.
   2. Business Associate shall have the meaning given to such term in 45 CFR § 160.103.
   3. CFR shall mean the Code of Federal Regulations.
   4. Designated Record Set shall have the meaning given to such term in 45 CFR § 164.501.
   5. Covered entity shall have the meaning given to such term in 45 CFR § 160.103.
   6. Protected Health Information or PHI shall have the meaning given to such term in 45 CFR § 164.501.

B. Obligations of Contractor
   1. Permitted Uses and Disclosures. Contractor may not use or disclose PHI received or created pursuant to this agreement except as follows: [Note: in order to avoid having to amend the Agreement if anything in the list changes, consider putting the list of permitted uses/disclosures of PHI in an exhibit.]
      a. <ordered list (use lower case letters) of permitted uses and disclosures by the Contractor; be specific in the description of what Contractor will do on behalf of the Company that relates to the creation, use, receipt, or disclosure of PHI,

include as the last numbered permitted uses/disclosures the following:>

  b. ___. Contractor's Operations — Permitted Uses of PHI. Contractor may use the PHI it receives in its capacity as a Business Associate for the proper management and administration of Contractor or to carry out Contractor's legal responsibilities.

  c. ___. Contractor's Operations — Permitted Disclosures of PHI. Contractor may disclose the PHI it obtains in its capacity as a Business Associate if such disclosure is necessary for the Contractor's proper management and administration or to carry out the Contractor's legal responsibilities, and:

    (i) the disclosure is required by law; or

    (ii) Contractor obtains reasonable assurances from the person to whom the PHI is disclosed that the PHI will be held confidentially and used or further disclosed only as required by law or for the purpose for which it was disclosed to the person, and the person notifies the Contractor (and Contractor in turn notifies Company) of any instances of which it is aware in which the confidentiality of the PHI has been breached.

2. Disclosure Accounting. [Note: Because disclosures of PHI made for purposes of payment, treatment, and healthcare operations are exempt from the disclosure accounting requirements and most business associates' disclosures of PHI are made for such purposes, it should be rare that an accounting of disclosures would be required, unless the disclosure is prohibited.] In the event that Contractor makes any disclosures of PHI that are subject to the accounting requirements of 45 CFR § 164.528, Contractor promptly shall report such disclosures to Company. The notice by Contractor to Company of the disclosure shall include the name of the individual and company affiliation to whom the PHI was disclosed and the date of the disclosure. Contractor shall maintain a record of each such disclosure, including the date of the disclosure, the name and, if available, the address of the recipient of the PHI, a brief description of the PHI disclosed, and a brief description of the purpose of the disclosure. Contractor shall maintain this record for a period of 6 years and make available to Company upon request in an electronic format so that Company may meet its disclosure accounting obligations under 45 CFR § 164.528.

3. Access by Covered entity. [Note: Access under HIPAA encompasses two ideas: (1) The Company's and the HHS Secretary's access to Contractor's books and records for the purpose of allowing Company to assess Contractor's compliance with the Agreement; and (2) the right of individuals to access their PHI as provided for in 45

CFR § 164.524. With respect to the first issue of access, the regulations do not require that the Contractor grant access to its books to Company, although Company, as the Covered entity, may wish to include this access by agreement. The second access issue requires Contractor to cooperate with Company to provide individuals access to their PHI. In the event that the requested PHI is held by the Contractor and not the Company, Company may wish to require that Contractor comply directly with 45 CFR § 164.524. Each of these issues is addressed in the Access provisions below.]

4. Access to PHI by Individuals. Contractor shall cooperate with Company to fulfill all requests by individuals for access to the individual's PHI that are approved by Company. Contractor shall cooperate with Company in all respects necessary for Company to comply with 45 CFR § 164.524. If Contractor receives a request from an individual for access to PHI, Contractor immediately shall forward such request to Company. Company shall be solely responsible for determining the scope of PHI and Designated Record Set with respect to each request by an individual for access to PHI. <If Contractor maintains PHI in a Designated Record Set on behalf of Company, Contractor shall permit any individual, upon notice by Company, to access and obtain copies of the individual's PHI in accordance with 45 CFR 164.524. Contractor shall make the PHI available in the format requested by the individual and approved by Company, unless the PHI is not readily producible in such format, in which case the PHI shall be produced in hard copy format. Contractor may not charge the individual any fees for such access to PHI.> Company shall reimburse Contractor a portion of the fee charged by Company to the individual that is proportional to the amount of PHI produced by Contractor in relation to the amount of PHI produced by Company.

5. Access to Contractor's Books and Records. Contractor shall make its internal practices, books, and records relating to the use and disclosure of PHI received from, or created or received by Contractor on behalf of Company, available to the Secretary of the Department of Health and Human Services for purposes of determining Company's compliance with the HIPAA laws and regulations. <Upon reasonable notice to Contractor and during Contractor's normal business hours, Contractor shall make such internal practices, books, and records available to Company to inspect for purposes of determining compliance with this Agreement.>

6. Amendment of PHI. As directed and in accordance with the time frames specified by Company, Contractor shall incorporate all amendments to PHI received from Company. Within five (5) business days following Contractor's amendment of PHI as directed

by Company, Contractor shall provide written notice to Company confirming that Contractor has made to amendments to PHI as directed by Company and containing any other information as may be necessary for Company to provide adequate notice to the individual in accordance with 45 CFR § 164.526.

7. Security Safeguards. Contractor shall implement a documented information security program that includes administrative, technical, and physical safeguards designed to prevent the accidental or otherwise unauthorized use or disclosure of PHI.

8. Reporting and Mitigating Unauthorized Uses and Disclosures of PHI. Immediately upon notice to Contractor, Contractor shall report to Company any uses or disclosures of PHI not authorized by this Agreement. Contractor shall use its best efforts to mitigate the deleterious effects of any use or disclosure of PHI not authorized by this Agreement. Further, in the notice provided to Company by Contractor regarding unauthorized uses and disclosures of PHI, Contractor shall describe the remedial or other actions undertaken or proposed to be undertaken regarding the unauthorized use or disclosure of PHI.

C. Affiliates, Agents, Subsidiaries, and Subcontractors. Contractor shall require that any agents, affiliates, subsidiaries, or subcontractors, to whom it provides PHI received from, or created or received by Contractor on behalf of Company, agree in writing to the same use and disclosure restrictions imposed on Contractor by this Agreement.

1. Term and Termination. This Agreement shall be for a term of ___ year(s), commencing on ___ and ending on ___ ("Initial Term"). This Agreement shall automatically renew for successive ___ year periods ("Renewal Term") unless one party notifies the other party of its intent not to renew within sixty (60) days prior to end of the Initial Term or any Renewal Term. [Note: The term should be the same as the underlying agreement.]

2. Termination by Breach. Company, at its sole option and without an opportunity to cure, immediately may terminate this Agreement if Company determines that Contractor has violated a material term of this Agreement.

3. Termination Without Cause. Either party to this Agreement may terminate the Agreement upon provision of thirty (30) days prior written notice. <Consider termination provisions for bankruptcy, breach by Company (with opportunity to cure and legislative changes.>

4. Effects of Termination; Disposal of PHI. Upon termination of this Agreement, Contractor shall recover all PHI that is in the possession of Contractor's agents, affiliates, subsidiaries, or subcontractors. Contractor shall return to Company or destroy all PHI that Contractor obtained or maintained pursuant to this Agreement

on behalf of Company. If the parties agree at that time that the return or destruction of PHI is not feasible, Contractor shall extend the protections provided under this Agreement to such PHI, and limit further use or disclosure of the PHI to those purposes that make the return or destruction of the PHI infeasible. If the parties agree at the time of termination of this Agreement that it is infeasible for the Contractor to recover all PHI in the possession of Contractor's agents, affiliates, subsidiaries, or subcontractors, Contractor shall provide written notice to Company regarding the nature of the unfeasibility and Contractor shall require that its agents, affiliates, subsidiaries, and subcontractors agree to the extension of all protections, limitations, and restrictions required of Contractor hereunder.

D. Insurance and Indemnification.
   1. Insurance. <Consider adding reciprocal insurance requirements.>
   2. Indemnification. Each party will indemnify and hold harmless the other party to this Agreement from and against all claims, losses, liabilities, costs, and other expenses incurred as a result of, or arising directly or indirectly out of or in conjunction with:
      a. any misrepresentation, breach of warranty or nonfulfillment of any undertaking on the part of the party under this Agreement; and
      b. any claims, demands, awards, judgments, actions, and proceedings made by any person or organization arising out of or in any way connected with the party's performance under this Agreement. [Note: The effectiveness of indemnification provisions is governed by state law and will vary from state to state. Also, the scope of the services performed under a business associate agreement should dictate the scope of the indemnification. Because neither of these variables can be known in drafting a form agreement, consider replacing this indemnification provision with one recommended by your own legal counsel.]

E. Miscellaneous.
   1. Contractor's Compliance with HIPAA. Company makes no warranty or representation that compliance by Contractor with this Agreement, HIPAA, or the HIPAA regulations will be adequate or satisfactory for Contractor's own purposes or that any information in Contractor's possession or control, or transmitted or received by Contractor, is or will be secure from unauthorized use or disclosure. Contractor is solely responsible for all decisions made by Contractor regarding the safeguarding of PHI.
   2. Notices. Any notice required to be given pursuant to the terms and provisions of this Agreement shall be in writing and may be either personally delivered or sent by registered or certified mail

in the United States Postal Service, Return Receipt Requested, postage prepaid, addressed to each party at the addresses which follow or to such other addresses as the parties may hereinafter designate in writing:

Company: _____

_____

_____

Contractor: _____

_____

_____

Any such notice shall be deemed to have been given, if mailed as provided herein, as of the date mailed.

3.  Change in Law. In the event that there are subsequent changes or clarifications of statutes, regulations, or rules relating to Agreement, Company shall notify Contractor of any actions it reasonably deems are necessary to comply with such changes, and Contractor promptly shall take such actions. In the event that there shall be a change in the federal or state laws, rules or regulations, or any interpretation or any such law, rule, regulation, or general instructions which may render any of the material terms of this Agreement unlawful or unenforceable, or materially affects the financial arrangement contained in this Agreement, Contractor may, by providing advanced written notice, propose an amendment to this Agreement addressing such issues. If, within fifteen (15) days following the notice, the parties are unable to agree upon such amendments, either party may terminate this Agreement by giving the other party at least thirty (30) days written notice.

4.  Amendments. By mutual consent of the parties, this Agreement may from time to time be modified or amended in writing and such written modifications signed by the parties shall be attached to and become part of this Agreement.

5.  Severability. In the event any provision of this Agreement is held to be unenforceable for any reason, the unenforceability thereof shall not affect the remainder of this Agreement, which shall remain in full force and effect and enforceable in accordance with its terms.

6. Counterparts. This Agreement may be executed in counterparts, any of which is considered to be an original agreement.

7. Governing Law. This Agreement shall be construed broadly to implement and comply with the requirements relating to the HIPAA laws and regulations. All other aspects of this Agreement shall be governed under the laws of the State of ___ and venue for any actions relating to this Agreement shall be in ___ County, ___.

8. Assignment/Subcontracting. This Agreement shall inure to the benefit of and be binding upon the parties hereto and their respective legal representatives, successors, and assigns. Contractor may not assign or subcontract the rights or obligations under this Agreement without the express written consent of Company. Company may assign its rights and obligations under this Agreement to any successor or affiliated entity.

9. Entire Agreement. This Agreement contains the entire agreement between parties and supersedes all prior discussions, negotiations, and services for like services.

10. No Third Party Beneficiaries. Nothing express or implied in this Agreement is intended to confer, nor shall anything herein confer, upon any person other than Covered entity, Business Associate, and their respective successors or assigns, any rights, remedies, obligations, or liabilities whatsoever.

11. Assistance in Litigation or Administrative Proceedings. Contractor shall make itself and any agents, affiliates, subsidiaries, subcontractors, or employees assisting Contractor in the fulfillment of its obligations under this Agreement, available to Company, at no cost to Company, to testify as witnesses, or otherwise, in the event of litigation or administrative proceedings being commenced against Company, its directors, officers, or employees based upon claimed violation of HIPAA, the HIPAA regulations or other laws relating to security and privacy, except where Contractor or its agents, affiliates, subsidiaries, subcontractors, or employees are a named adverse party.

IN WITNESS WHEREOF, the parties hereto have duly executed this agreement to be effective as of <effective date of the agreement>.

_____     _____
COMPANY                          CONTRACTOR


_____     _____
By                               By

| | |
|---|---|
| Printed Name | Printed Name |

| | |
|---|---|
| Title | Title |

| | |
|---|---|
| Date | Date |

## HIPAA Privacy and Security-Specific Policies

You must formally document, communicate, and maintain the policies and procedures you create and implement to comply with the HIPAA Privacy Rule and Security Rule requirements. Policy statements are fairly high-level directives that indicate WHAT actions and results will occur. Procedures are much more detailed explanations of HOW to reach the results required by the policies. Keep this in mind as you are developing your policies so you will not get caught up in trying to put details into your policy statements that you really should be placing within the supporting procedure documents.

Start by creating a privacy policy for your organization that directs personnel how to handle and process PHI, and what practices are allowed and disallowed. Then, identify the privacy and security requirements applicable for your organization and create policies, and subsequent supporting procedures. Here are a few example policy statements to help get you started. Remember, you will need to modify these to best meet your organization's business environment.

### *Sample Privacy Policies*

**Uses and Disclosures of Protected Health Information.** Company XYZ customer and patient information will only be used or disclosed in the following situations:

1. The individual who is the subject of the information has authorized the use or disclosure.
2. The individual who is the subject of the information has received the Company XYZ Notice of Privacy Practices and has acknowledged receipt of the Notice. This allows use or disclosure for treatment, payment, or healthcare operations.
3. The individual who is the subject of the information agrees or does not object to the disclosure to persons involved in the healthcare of the individual.

4. The disclosure is to the individual who is the subject of the information, or to HHS for compliance-related purposes.
5. The use or disclosure is for a HIPAA "public purposes" exception.

### Notice of Privacy Practices

Company XYZ will publish a Notice of Privacy Practices and provide it to all individuals at the earliest practicable time. All uses and disclosures of protected health information (PHI) will be done according to the Company XYZ Notice of Privacy Practices. Company XYZ will attempt to gain written acknowledgement of the receipt of the Notice from all individuals receiving the Notice of Privacy Practices. Company XYZ will document attempts to gain this acknowledgement if we cannot successfully obtain written receipt of the Notice.

### Restriction Requests

Company XYZ will give serious consideration to all requests for restrictions on uses and disclosures of protected health information as published in the Notice of Privacy Practices and follow Company XYZ procedures for addressing such requests. When Company XYZ agrees to a restriction, personnel with Company XYZ will observe and comply with the restriction.

### Minimum Necessary Disclosure of Protected Health Information

Except for disclosures made for treatment purposes, all disclosures of protected health information (PHI) will be limited to the minimum amount of information necessary to accomplish the purpose of the disclosure. All requests for PHI (except requests made for treatment purposes) will be limited to the minimum amount of information needed to accomplish the purpose of the request.

### Access to Protected Health Information

Company XYZ will grant access to protected health information (PHI) to each employee or contractor based on the assigned job responsibilities. The access privileges will not exceed those necessary to accomplish the assigned job responsibilities.

### Access to Protected Health Information by the Individual

Company XYZ will provide access to protected health information (PHI) to the person who is the subject of such information when the individual requests access within the timeframes required by the HIPAA Privacy Rule. Company XYZ will inform the person requesting access of the location of their PHI if Company XYZ does not physically possess the PHI but knows where it is located.

## Amendment of Incomplete or Incorrect Protected Health Information

Company XYZ will respond to all requests for amendment of protected health information (PHI) in a timely manner following Company XYZ procedures for updating PHI. If requests reveal the PHI is incorrect, Company XYZ amend the PHI appropriately within the timeframe dictated by the HIPAA Privacy Rule and will document the amendment. A notice of corrections will be given to any organization with which the PHI has been shared.

## Disclosure Accounting

Company XYZ will provide an accounting of all disclosures of PHI subject to HIPAA Privacy Rule requirements to an individual upon their request.

## Marketing Activities

Company XYZ will use or disclose PHI for marketing activities only after obtaining a valid authorization. Company XYZ considers marketing as any communication to purchase or use a product of service where an arrangement exists in exchange for direct or indirect payment, or where Company XYZ encourages purchase or use of a product or service. Company XYZ does not consider the communication of alternate forms of treatment, or the use of products and services in treatment to be marketing. Company XYZ will not obtain an authorization when a face-to-face communication is made by us to the patient, or when giving an individual a promotional gift of nominal value.

## Prohibited Activities

No Company XYZ employee or contractor may engage in any intimidating or retaliatory acts against persons who file complaints or otherwise exercise their rights under HIPAA regulations. No Company XYZ employee or contractor may condition treatment, payment, enrollment, or eligibility for benefits on the provision of an authorization to disclose protected health information.

## Business Associates

Company XYZ business associates will be contractually required to protect health information to the same degree as Company XYZ personnel. Company XYZ will deal with business associates who violate their agreement by first attempting to correct the situation; if the situation cannot be resolved, the business associate agreement will be terminated, and the services provided by the business associate will be discontinued.

### Training and Awareness

Company XYZ will train all personnel on the policies and procedures related to HIPAA Privacy Rule requirements. New personnel will receive training within two weeks of their start date. Existing personnel will receive ongoing awareness messages covering the privacy and security requirements for customer and patient information, and will attend formal training soon after the Company XYZ privacy policies are changed, and at least once a year. Company XYZ will document the training for which each personnel member participates, including the date and topic of the training.

### Sanctions

Company XYZ will apply disciplinary sanctions for any personnel member who violates these policies, or any procedures implemented to support these policies. Sanctions include disciplinary actions up to and possibly including termination of employment and possible criminal prosecution.

### Retention of Records

Company XYZ will retain, secure, and maintain all records identified within the HIPAA Privacy Rule for at least 6 years using procedures that allow for access when necessary within a reasonable amount of time as determined by the Privacy Officer. Company XYZ will extend the records retention time requirement as necessary to comply with other governmental regulations, laws, or requirements made by the Company XYZ professional liability carrier.

### Sample Security Policies

### Contingency Plans

Company XYZ will create and implement contingency plans for all systems and networks processing or storing protected health information (PHI).

### Criticality Analysis

Company XYZ will establish procedures to formally analyze the criticality of all software applications and data. The results of the Company XYZ application and data criticality analysis will be documented within the Company XYZ contingency plan.

### Emergency Mode Operation

Company XYZ will create an emergency mode operation plan to continue operations in the event of fire, vandalism, natural disaster, or system failure.

### Access Authorization to Systems Components

Company XYZ will grant users access to terminals, transactions, software programs, other users, and related network systems components based on minimum necessary to perform job responsibilities.

### Access Authorization

Company XYZ will verify access authorizations to PHI, computer systems, and network components before creating a user account and granting access.

### Computer Systems Access Controls

All computer-resident protected health information (PHI) will have system access controls to ensure that it is not improperly disclosed, modified, deleted, or rendered unavailable.

### Internal Audits

Company XYZ will ensure regular and frequent internal audits of protected health information (PHI) systems activities. Company XYZ audit activities will include reviews of login activities, file accesses, and security incidents.

### Background Checks

Company XYZ will provide access to protected health information (PHI) only to personnel who have the appropriate security clearances and authorizations and need PHI access to fulfill their job responsibilities.

### Personnel Security: Visitor Escorts

Visitors to Company XYZ offices including, but not limited to, customers, former employees, worker family members, equipment repair contractors, package delivery company staff, and police officers will be escorted at all times by an authorized workforce member.

### Security Configuration Management

Company XYZ will establish security configuration management procedures to ensure the security of information systems.

### Computer Emergency Response

Management will organize and maintain an in-house computer emergency response team that will provide accelerated problem notification, damage control, and problem correction services in the event of computer related emergencies such as virus infestations and hacker break-ins.

377

APPENDICES

### Risk Assessments

Company XYZ will perform risk and vulnerability assessments and implement correspondingly appropriate security measures for all protected health information (PHI) in possession.

### Contractor Termination Procedures

Upon the termination or expiration of their contracts, all contractors, consultants, and temporaries will give their project manager all copies of Company XYZ information received or created during the execution of the contract.

### Media Removal

All computer storage media leaving Company XYZ offices will be accompanied by a properly authorized pass and will be logged at the building's front desk.

# Appendix C
# HIPAA Resources

---

## LINKS TO HIPAA REGULATORY TEXTS

### HIPAA Privacy Rule:

http://www.cms.hhs.gov/hipaa/hipaa2/regulations/privacy/default.asp
http://www.hhs.gov/ocr/combinedregtext.pdf

### HIPAA Security Rule:

http://www.cms.hhs.gov/hipaa/hipaa2/regulations/security/default.asp

### HIPAA Transaction Standards and Code Sets:

http://www.cms.hhs.gov/hipaa/hipaa2/regulations/transactions/default.asp

### HIPAA Identifiers Standards

http://www.cms.hhs.gov/hipaa/hipaa2/regulations/identifiers/default.asp

### OCR Civil Money Penalties: Procedures for Investigations, Imposition of Penalties, and Hearings

http://www.hhs.gov/ocr/moneypenalties.html


## HIPAA WEB SITES AND RELATED ORGANIZATIONS

### Centers for Medicare and Medicaid Services

http://www.cms.gov/hipaa/hipaa2/default.asp

### DHHS — Administrative Simplification

http://aspe.os.dhhs.gov/admnsimp/

### DHHS — Health Insurance and Portability Act of 1996

http://aspe.os.dhhs.gov/admnsimp/pl104191.htm

---

The information and opinions provided in this book do not constitute or substitute for legal or other professional advice.

APPENDICES

## Administrative Simplification Under HIPAA National Standards for Transactions, Security and Privacy (Fact Sheet)

http://www.hhs.gov/news/press/2002pres/hipaa.html

## Covered Entity Decision Support Tool Home Page

http://www.cms.gov/hipaa/hipaa2/support/tools/decisionsupport/default.asp

## Final Privacy Rule Preamble — Discussion of Comments

http://www.hhs.gov/ocr/part3.html

## Final Privacy Rule Preamble — Final Regulatory Analyses

http://www.hhs.gov/ocr/part4.html

## Health Insurance Association of America

http://www.hiaa.org

## HHS Data Council Privacy Committee

http://aspe.hhs.gov/datacncl/privcmte.htm

## HIPAA Resources for Financial Institutions and Payment Professionals

http://www.hipaabanking.org

## Workgroup for Electronic Data Interchange Strategic National Implementation Process

http://snip.wedi.org

## California Department of Mental Health HIPAA Home Page

http://www.dmh.ca.gov/hipaa/

## HIPAA Privacy Rule and Its Impact on Research

http://privacyruleandresearch.nih.gov/resources.asp

## HIPAAdvisory

http://www.hipaadvisory.com

## HIPAASource Links

http://www.himss.org/hipaasource/hipaalinks-RegionalGroups.asp

**HIPAAComply**

http://www.hipaacomply.com

**HIPAA Security Categories**

http://www.aamc.org/members/gir/gasp/securitycategories.pdf

**Workers Compensation Guidelines**

http://www.hhs.gov/ocr/hipaa/guidelines/workerscompensation.pdf

**IOMA HIPAA HELP**

http://www.ioma.org/PDF/HIPAA/IOMAHIPAAHELP.pdf

**WEDI SNIP Privacy Policies and Procedures: A Resource Document**

http://www.wedi.org/snip/public/articles/privacy_pp1115_02.pdf

**Massachusetts Health Data Consortium**

http://www.mahealthdata.org

**HHS Initial Regulatory Flexibility Analysis for the HIPAA Privacy Rule**
http://aspe.hhs.gov/admnsimp/nprm/pvc53.htm

**Office for Civil Rights — Privacy of Health Records**

http://www.hhs.gov/ocr/hipaa/privacy.html

**Practice Brief Defining the Designated Record Set**

http://library.ahima.org/xpedio/groups/public/documents/ahima/pub_bok1_017122.html

**The Top Fifteen Privacy Concerns Quiz — DHHS**
http://www.regreform.hhs.gov/HIPAAQUIZ_0204171/sld001.htm

**Southern HIPAA Regional Administrative Process**

http://www.sharpworkgroup.com

**NCVHS — National Committee on Vital and Health Statistics**

http://www.ncvhs.hhs.gov

**U.S. Government Printing Office**

http://www.access.gpo.gov

**Model HIPAA Privacy and Security Audit for Small Practices**

http://www.edss.com/download/HIPAA/Model%20HIPAA%20Provider%20
Security%20and%20Privacy.pdf

**HIMSS — Healthcare Information and Management Systems Society**

http://www.himss.org

**AHIMA — American Health Information Management Association**

http://www.ahima.org

**URAC/NIST HIPAA Privacy and Security Accreditation**

http://www.urac.org/urac.asp?id=87

**RELATED HIPAA RESOURCE BOOKS BY THE AUTHORS**

*The Privacy Papers*; Rebecca Herold; Auerbach Publishing
*Healthcare Information Systems, 2nd ed.*; Kevin Beaver; Auerbach Publishing
*The Definitive Guide to Email Management and Security*; Kevin Beaver;
Realtimepublishers.com

**PERIODICALS, E-MAIL SUBSCRIPTIONS, AND HIPAA-RELATED FORUMS**

**Auerbach Publications: *Information Systems Security***

http://www.auerbach-publications.com

**Auerbach Publications: *EDP Audit, Control, and Security newsletter***

http://www.auerbach-publications.com

**HCPro's HIPAA Weekly Advisor and HIPAA Training Advisor e-mails**

http://www.hcmarketplace.com/free/emailnls

**HCPro's Healthcare Information Security newsletter**

http://www.hcmarketplace.com/prod.cfm?id=708

**HIPAA-CISSP Yahoo! Group**

http://groups.yahoo.com/group/HIPAA-CISSP

**DelCreo Risk Management and Privacy eZine Newsletter**

http://www.delcreo.com/delcreo/information.cfm

## SOFTWARE TOOLS SUPPORTING HIPAA COMPLIANCE

**PrivaPlan**

http://www.privaplan.com

**NetIQ HIPAA VigilEnt Policy Center HIPAA Content Module
by Rebecca Herold**

http://www.netiq.com/products/vpc/hipaa.asp

**WorkSmart MD HIPAA RX Compliance Toolkit
http://www.worksmartmd.com**

**Omtool Enterprise Document Management Exchange Products**

http://www.omtool.com

**HIMSS CPRI Toolkit for Health Care Security Management**

http://www.himss.org/asp/cpritoolkit_toolkit.asp

## SECURITY POLICY PRODUCTS AND RESOURCES

**NetIQ VigilEnt Policy Center**

http://www.netiq.com/products/vpc/default.asp

**Bindview Policy Center**

http://www.bindview.com

**Security Policies Made Easy by Charles Cresson Wood**

http://www.netiq.com/products/pub/ispme.asp

**The SANS Security Policy Project**

http://www.sans.org/resources/policies

**IETF Site Security Handbook**

ftp://ftp.isi.edu/in-notes/rfc2196.txt

## HIPAA AND INFORMATION SECURITY AND PRIVACY TRAINING, EDUCATION, AND AWARENESS-RELATED ORGANIZATIONS AND VENDORS

### Classes and Certifications

*DelCreo, Inc.*
http://www.delcreo.com

*Principle Logic, LLC*
http://www.principlelogic.com

*HIMSS*
http://www.himss.org

*AHIMA*
http://www.ahima.org

*ISC²*
http://www.isc2.org

*ISACA*
http://www.isaca.org

*MIS Training Institute*
http://www.misti.com

*Computer Security Institute*
http://www.gocsi.com

*SANS*
http://www.sans.org

*Southeast Cybercrime Institute*
http://cybercrime.kennesaw.edu

### Training Tools

*Green Idea, Inc. Awareness Screen Savers*
http://www.greenidea.com

*Security Awareness, Inc. Awareness Resources*
http://www.securityawareness.com

*HCPro's HCProfessor online HIPAA training modules*
http://www.hcprofessor.com

# GENERAL IT AND INFORMATION SECURITY BOOKS AND RESOURCES

*Information Security Policies, Procedures, and Standards: Guidelines for Effective Information Security Management* by Thomas R. Peltier — Auerbach Publications

http://www.crcpress.com

**Information Security Management Handbook edited by Harold F. Tipton and Micki Krause — Auerbach Publications**

http://www.crcpress.com

**Information Security Roles & Responsibilities Made Easy by Charles Cresson Wood — NetIQ**

http://www.netiq.com/products/pub/israr.asp

**Network Security for Dummies by Chey Cobb — Wiley Publishing**

http://www.dummies.com

**National Institute of Standards and Technology (NIST) Security Publications**

http://csrc.nist.gov/publications/nistpubs/index.html

## RISK ANALYSIS RESOURCES

**Information Security Risk Analysis by Thomas R. Peltier — Auerbach Publications**

http://www.crcpress.com

**Managing a Network Vulnerability Assessment by Thomas R. Peltier, John A. Blackley, and Justin Peltier — Auerbach Publications**

http://www.crcpress.com

**CERT OCTAVE^SM Methodology**

http://www.cert.org/octave

**Managing Information Security Risks: The OCTAVE^SM Approach by Christopher Alberts and Audrey Dorofee — Pearson Technology Group**

http://www.pearsonptg.com

**ISO 17799 Information Technology — Code of Practice for Information Security Management**

http://www.iso.ch

**NIST Special Publication 800-26 — Security Self-Assessment Guide for Information Technology Systems**

http://csrc.nist.gov/publications/nistpubs/800-26/sp800-26.pdf

**Privacy and Security Technologies**

The following Web sites provide links to various security and privacy tools — sometimes called Privacy Enhancing Technologies or PETs — that can control and manage how information is gathered, used, shared, and secured. These technologies can be used to protect PHI as it is transmitted across a public network, while it is stored on internal computer systems, etc. These are not necessarily comprehensive lists. There are so many possible solutions we encourage you to perform an Internet search if you cannot find a good match for your specific needs.

**Information Security Magazine's Buyers' Guide**

http://www.infosecuritymag.com

**SC Magazine's Online Product Reviews**

http://www.scmagazine.com/scmagazine/sc-online/archives/index.html

**CSI's Annual Buyer's Guide**

http://www.gocsi.com/bg/csibgp1.html

# Appendix D
# Answers to Chapter Quizzes

**Section 1: HIPAA Essentials Quiz**

1. What section of HIPAA was designed to help decrease the costs of healthcare administration with the goal of spending that money instead on increasing the quality of healthcare?
   A. Accounting and Budget
   **B. Administrative Simplification**
   C. Costs and Analysis
   D. Low Price Healthcare

As indicated in Chapter 1, Introduction to HIPAA, the Administrative Simplification section of HIPAA was designed to help decrease the costs of healthcare administration with the goal of spending that money instead on increasing the quality of healthcare. This includes standardizing on electronic transactions, national identifiers, and ensuring the privacy and security of confidential health information.

Choice B is the correct answer.

2. What organization is responsible for establishing the HIPAA standards?
   A. CIA
   B. CMS
   **C. HHS**
   D. FCC

As indicated in Chapter 1, Introduction to HIPAA, the Department of Health and Human Services (HHS) is the organization responsible for establishing the HIPAA standards.

Choice C is the correct answer.

3. HHS reports that if all healthcare entities follow the electronic transaction standards, the healthcare industry will realize what amount of savings over a 10-year period?
   A. $1.2 million
   **B. $29.9 billion net**

---

The information and opinions provided in this book do not constitute or substitute for legal or other professional advice.

    C. Over $500,000

    D. 42 cents

As indicated in Chapter 1, Introduction to HIPAA, HHS reports that if all healthcare entities follow these standards, the healthcare industry will realize a $29.9 billion net savings over a 10-year period by eliminating inefficient paper forms.

Choice B is the correct answer.

4. What are the two rules proposed for identifiers?
    **A. National Provider Identifier and the National Employer Identifier**
    B. Certified Physician Identifier and the Patient Privacy Set
    C. Federated Healthcare Identifier and the Home Health Identifier
    D. National Safety and Privacy Codes and the Employer Regulations Identifier

As indicated in Chapter 1, Introduction to HIPAA, so far there have been two rules proposed for identifiers: the National Provider Identifier and the National Employer Identifier. The proposed National Provider Identifier is a new 8-character alphanumeric or 10-digit numeric with a check digit. The National Employer Identifier is the same as the Federal Employer Identification Number (EIN), which is composed of nine digits separated by a hyphen (for example, 00-0000000).

Choice A is the correct answer.

5. Successful HIPAA change management will involve which of the following?
    A. A large budget
    **B. A strong leadership role**
    C. A 10-person technical team
    D. Outside consultants

As indicated in Chapter 2, Preparing for the HIPAA Changes, successful HIPAA change management will involve a strong leadership role, the decision to move forward with your compliance efforts, and proactive planning and implementation.

Choice B is the correct answer.

6. Which of the following is one key factor in helping to create a new way of "HIPAA" thinking?
    A. Bribery
    B. Signed contracts
    C. The right software
    **D. Persuasion**

As indicated in Chapter 2, Preparing for the HIPAA Changes, the new ways of providing healthcare mandated by HIPAA are a lot to take on. One key factor in helping to create a new way of "HIPAA" thinking is persuasion.

Choice D is the correct answer.

7. Instilling the proper HIPAA-aware mindset begins with which of the following?
   **A. Creating the proper culture**
   B. Convincing the patients
   C. Handing out flyers
   D. Online research

As indicated in Chapter 2, Preparing for the HIPAA Changes, instilling the proper HIPAA-aware mindset begins with creating the proper culture. Upper management and HIPAA officers who lead by example must embrace this culture.

Choice A is the correct answer.

8. What is one of the best ways to get buy-in for HIPAA in your organization?
   A. Enforcement of rules
   B. A three-day seminar
   **C. Demonstrate the business value**
   D. Long-term planning

As indicated in Chapter 2, Preparing for the HIPAA Changes, one of the best ways to get buy-in on HIPAA in your organization is to demonstrate the business value that it brings. Embrace HIPAA with the future in mind and give examples of how HIPAA will pay off long term.

Choice C is the correct answer.

9. How much are hospitals nationwide planning to spend during the first 5 years to comply with applicable HIPAA laws?
   **A. As much as $22 billion**
   B. An estimated $400,000
   C. Close to 1 million
   D. Under $50,000

As indicated in Chapter 3, HIPAA Cost Considerations, according to AHA funded research, hospitals nationwide are planning to spend as much as $22 billion during the first five years to comply with applicable HIPAA laws. For example, they project that implementing minimum necessary requirements will cost a minimum $1.3 billion over five years for hospitals, and up to $19.8 billion if hospitals must invest in new or upgraded computer systems.

Choice A is the correct answer.

10. Peter Swire, the Chief Privacy Counsel for the administration in the year 2000, projected compliance with which of the following would equate to $6.25 per year for every insured American?
    A. EDI
    **B. Privacy Rule**
    C. Administrative Simplification Act
    D. Disability Insurance

As indicated in Chapter 3, HIPAA Cost Considerations, in December 2000 Clinton administration officials did some number crunching to determine what costs may be involved. Peter Swire, the Chief Privacy Counsel for the administration at that time, projected the Privacy Rule cost would equate to $6.25 per year for every insured American.

Choice B is the correct answer.

11. AHIMA indicates the salary range for a privacy officer will be in what range?
    A. $20,000 to $30,000
    B. $8.00 to $12.00 hourly
    **C. $80,000 to $140,000**
    D. Will vary widely

As indicated in Chapter 3, HIPAA Cost Considerations, in larger organizations it will probably be necessary to assign a person to dedicate their entire time to addressing the privacy requirements. AHIMA indicates the salary range for a privacy officer will be in the $80,000 to $140,000 range.

Choice C is the correct answer.

12. What is a really positive aspect of the Security Rule?
    A. The enforcement deadlines
    B. The lack of technical requirements
    C. The control given to the patients
    **D. The flexibility regarding costs and implementation requirements**

As indicated in Chapter 3, HIPAA Cost Considerations, a really positive aspect of the Security Rule is that it is flexible regarding costs. There are many security standards that are "addressable," meaning that CEs have some wiggle room depending on their specific situation.

Choice D is the correct answer.

13. Which of the following best describes security (as opposed to privacy)?
    A. Enables consumers to find out how financial information is going to be protected
    B. Limits release of information to the minimum reasonably needed for the purpose of the disclosure

C. **Is the implementation of reasonable and prudent policies, processes, steps, and tools that are used to maintain confidentiality**

D. Enables patients to find out how their information may be used and what disclosures of their information have been made

As indicated in Chapter 4, The Relationship Between Security and Privacy, security with respect to HIPAA constitutes those reasonable and prudent policies, processes, steps, and tools that are used to maintain confidentiality and privacy. It involves all methods, processes, and technology used to ensure the confidentiality and safety of the private information that has been entrusted to the covered entity by the customer or patient.

Choice C is the correct answer.

14. The Privacy Rule generally does not refer directly to security requirements, but instead uses another term that basically means the same thing as security. Which of the following terms is used to represent all types of security in this way within the Privacy Rule?

A. Administrative Requirements

B. **Safeguard Requirements**

C. Technical Requirements

D. Physical Requirements

As indicated in Chapter 4, The Relationship Between Security and Privacy, the Privacy Rule explicitly requires several safeguard requirements. These are the statements that specifically require security.

Choice B is the correct answer.

15. Which of the following is the most apparent difference between the Privacy Rule and the Security Rule?

A. The Security Rule will cost more to implement

B. The Privacy Rule applies to international locations

C. **The Security Rule applies only to electronic PHI, and the Privacy Rule applies to PHI in any form**

D. The Security Rule contains very specific technology requirements and vendor specifications, and the Privacy Rule contains only broad requirement specifications

As indicated in Chapter 4, The Relationship Between Security and Privacy, the Privacy Rule requires CEs to safeguard all PHI it has, regardless of the form the PHI is in, such as on paper, electronic, or spoken. The Security Rule applies to PHI in electronic form only.

Choice C is the correct answer.

## Section 2: HIPAA Privacy Rule Quiz

1. Which of the following is an intention of the Privacy Rule?
   A. Remove limitations on the use and disclosure of health records
   B. **Enable patients to learn how their information can be used along with the disclosures of other information**
   C. Give employers the right to examine their employees' personal health records
   D. Give individual patients complete control in deciding who gets access to their information, regardless of the situation

As detailed within Chapter 5, HIPAA Privacy Rule Requirements Overview, the Privacy Rule intends to protect personal health information by:

- Giving patients more control over their health information
- Setting limitations on the use and release of health records
- Establishing safeguards covered entities must implement to protect the privacy of health information
- Holding those in noncompliance responsible through civil and criminal penalties for privacy violations
- Attempting to create a balance between public responsibility for disclosure of some forms of information and the personal information of individual patients
- Giving patients the opportunity to make informed choices when seeking care and reimbursement for care based on considering how personal health information can be used
- Enabling patients to learn how their information can be used along with the disclosures of their information
- Limiting release to only the minimal amount of information needed for required disclosures
- Giving patients the right to examine and correct any mistakes in their personal health records

Choice B is the correct answer.

2. Which of the following best describes what "use" of PHI means?
   A. **The sharing, employment, application, utilization, examination, or analysis of individually identifiable health information within a covered entity**
   B. The release, transfer, provision of access to, or divulging of information outside the entity holding the information
   C. The utilization of health information to assist with investigations related to public health issues
   D. The sharing, utilization, or examination of individually identifiable health information with a third party

As indicated in Chapter 5, HIPAA Privacy Rule Requirements Overview, within the General Rules for PHI Uses and Disclosures, "use" means the sharing, employment, application, utilization, examination, or analysis of individually identifiable health information within a covered entity.

Choice A is the correct answer.

3. In which of the following situations may PHI be used without authorization?
   A. To publish the names of people who have been admitted to a hospital, and their accompanying malady, in the local newspaper
   B. To send names and addresses to a company marketing a birth announcement service
   C. For including PHI within a research study
   **D. For treatment activities of a healthcare provider**

As indicated in Chapter 5, HIPAA Privacy Rule Requirements Overview, PHI may be used by covered entities without an authorization in the following situations:

- For a covered entity's own TPO
- For treatment activities of a healthcare provider
- By another covered entity or healthcare provider for payment processes of the entity that receives the PHI
- For another covered entity that has, or had, a relationship with the individual
- By another covered entity that participates in an organized healthcare arrangement
- Use and disclosure for public health activities
- Use and disclosure for health oversight activities
- Use and disclosure for judicial and administrative proceedings
- Disclosure to coroners and medical examiners
- Disclosure for law enforcement
- Use and disclosure for governmental health data systems
- Disclosure for directory information
- Disclosure for banking and payment processes
- Use and disclosure for research, emergency circumstances, next-of-kin, and as required by other laws

Choice D is the correct answer.

4. An incidental use or disclosure is not permitted if it results from a violation of the Privacy Rule. What is an incidental use or disclosure?
   A. A primary use or disclosure that is too expensive to address adequately
   **B. A secondary use or disclosure that cannot reasonably be prevented as a result of an acceptable use or disclosure, and is limited in nature**
   C. A secondary use or disclosure that occurs within a business associate network

D. A primary use or disclosure that results as a result of lack of privacy training

As indicated in Chapter 5, HIPAA Privacy Rule Requirements Overview, an incidental use or disclosure is a secondary use or disclosure that cannot reasonably be prevented as a result of an acceptable use or disclosure, and is limited in nature. An incidental use or disclosure is not permitted if it results from a violation of the Privacy Rule.

Choice B is the correct answer.

5. When can a covered entity deny an individual's PHI amendment request?
   A. If the individual has not kept their health insurance coverage premiums paid to date
   B. If the cost of updating the PHI would cause financial hardship for the covered entity
   **C. If the PHI is in actuality accurate and complete**
   D. If the PHI was created more than three years prior to the amendment request

As indicated in Chapter 5, HIPAA Privacy Rule Requirements Overview, the covered entity must permit an individual to request amendment to PHI maintained in a designated record set. The entity may require the requests to be in writing and require a reason to support a requested amendment. A covered entity must honor requests to amend PHI for individuals for as long as they maintain PHI records. A covered entity can deny an individual's amendment request if the PHI was not created by the covered entity (unless the originator of PHI is no longer available), if the PHI is not part of the designated record set, or if the PHI is determined to be accurate and complete.

Choice C is the correct answer.

6. What is the best way for you to determine where HIPAA compliance requirements must be addressed within your organization?
   A. Perform a penetration test
   **B. Perform a gap analysis**
   C. Perform a cost analysis
   D. Perform a social engineering test

As indicated in Chapter 6, Performing a Privacy Rule Gap Analysis, to determine where HIPAA compliance requirements must be addressed, or your HIPAA gaps, you must perform a HIPAA Privacy Rule gap analysis and risk assessment. Using the results of the analysis and assessment, along with any existing business and financial plans, your organization will be ready to develop a HIPAA compliance plan, including a listing of compliance priorities.

Choice B is the correct answer.

7. Which of the following headers must appear in your Notice of Privacy Practices?

**A. THIS NOTICE DESCRIBES HOW MEDICAL INFORMATION ABOUT YOU MAY BE USED AND DISCLOSED AND HOW YOU CAN GET ACCESS TO THIS INFORMATION. PLEASE REVIEW IT CAREFULLY.**

B. THIS NOTICE ADVISES YOU OF YOUR LEGAL RIGHTS WITH RESPECT TO HOW MEDICAL INFORMATION ABOUT YOU MAY BE USED. PLEASE REVIEW THIS CAREFULLY.

C. THIS NOTICE DESCRIBES YOUR OBLIGATIONS TO ENSURE THE PROTECTION OF YOUR OWN MEDICAL INFORMATION THAT IS PROCESSED BY THIS ORGANIZATION. PLEASE REVIEW THIS INFORMATION CAREFULLY.

D. THIS NOTICE DETAILS YOUR RIGHTS, OBLIGATIONS, AND COURSE OF ACTIONS RELATED TO YOUR HEALTH INFORMATION. REVIEW THIS CAREFULLY.

As indicated in Chapter 7, Writing Effective Privacy Policies, the HIPAA Privacy Rule requirements are very specific and straightforward when it comes to specifying the wording for the heading of the privacy notice (45 CFR 164.520(b)(1)(i)). The header, or a prominently displayed message, must be written exactly as follows:

*THIS NOTICE DESCRIBES HOW MEDICAL INFORMATION ABOUT YOU MAY BE USED AND DISCLOSED AND HOW YOU CAN GET ACCESS TO THIS INFORMATION. PLEASE REVIEW IT CAREFULLY.*

Choice A is the correct answer.

8. There are three requirements related to the content of a Notice of Privacy Practices. Which of the following is one of these three requirements?

A. A listing of your business associates

**B. Your organization's legal duties for handling PHI**

C. The technical safeguards you have in place to protect PHI

D. The background check practices you follow for your personnel

As indicated in Chapter 7, Writing Effective Privacy Practices, there are some requirements related to the content of a notice of privacy practices:

- Your notice of privacy practices must be written clearly, in plain language, describing:
  - How your organization may use and disclose PHI. Include an example of each use and disclosure.
  - All the individuals' rights with regard to their corresponding PHI, and how individuals may execute their rights, including their

right to submit formal complaints to your organization. This section may be quite lengthy depending upon your other state laws that have more stringent requirements for related to health information privacy.

- Your organization's legal duties for handling PHI, including a statement clearly stating your organization is required by law to maintain the privacy of PHI.
- Who individuals should contact for more information about your organization's privacy policies.
- Your organization's notice must include an effective date.
- Your organization must revise and distribute its notice promptly following material changes to its privacy practices.

Choice B is the correct answer.

9. Which of the following describes a situation in which a state law is considered "contrary to" a HIPAA privacy standard, requirement, or implementation specification?
   A. Where the penalties for the state requirements are more excessive than those for the HIPAA requirements
   B. Where the state law is similar in all respects to the HIPAA requirements
   C. Where the state law has an expiration date
   **D. Where the covered entity cannot comply with both the state and HIPAA requirements**

As indicated in Chapter 8, State Preemption, a state law is considered "contrary to" a HIPAA privacy standard, requirement, or implementation specification in one of two situations (45 CFR §160.202), where:

- The covered entity cannot possibly comply with both the state and federal requirements. So, compliance with a state requirement would prevent compliance with the HIPAA requirement.
- A provision of state law stands as "an obstacle" to the accomplishment and execution of the full purposes of the HIPAA legislation related to Administrative Simplification. This language is far from clear cut but anticipates situations in which state and federal law do not directly conflict but state and federal requirements nevertheless compete with one another.

Choice D is the correct answer.

10. Which of the following is a state preemption category?
    **A. Health plan regulation and monitoring**
    B. International requirements
    C. Litigation activities
    D. Determination by the HIMSS president

As indicated in Chapter 8, State Preemption, the following are the state law HIPAA and Privacy Rule preemption exception categories:

- Public health and vital statistics. This allows for reporting diseases or injuries, child abuse, births, or deaths or that authorize public health surveillance, or public health investigation or intervention.
- Health plan regulation and monitoring. This allows for the application of state laws that require a health plan to report, or provide access to, information for regulatory management audits, financial audits, program monitoring and evaluation, facility licensure or certification, or individual licensure and certification.
- Determination by HHS Secretary. The Secretary has the discretion to determine that HIPAA will not preempt contrary state laws that are necessary to prevent fraud and abuse related to healthcare payment; to ensure appropriate state regulation of insurance and health plans; to permit state reporting on healthcare delivery or cost; or to server a compelling need related to public health, safety, or welfare.
- More stringent health privacy protections. HIPAA does not preempt provisions of state law covering the privacy of individually identifiable health information and impose requirements that are more stringent than the requirements, standards, or specifications imposed under HIPAA privacy rule.

Choice A is the correct answer.

11. Which of the following should be included within your HIPAA Privacy Rule implementation plan?
    **A. Planning remediation strategies**
    B. Implementing PKI
    C. Upgrading all your systems
    D. Creating consents for all individuals to sign

As indicated in Chapter 9, Crafting a Privacy Implementation Plan, you need to plan and document your remediation strategies.

Choice A is the correct answer.

12. When is an authorization defective?
    A. If it was obtained within a provider's facility
    B. If it was signed just prior to April 14, 2003
    C. When it contains the names of hybrid entities
    **D. If it has expired**

As indicated in Chapter 10, Privacy Rule Compliance Checklist, a covered entity may not use or disclose protected health information using a defective authorization. Authorization is defective if it has expired, it is incomplete, it has been revoked, it is known to be false, it is part of a compound authorization or treatment, or if payment, enrollment, or eligibility has been conditioned on obtaining the individual's signature.

Choice D is the correct answer.

13. Which of the following is an example of when a covered entity is applying the minimum necessary requirement?
    A. A covered entity denies an individual's request to amend PHI
    **B. A covered entity identifies classes of persons who need access to PHI to carry out job responsibilities**
    C. A covered entity permits an individual to opt-out of having certain pieces of their PHI used in the facility directory
    D. A covered entity does not give law enforcement access to the PHI they want to see

As indicated in Chapter 10, Privacy Rule Compliance Checklist, a covered entity must identify classes of persons who need access to protected health information to carry out their duties and must establish the levels of access needed by each. A covered entity must make reasonable efforts to limit access to the minimum information required to perform an assigned job function.

Choice B is the correct answer.

14. When may a CE choose not to treat a parent as a personal representative of a minor?
    A. When the parent has a criminal record
    B. When the minor signs an authorization
    C. When the parent lives in a different state as where the treatment occurs
    **D. When the minor may lawfully obtain healthcare without parental consent**

As indicated in Chapter 5, HIPAA Privacy Requirements Overview, a covered entity must treat a parent, guardian, or person acting with parental rights of an unemancipated minor as a personal representative of that minor, unless the minor may lawfully obtain the healthcare without parental consent. If the minor may lawfully obtain the healthcare without parental consent, then the covered entity must follow state law with respect to disclosures to parents, guardians, and persons acting with parental rights.

Choice D is the correct answer.

15. Access controls are fundamentally what kind of mechanisms?
    A. Legal
    **B. Security**
    C. Technology
    D. Administrative

As indicated in Chapter 5, HIPAA Privacy Rule Requirements Overview, the Privacy Rule contains many access control requirements, and access controls are fundamentally security mechanisms.

Choice B is the correct answer.

### Section 3: HIPAA Security Rule Quiz

1. Which of the following does NOT characterize the Security Rule?
   A. A set of information security best practices that make good business sense
   B. A minimum security baseline which is intended to help prevent unauthorized access of PHI
   C. **An inflexible and unscalable set of rules that healthcare organizations must comply with**
   D. An outline of what to do

As indicated in Chapter 11, Security Rule Requirements Overview, the Security Rule can be characterized as:

- A set of information security best practices that make good business sense
- A minimum security baseline which is intended to help prevent unauthorized access of PHI
- An outline of what to do
- Something that encourages healthcare organizations to embrace E-business and leverage the benefits that an improved technology infrastructure can provide
- Standards to reduce the threats and vulnerabilities and overall risks to PHI along with their associated costs and negative impact on the organization

Choice C is the correct answer.

2. The Security Rule was designed to be which of the following?
   A. Technology neutral
   B. Scalable
   C. Flexible
   D. **All of the above**

As indicated in Chapter 11, Security Rule Requirements Overview, the Security Rule was designed to be:

- Technology neutral: Focuses on what needs to be done rather than how to do it or what technologies to use
- Scalable: Does not require all organizations to implement the same exact policies, procedures, and technologies; a CE's information systems' complexity will define its Security Rule implementation complexity.

- Flexible: Allows CEs to take size, capabilities, risks, and costs into consideration when trying to determine whether or not to implement certain security systems.
- Comprehensive: Covers the technical, business, and behavioral issues related to securing PHI.

Choice D is the correct answer.

3. Have there been any changes to the Security Rule since it was first proposed?
    A. Yes, the entire original rule was scrapped and a new one was created
    B. No, the document was so comprehensive that no changes were needed
    **C. Yes, numerous changes were made to the Security Rule before its final form**
    D. There have not been any changes yet, but new ones are expected in the Fall of 2005

As indicated in Chapter 11, Security Rule Requirements Overview, numerous changes were made to the Security Rule before its final form. The proposed rule contained several terms that were unclear and there were several areas of overlap among the four different safeguard sections. HHS clarified these confusing terms and removed the redundancies so that there are now 18 standards in the final rule instead of the original 24.

Choice C is the correct answer.

4. How many required implementation specifications does the Security Rule have?
    A. Over 300
    B. None
    **C. 20**
    D. Each CE must find out after doing a risk analysis

As indicated in Chapter 11, Security Rule Requirements Overview, there are a total of 20 required implementation specifications that must be implemented by all CEs regardless of the outcome of their risk analysis.

Choice C is the correct answer.

5. What can be used to assist meeting the Access Authorization (Addressable) specification in the Security Rule?
    A. HR, supervisor, and manager education on this matter
    B. Strong line of communication between HR and IT
    C. Internal employee to develop the specific procedures
    **D. All of the above**

As Chapter 11, Security Rule Requirements Overview, indicates, in Access Authorization (Addressable) the rule says:

- Implement policies and procedures for granting access to electronic protected health information, for example, through access to a workstation, transaction, program, process, or other mechanism.
- The following can be used to assist in meeting this specification:
  - HR, supervisor, and manager education on this matter
  - Strong line of communication between HR and IT
  - Internal employee to develop the specific procedures

Choice D is the correct answer.

6. What do security policies and supporting documents outline?
   A. Roles and responsibilities
   B. Standards for all employees to adhere to
   **C. Both A and B**
   D. None of the above

As indicated in Chapter 13, Writing Effective Information Security Policies, security policies are comprised of sets of documents that define who, what, when, where, why, and how of your organization's electronic information (PHI) protection strategy. They outline roles and responsibilities, who has access to what information, acceptable usage for your employees, standards for all employees to adhere to, and procedures to actually carry out the specific policies, standards, and guidelines.

Choice C is the correct answer.

7. How often should you consider performing a review of your security policies?
   A. Never; once you finish, it should work forever
   B. Every five years
   C. Right before you are audited
   **D. Annually**

As indicated in Chapter 13, Writing Effective Information Security Policies, you should consider performing an annual review of your policies to ensure they are still appropriate for your information systems and business needs.

Choice D is the correct answer.

8. What should you establish that will plan, oversee, and guide your HIPAA security efforts?
   A. A Vendor-Neutral Task Force
   **B. A Steering Committee**
   C. A Yearly Calendar
   D. Rules and Regulations

As indicated in Chapter 14, Crafting a Security Implementation Plan, you should establish a steering committee that will plan, oversee, and guide your HIPAA security efforts. You do not want to go at this alone. Even if you are a small covered entity, get at least one other person involved.

Choice B is the correct answer.

9. What is helpful in performing a Security Rule Gap Analysis?
   **A. Collecting the inventory of the electronic PHI that you compiled for your Privacy Rule initiatives**
   B. Making sure that all computers on your network are using Windows 2000
   C. Deleting old transaction logs
   D. Compiling a list of all current and former patients

As indicated in Chapter 14, Crafting a Security Implementation Plan, you should collect the inventory of the electronic PHI that you compiled for your Privacy Rule initiatives. Verify that this inventory is still accurate and comprehensive.

Choice A is the correct answer.

10. At what point can you achieve 100 percent security for your organization?
    A. Six months into the HIPAA Security Compliance Process
    B. After all recommended Security measures have been taken
    **C. Never**
    D. When you have installed all necessary software

As indicated in Chapter 14, Crafting a Security Implementation Plan, there is no such thing as 100 percent security. Covered entities are just expected to follow the Security Rule standards, implement the proper policies, procedures, and technologies, and reasonably show that the organization is making an effort to protect against common threats and vulnerabilities.

Choice C is the correct answer.

11. Security Rule compliance is only possible with which of the following?
    A. A large HIPAA compliance budget
    B. Outside help from HIPAA experts
    C. A complete copy of the Security Policy in hand
    **D. An appropriate risk analysis is performed on your information systems**

As indicated in Chapter 12, Performing a Security Rule Gap Analysis and Risk Assessment, Security Rule compliance is only possible when an appropriate risk analysis is performed on your information systems. Stated another way, you must know what you are trying to protect and what you are trying to protect against before you can actually protect anything.

Choice D is the correct answer.

12. A risk analysis will help you determine which of the following?
    A. How confidential the PHI needs to be
    B. When and how the PHI needs to be protected
    C. Where the PHI is stored and transmitted
    **D. All of the above**

As indicated in Chapter 12, Performing a Security Rule Gap Analysis and Risk Assessment, a risk analysis will help you determine:

- What PHI your organization has
- Where the PHI is stored and transmitted
- What the specific threats and vulnerabilities are associated with the PHI
- What could happen to the PHI if unauthorized uses or disclosures occur
- How confidential the PHI needs to be
- When and how the PHI needs to be protected

Choice D is the correct answer.

13. Is it possible for a CE to come to the conclusion that their PHI is not at risk whatsoever?
    A. Yes, if they already had the proper safeguards in place
    **B. No**
    C. Perhaps once the Risk Analysis is complete
    D. None of the above

As indicated in Chapter 12, Performing a Security Rule Gap Analysis and Risk Assessment, we cannot imagine any scenario where a CE would come to the conclusion that their PHI is not at risk whatsoever. There are bound to be certain threats or vulnerabilities that exist that just may not be so obvious.

Choice B is the correct answer.

14. The Security Rule requires CEs to perform an initial risk analysis to determine which of the following?
    A. Specific unauthorized uses
    B. Disclosures
    C. Data integrity losses that could occur to PHI
    **D. All of the above**

As indicated in Chapter 12, Performing a Security Rule Gap Analysis and Risk Assessment, the Security Rule requires CEs to perform an initial risk analysis to determine specific unauthorized uses, disclosures, and data integrity losses that could occur to PHI if certain systems are not in place. This is part of the Security Management standard that falls under Administrative Safeguards in the Security Rule.

Choice D is the correct answer.

15. The Security Rule does not apply to information in any risk analysis documentation except in which of the following situations?
    A. It involves information stored on your computer
    B. The information is used to diagnose medical problems
    **C. It specifically contains PHI**
    D. None of the above

As indicated in Chapter 12, Performing a Security Rule Gap Analysis and Risk Assessment, the Security Rule does not apply to information in any risk analysis documentation unless it specifically contains PHI. Just make sure that you secure these records as you should any other critical business document.

Choice C is the correct answer.

## Section 4: Covered Entity Issues Quiz

1. Which of the following is typically not required by HIPAA to provide a Notice of Privacy Practices to individuals?
    A. Family physician
    B. Chiropractor
    C. Health insurance company
    **D. Healthcare clearinghouse**

As indicated in Chapter 17, Healthcare Clearinghouse Issues, unlike healthcare providers and plans, healthcare clearinghouses do not have to develop a notice of privacy practices if the only PHI they create or receive is as a business associate of another covered entity (provider or plan).

Choice D is the correct answer.

2. When must a direct healthcare treatment provider give an individual a Notice of Privacy Practices?
    A. By December 31, 2003
    **B. The date of first service delivery, with exceptions**
    C. The date of first service delivery, with no exceptions
    D. By April 14, 2003, and upon each office visit

As indicated in Chapter 16, Healthcare Provider Issues, covered direct healthcare treatment providers must provide a notice of privacy practices to an individual on the date of first service delivery and, except for in emergencies, attempt to obtain the individual's written acknowledgment of receipt of the notice. When an acknowledgment cannot be obtained, the provider must document the efforts to obtain the acknowledgment and provide an explanation why it was not obtained. If first service delivery to an individual is provided over the Internet, through e-mail, or using some other electronic method, the provider must send an electronic notice automatically at the same time of the individual's first request for service. The provider must try to obtain a return receipt or some other recognition from the individual in response to receiving the notice.

Choice B is the correct answer.

3. In which of the following situations is an employer directly impacted by HIPAA requirements?
   A. When workers' compensation claims are filed
   B. When a workforce member uses the benefits allowed by FMLA
   **C. When the employer sponsors an on-site clinic**
   D. When the employer provides Medigap coverage to retirees

As indicated in Chapter 19, Employer Issues, most employers now offer their employees wellness programs, on-site clinics, employee assistance programs, and similar health-related benefits. Employers are generally not considered covered entities under HIPAA definitions; however, they qualify when they sponsor healthcare components such as self-insured health plans, wellness programs, on-site clinics, or employee assistance programs. The Privacy Rule impacts the use and disclosure of protected health information by the healthcare component of the employer and the applicable personnel, and requires the establishment of "firewalls," or procedural and operational separations, to keep health-related functions separate from general, employment-related functions and personnel.

Choice C is the correct answer.

4. Many to most employers need to implement HIPAA requirements on behalf of which of the following?
   A. Their long-term care participants
   **B. Their covered health insurance benefit plans**
   C. Their long-term disability personnel
   D. Their casualty and fire insurance plans

As indicated in Chapter 19, Employer Issues, as plan sponsors or plan fiduciaries, most employers need to implement the HIPAA requirements on behalf of their covered benefit plans, or ensure that the insurance provider implements the HIPAA requirements. These covered plans were required to comply with the HIPAA standard transactions by October 16, 2002 (October 16, 2003, for small health plans).

Choice B is the correct answer.

5. Employer health plan sponsors are typically allowed by HIPAA to have access to what type of information?
   **A. Summary health information**
   B. Individually identifiable health information
   C. Protected health information
   D. Health history information

As indicated in Chapter 19, Employer Issues, employer health plan sponsors are typically allowed to have access under HIPAA to summary health information.

Choice A is the correct answer.

6. Which of the following is an example of a government-funded health plan?
   A. A Pacificare Plan
   **B. An Indian Health Service Program**
   C. An FDA Program
   D. A Voluntary Blood Bank Program

As indicated in Chapter 18, Healthcare Payer Issues, government-funded health plans include:

- Medicare program under Title XVIII of the Social Security Act (Parts A, B, and C) (42 U.S.C. 1395, et seq.)
- Medicaid program under Title XIX of the Social Security Act (42 U.S.C. 1396, et seq.)
- Healthcare program for active military personnel (10 U.S.C. 1074, et seq.)
- Veterans healthcare program (38 U.S.C. Ch.17)
- Civilian Health and Medical Program of the Uniformed Services (CHAMPUS) (10 U.S.C. 1061, et seq.)
- Indian Health Service program under the Indian Healthcare Improvement Act (25 U.S.C. 1601)
- Federal Employees Health Benefit Program (5 U.S.C. Ch. 89); and approved state child health programs under Title XXI of the Social Security Act (42 U.S.C. 1397, et seq.) (SCHIP)

Choice B is the correct answer.

7. By what date must a qualified small health plan be in compliance with the HIPAA Privacy Rule?
   A. April 21, 2005
   B. October 17, 2003
   C. April 14, 2003
   **D. April 14, 2004**

As indicated in Chapter 18, Healthcare Payer Issues, HIPAA defines a small health plan as one that has annual receipts of $5 million or less. Small health plans have an additional year to comply with the Privacy Rule; April 14, 2004.

Choice D is the correct answer.

8. A group health plan must require a plan sponsor to amend the plan documents to include which of the following provisions?
   A. Allow disclosures to employers for employment-related actions only after receiving a signed consent
   B. **Do not allow disclosures to employers for employment-related actions**
   C. Allow disclosures to employers for employment-related decisions related to any other benefit
   D. Do not allow disclosures to employers for plan-related sponsor actions

As indicated in Chapter 18, Healthcare Payer Issues, a group health plan must disclose protected health information to the plan sponsor only upon receipt of a certification by the plan sponsor that the plan documents have been amended to incorporate several provisions, including not using or disclosing the information for employment-related actions and decisions or in connection with any other benefit or employee benefit plan of the plan sponsor.

Choice B is the correct answer.

9. Which of the following is an example of marketing that requires an authorization?
   A. A face-to-face discussion with a patient where the doctor describes drugs available to treat a symptom
   B. **A mailing from a health insurer promoting a mortgage product offered by the same company**
   C. A mailing from a health insurer to a policyholder listing the physicians participating in the health plan network
   D. An insurer sends a mailing to subscribers nearing Medicare eligible age with information about its Medicare supplemental plan and an application form

As indicated in Chapter 18, Healthcare Payer Issues, the Privacy Rule defines marketing as "a communication about a product or service that encourages recipients of the communication to purchase or use the product or service." The following are examples of marketing communications that require authorization:

- A communication from a health insurer to plan subscribers informing them about a clinic that can provide a physical for $39
- A communication from a health insurer promoting a mortgage product offered by the same company

- A health plan selling a list of its members to a company that plans to send the members brochures advertising the benefits of purchasing and using their blood pressure monitors
- A health plan receives remuneration from a drug manufacturer after sending it a list of plan members who have made claims for anti-depressant medication, then the drug manufacturer sends coupons for their drugs directly to the listed plan members

Choice B is the correct answer.

10. How soon following a material revision of a notice of privacy practices must a health plan provide the revised notice to individuals who subscribe to the plan?
    A. Within 6 days
    B. At least once every 3 years
    C. Within 30 days
    **D. Within 60 days**

As indicated in Chapter 18, Healthcare Payer Issues, health plans must also provide a revised notice to individuals then covered by the plan within 60 days of a material revision, and they must notify individuals then covered by the plan of the availability of the privacy practices notice, and how to obtain the notice at least once every 3 years.

Choice D is the correct answer.

11. Which of the following is a distinguishing feature of a healthcare clearinghouse?
    **A. Processing health information from a nonstandard format to a standard format**
    B. Selling software that converts the format of health information
    C. Creating software that concerts the format of health information
    D. Electronically transferring health information from a health plan to a bank system

As indicated in Chapter 17, Healthcare Clearinghouse Issues, if your organization processes, or facilitates the processing of, health information from nonstandard format or content into standard format or content or from standard format or content into nonstandard format or content, then you are likely a healthcare clearinghouse.

Choice A is the correct answer.

12. Which of the following is an example of a HIPAA-covered service provided by a healthcare provider?
    A. Body piercing
    B. Sponsoring a weight-loss plan
    C. Storing blood bank supplies
    **D. Dispensing drugs for a prescription**

As indicated in Chapter 16, Healthcare Provider Issues, a healthcare provider provides healthcare services or supplies related to the health of an individual. It includes, but is not limited to, the following:

- Preventive, diagnostic, rehabilitative, maintenance, or palliative care, and counseling, service, assessment, or procedure with respect to the physical or mental condition, or functional status, of an individual or that affects the structure or function of the body; and
- Sale or dispensing of a drug, device, equipment, or other item in accordance with a prescription.

Choice D is the correct answer.

13. Which of the following can a covered entity charge an individual for when providing a copy of their corresponding PHI?
    A. Postage, copying, preparing a summary, and the time involved with gathering all this information
    B. **Postage, copying, and the costs directly involved with preparing a requested summary of PHI if applicable**
    C. The total amount of time it takes to gather all information charged at the current federal minimum hourly wage
    D. Postage costs only

As indicated in Chapter 16, Healthcare Provider Issues, individuals must be given a copy of their corresponding PHI within a reasonable period of time after they request it. If the individual agrees to a summary or explanation of the information, a covered entity can request a reasonable fee based upon the cost of providing that information. The fee must only consist of the costs involved in:

- Copying the PHI, including the cost of the supplies for the copy and the labor used for the copy
- Postage, if the individual has asked for the copy of PHI or the summary or explanation to be mailed
- Preparing the explanation or summary of the PHI, if the individual is told of this cost and agrees to it prior to preparing it

Choice B is the correct answer.

14. Which of the following is not allowed and is not considered an incidental disclosure under HIPAA?
    A. Calling a person's full name in a provider's waiting room
    B. A patient in a shared hospital room overhearing a doctor discuss medical treatment with the other patient in the room
    C. **Placing lab test descriptions by the corresponding individual on sign-in sheets**
    D. Placing a patient's file in a slot outside a hospital room with name and admission date in full view of everyone passing

As indicated in Chapter 16, Healthcare Provider Issues, physicians' offices can use patient sign-in sheets or call out the names of patients in their waiting rooms. Be careful that the information disclosed is limited. The Privacy Rule permits certain incidental disclosures, such as in waiting rooms when patient names are called. However, they are allowed only as long as your office has implemented reasonable safeguards to implement the minimum necessary standard. For example, consider calling out only the first name of the patient instead of the full name. And, do not place medical information on the sign-in sheet that is not necessary for sign-in purposes.

Choice C is the correct answer.

15. Which of the following is most likely a Business Associate as defined by HIPAA?
    A. Temporary receptionist
    **B. Collection agency**
    C. Security guard for a medical clinic
    D. Trash collection service hauling shredded documents

As indicated in Chapter 20, Business Associate Issues, a BA is basically any individual or organization that performs an activity involving the use or disclosure of PHI on behalf of a CE. Collection agencies typically have access to PHI to perform their contracted job responsibilities. Receptionists and security guards are typically considered workforce members. If the documents are already shredded, the trash collection service will not have access to PHI.

Choice B is the correct answer.

## Section 5: HIPAA Technology Considerations Quiz

1. Which of the items below is NOT a technical component that HIPAA mandates based upon the risk analysis results?
   A. Physical access controls
   B. Authentication controls
   **C. Barcode Scanner methodologies**
   D. Data encryption mechanisms

As Chapter 21, Building a HIPAA-Compliant Technology, indicates, there are certain technical components that HIPAA mandates, such as:

- Logical access controls
- Physical access controls
- Authentication controls
- Authorization controls
- Audit controls
- Data encryption mechanisms

Choice C is the correct answer

2. Why should you use network address translation (NAT) on your network firewall?
   A. This is a guaranteed measure to stop spam
   **B. Helps to conceal your internal network configuration**
   C. Because it forwards inbound traffic to the proper host
   D. It can help prevent IP spoofing

As indicated in Chapter 21, Building a HIPAA-Compliant Technology, you can use network address translation (NAT) to help conceal your internal network configuration and to help restrict incoming and outgoing traffic.

Choice B is the correct answer.

3. You should look for IDS that have which of the following beneficial features?
   A. Can cut off an attack immediately
   B. Can monitor network bandwidth usage
   C. Can detect specific network events
   **D. All of the above**

As indicated in Chapter 21, Building a HIPAA-Compliant Technology, you should look for Intrusion Detection Systems (IDS) that have some or all of the following beneficial features:

- Do not rely solely on attack signature but can also detect network protocol anomalies and behavior-based attacks
- Can cut off an attack immediately (referred to as intrusion detection and prevention or IDP)
- Can monitor network bandwidth usage
- Can detect:
  - Trends
  - Malicious software
  - Unauthorized hardware or software
  - Specific network events
  - Network analyzers
- Can be distributed with multiple sensors across the various segments of your network
- Can track the attack to its source
- Can reconstruct and play back network attacks
- Have good alerting capabilities such as e-mail, pager, etc.
- Have good reporting capabilities — preferably through one centralized management console

Choice D is the correct answer.

4. Where should you use personal firewall/IDS software?
   A. On management's computers
   B. On those computers that receive the most e-mail

**C. On every computer possible inside the network**
D. You do not need a personal firewall

As indicated in Chapter 21, Building a HIPAA-Compliant Technology, use personal firewall/IDS software on every computer possible inside the network. We cannot stress enough how critical it is to have this software in addition to your regular firewall — it will help catch attacks destined for specific computers and applications that most network firewalls cannot.

Choice C is the correct answer.

5. Access controls consist of what?
   **A. Identification, authentication, and authorization**
   B. Modification, cancellation, and hyper scripting
   C. Messaging, alerts, and random checks
   D. All of the above

As indicated in Chapter 21, Building a HIPAA-Compliant Technology, access controls consist of identification, authentication, and authorization — these are all integral functions of OSs, applications, and databases.

Choice A is the correct answer.

6. Which of the following is NOT an acceptable technical way to authenticate a person or entity?
   A. Password
   B. Secure token
   C. Biometric
   **D. Recognize**

As Chapter 21, Building a HIPAA-Compliant Technology, indicates, there are three ways to authenticate a person or entity — something they know (password), something they have (secure token), and something they are (biometric).

Choice D is the correct answer.

7. What are often the most highly targeted yet the most vulnerable part of your information systems?
   **A. Databases**
   B. Firewalls
   C. Servers
   D. E-mail accounts

As indicated in Chapter 21, Building a HIPAA-Compliant Technology, you should treat databases as one of your most critical assets — this is where the "good stuff" is — this is where your PHI spends most of its waking hours.

- Databases are often the most highly targeted yet the most vulnerable part of your information systems
- Specific attention must be given to your databases during and after your risk analysis

Choice A is the correct answer.

8. Although encryption is an "addressable" Security Rule implementation specification, when must your data be encrypted?
   A. After two or more security breeches
   B. If you have a wireless network
   **C. If your risk analysis turns up specific threats and vulnerabilities to PHI at rest or in transit**
   D. If your organization decides to transmit PHI electronically

As Chapter 21, Building a HIPAA-Compliant Technology, indicates, although encryption is an "addressable" Security Rule implementation specification, data must be encrypted if your risk analysis turns up specific threats and vulnerabilities to PHI at rest or in transit.

Choice C is the correct answer.

9. Which of the following is NOT a reason security incident occurrences are becoming more frequent?
   A. The simplicity of performing computer attacks and not getting caught
   B. The increasing number of vulnerabilities found in the software we use
   **C. New government regulations that require computer accessibility for all U.S. citizens**
   D. The widespread use of the Internet

As Chapter 22, Crafting Security Incident Procedures and Contingency Plans, indicates, security incident occurrences are becoming more frequent due to the simplicity of performing computer attacks and not getting caught, the increasing number of vulnerabilities found in the software we use, and also because of the widespread use of the Internet.

Choice C is the correct answer.

10. What should you be sure to include in your communications plan?
    A. Who will communicate the message of a security incident
    B. When it will be communicated
    C. What will be said
    **D. All of the above**

As Chapter 22, Crafting Security Incident Procedures and Contingency Plans, indicates, you should prepare a communications plan in advance of a security incident so that everyone is not scrambling in an unprofessional light to figure what to do and what to say. Be sure to include:

- Who will communicate the message of a security incident (internal or external PR, HIPAA Security Officer, etc.)
- When it will be communicated
- What will be said
- What is being done to resolve the issue and prevent further damage

Choice D is the correct answer.

11. The Security Rule defines the data backup plan requirement as what?
    A. A set of standards for how you save files on your computers
    B. The ability to save hard copies of all PHI
    C. A plan for how you will back up your files if a security incident occurs
    **D. Procedures to create and maintain retrievable exact copies of electronic protected health information**

As Chapter 22, Crafting Security Incident Procedures and Contingency Plans, indicates, the Security Rule defines the data backup plan requirement as "establish and implement procedures to create and maintain retrievable exact copies of electronic protected health information."

Choice D is the correct answer.

12. Who of the following does NOT need to be part of your security incident team?
    A. CIO
    B. Legal Counsel
    C. HIPAA Security Officer
    **D. ER Nurse**

As Chapter 22, Crafting Security Incident Procedures and Contingency Plans, indicates, anyone that plays a key role in your information systems and healthcare operations should be included. The following is a list of people you need to consider having on your team:

- HIPAA Security Officer
- Network and/or Security Administrator
- Security Manager or Executive
- Risk Management Executive
- Operations Manager

Choice D is the correct answer.

13. An Intrusion Detection System (IDS) is used to do what?
    **A. Monitor for well-known and suspected attacks on your network**
    B. Keep strangers out of your office

C. Stop spam e-mail

D. Alert you when you send out PHI

As Chapter 22, Crafting Security Incident Procedures and Contingency Plans, indicates, an intrusion detection system can monitor for well-known and suspected attacks on your network (network-based IDS) or computers (host-based IDS). Newer technologies focus on intrusion detection and prevention, meaning that attacks can be cut off as soon as they are detected.

Choice A is the correct answer.

14. According to the Spring 2003 U.S. Healthcare Industry Quarterly HIPAA Compliance Survey, what percentage of respondents were currently outsourcing various HIPAA initiatives?
    A. 2
    B. 25
    C. All
    **D. 44**

As indicated in Chapter 23, Outsourcing Information Technology Services, in the Winter 2003 U.S. Healthcare Industry Quarterly HIPAA Compliance Survey published by HIMSS and Phoenix Health Systems, 42 percent of respondents are currently outsourcing various HIPAA initiatives.

Choice D is the correct answer.

15. Which of the following certifications should NOT be considered as a baseline requirement for an outsourcing firm?
    A. GIAC
    B. CHS
    **C. PA**
    D. CISSP

As indicated in Chapter 23, Outsourcing Information Technology Services, you should consider the following certifications as a baseline requirement:

- CISSP (Certified Information Systems Security Professional sponsored by ISC2)
- CISA (Certified Information Systems Auditor sponsored by ISACA)
- CISM (Certified Information Security Manager sponsored by ISACA)
- CHS (Certified in Healthcare Security sponsored by HIMSS)
- GIAC (Global Information Assurance Certification sponsored by SANS)
- IAM (INFOSEC Assessment Methodology sponsored by the National Security Agency)
- Security+ (sponsored by The Computing Technology Industry Association)

Choice C is the correct answer.

## Section 6: Managing Ongoing HIPAA Compliance Quiz

1. Which of the following should be a goal of your HIPAA awareness and training program?
   **A. Instill privacy and security requirements and concerns into the organizational culture**
   B. Describe the history and background of HIPAA
   C. Identify those within your organization who have been in non-compliance with the HIPAA regulations
   D. Describe how to coerce individuals into waiving their rights under HIPAA

As indicated in Chapter 24, HIPAA Training, Education, and Awareness, healthcare organizations must develop and implement an awareness program that meets the following goals:

- Ensures compliance with HIPAA privacy and security regulations.
- Is supported by executive management. Establish an executive owner or sponsor to champion, maintain, and ensure senior level involvement. This will be necessary to get the message across and secure support of the HIPAA compliance activities throughout the organization.
- Instills the privacy and security requirements and concerns into the organizational culture.
- Clearly communicates the HIPAA privacy and security issues and challenges.
- Supports your strategic and tactical HIPAA implementation strategies.

Choice A is the correct answer.

2. Which of the following should be included within your training and awareness strategy?
   A. A strategy to use marketing techniques to raise training budget
   B. Identify states to create preemption procedures
   **C. A procedure for measuring the overall effectiveness of the awareness and education program**
   D. A procedure for answering complaints related to HIPAA compliance

As indicated in Chapter 24, HIPAA Training, Education, and Awareness, your awareness strategy should include the following:

- An awareness budget that accounts for the communications, planning, and implementation activities that will be proportionate to this piece of the total amount of the HIPAA compliance budget.
- A timeline indicating target dates for all phases of the awareness and training program.

- A procedure and/or tool for measuring the overall effectiveness of the awareness program.
- Identification of integration points and implementation windows to effectively coordinate the privacy and security awareness and education practices within the overall HIPAA compliance plan.
- A strategy to integrate the awareness processes throughout all departments and teams of the organization to help ensure a successful awareness program.
- Execution of an awareness risk assessment to identify awareness compliance gaps and form the baseline to use for measuring future awareness compliance success.
- A description of the tactical objectives of the awareness and education program.
- The development, implementation, communication, and enforcement of policies and procedures to mitigate risk and ensure on-going compliance with HIPAA privacy and security regulations.

Choice C is the correct answer.

3. Which of the following most accurately describes the difference between training and awareness?
   A. Training is less formal and interactive than an awareness program
   B. **Training is more formal and interactive than an awareness program**
   C. A training program is more expensive than an awareness program
   D. An awareness program is more expensive than a training program

As indicated in Chapter 24, HIPAA Training, Education, and Awareness, training is more formal and interactive than an awareness program.

Choice B is the correct answer.

4. Which of the following is the most likely group to target for HIPAA privacy and security training?
   A. **Customer services and call centers**
   B. Personnel who have received recent promotions
   C. Third parties
   D. Trash removal contractors

As indicated in Chapter 24, HIPAA Training, Education, and Awareness, you should specialize training content for target groups based upon specific issues for which they must understand and with which they must comply. Match the course content to job responsibilities and roles as much as possible to be most effective. For instance, assume you have the following defined roles:

- R1: Healthcare delivery personnel (for example, physicians, nurses, and so on.)
- R2: Clinic and Provider Facility Managers
- R3: Health Plan Claims Examiners
- R4: Information Technology Personnel
- R5: Privacy and Security Officers
- R6: Plan Member Service Representatives
- R7: Billing Personnel
- R8: Health Plan Enrollment Personnel
- R9: Legal Counsel and Human Resources
- R10: Marketing and Sales
- R11: Customer Services and Call Centers

Choice A is the correct answer.

5. Training delivery should best be created based upon which of the following?
   A. The preferences of your upper management
   B. The time of year
   C. The number of personnel
   **D. The best way to achieve your objectives**

As indicated in Chapter 24, HIPAA Training, Education, and Awareness, the training delivery method should be based upon the best way to achieve your objectives. In choosing a delivery method, select the best method for the learning objectives, the number of students, and your organization's ability to efficiently deliver the material.

Choice D is the correct answer.

6. Which of the following most accurately describes a characteristic of awareness activities?
   A. Should only occur during new-employee orientation
   B. Should be detailed within business associate contracts
   **C. Should occur on an ongoing basis**
   D. Should be very formal and structured

As indicated in Chapter 24, HIPAA Training, Education, and Awareness, awareness activities should:

- Occur on an ongoing basis
- Use a wide range of delivery methods
- Catch the attention of the target audience
- Be less formal than training
- Take less time than training
- Be creative and fun
- Reinforce the lessons learned during formal training

Choice C is the correct answer.

7. Your evaluation of training and awareness effectiveness has four distinct purposes, including which one of the following?
   A. Determine the total budget for HIPAA compliance efforts
   B. Identify privacy and security officers
   C. Compare your organization with other healthcare organizations
   **D. Determine what the student learned from a specific course**

As indicated in Chapter 24, HIPAA Training, Education, and Awareness, your evaluation of training and awareness effectiveness has four distinct purposes, to measure:

* The extent that conditions were right for learning and the learner's subjective satisfaction
* What the student learned from a specific course
* A pattern of student outcomes following a specified course
* The value of the class compared to other training and awareness options

Choice D is the correct answer.

8. According to research by HHS, ongoing Privacy Rule compliance efforts will cost CEs how much of their projected national health expenditures by 2008?
   A. 0.007 percent
   **B. 0.07 percent**
   C. 0.7 percent
   D. 7 percent

As indicated in Chapter 25, Performing Ongoing HIPAA Compliance Reviews and Audits, analysis by HHS determined that the average cost of ongoing Privacy Rule compliance would be approximately 0.05 percent of each small entity's annual expenditures. HHS estimates that by 2008, the Privacy Rule will cost an estimated 0.07 percent of projected national health expenditures for ongoing compliance by all CEs.

Choice B is the correct answer.

9. Which of the following is the best way to ensure that privacy processes are addressed during process planning?
   **A. Incorporating a privacy architecture within your applications and business process development process**
   B. Performing a periodic risk analysis
   C. Hiring a third-party reviewer
   D. Implement a privacy software implementation package

As indicated in Chapter 25, Performing Ongoing HIPAA Compliance Reviews and Audits, incorporating a privacy architecture within your applications and business process development projects is the best way to ensure that privacy processes are addressed from the very beginning of planning a new process.

Choice A is the correct answer.

10. In a recent study by Harris Interactive, what percentage of respondents said they would stop doing business with a company if they found out the company has misused customer information?
    **A. 83 percent**
    B. 100 percent
    C. 2 percent
    D. None of the above

As indicated in Chapter 25, Performing Ongoing HIPAA Compliance Reviews and Audits, in a recent study by Harris Interactive, 83 percent of respondents said they would stop doing business with a company if they found out the company has misused customer information. Performing ongoing reviews and audits will not only ensure HIPAA compliance, but they can also help build customer and business partner confidence and ultimately lower operating costs due to streamlined operations.

Choice A is the correct answer.

11. What sort of information should you gather before starting any HIPAA compliance audits?
    A. Privacy policies and procedures
    B. Security policies and procedures
    C. The methods and systems in place to protect PHI
    **D. All of the above**

As indicated in Chapter 25, Performing Ongoing HIPAA Compliance Reviews and Audits, before starting any HIPAA compliance audits, you will need to gather as much information as possible, including:

- Privacy policies and procedures
- Security policies and procedures
- All forms of PHI that are stored or transmitted both in hard copy and electronic formats
- The methods and systems in place to protect PHI

Choice D is the correct answer.

12. What is the first step of security audits and reviews?
    A. Hire a consultant with a strong security background
    B. Gather your HIPAA compliance team and brainstorm how to protect PHI
    **C. Understand the business objectives and HIPAA requirements for what is being audited**
    D. Isolate known vulnerabilities on your network

As indicated in Chapter 25, Performing Ongoing HIPAA Compliance Reviews and Audits, the first step of security audits and reviews is to understand the business objectives and HIPAA requirements for what is being audited.

Choice C is the correct answer.

13. How many new vulnerabilities have been have been reported to the Carnegie Mellon CERT Coordination Center between the years 2000 and 2003?
    **A. Over 8600**
    B. 1+ million
    C. 25,000
    D. 42

As indicated in Chapter 25, Performing Ongoing HIPAA Compliance Reviews and Audits, over 8600 security vulnerabilities have been reported to the Carnegie Mellon CERT Coordination Center since the year 2000! This number alone should help justify why security needs to be reassessed so often.

Choice A is the correct answer.

14. What should you do if your audit turns up clean?
    A. Relax until next year
    **B. Consider that perhaps the audit is not detailed enough**
    C. Hire an outside consultant to do the audit again
    D. None of the above

As indicated in Chapter 25, Performing Ongoing HIPAA Compliance Reviews and Audits, the results of your audits will, and probably should, vary from year to year. If everything turns up clean, perhaps the audit is not detailed enough. If your results get progressively worse over time, perhaps there is an internal process or management issue.

Choice B is the correct answer.

15. What are some things you should consider if the audits are performed by outside entities?
    A. Make sure that they have your organization's best interests in mind
    B. Keep an eye out for auditors recommending that you fix all problems regardless of their significance or impact to your organization or the privacy and security of PHI
    **C. Both A and B**
    D. None of the above

As indicated in Chapter 25, Performing Ongoing HIPAA Compliance Reviews and Audits, if the audits are performed by outside entities, make sure that they have your organization's best interests in mind. You will want to keep an eye out for auditors recommending that you fix all problems regardless of their significance or impact to your organization or the privacy and security of PHI. You will have to consider the cost of remediation for each issue vs. the benefits remediation will provide.

Choice C is the correct answer.

# Appendix E
# HIPAA Glossary

## General and Miscellaneous Terms

**ACL:**  Access Control Lists. Generally a list of users with privileges to a system.

**Audit Trail:**  Record of events, usually tracked by subject or object. For example, users' failed log-on attempts.

**Authentication:**  Verification of the identity of a user or other entity as a prerequisite to allowing access to computer resources.

**Authorization:**  Granting a user the right of access to computing resources, programs, processes, and data.

**Business Associate:**  Under HIPAA, a person who is not a member of a covered entity's workforce (see Workforce), and who performs any function or activity involving the use or disclosure of individually identifiable health information, such as temporary nursing services, or who provides services to a covered entity that involves the disclosure of individually identifiable health information, such as legal, accounting, consulting, data aggregation, management, accreditation, etc. A covered entity may be a business associate of another covered entity.

**Certification:**  Formal written assurance that a system meets specified security controls.

**CIA:**  With regard to information security: Confidentiality, Integrity, and Availability.

**CISSP:**  Certified Information Systems Security Professional.

**Covered Entity:**  The specific types of organization to which HIPAA applies, including providers, health plans (payers), and clearinghouses (who process nonstandard claims from providers and distribute them to the payers in their required formats — a process that will not be necessary if providers adopt the HIPAA transactions standards).

**CPRI:**  Computer-Based Patient Record Institute — organization formed in 1992 to promote adoption of healthcare information systems. Has created a Security Toolkit with sample policies and procedures (www.cpri-host.org).

---

**Disclosure:** The release, transfer, provision of access to, or divulging in any other manner, information outside the entity holding the information. (See Use, in contrast.)

**DSL:** Digital Subscriber Line. A technology that dramatically increases the digital capacity of ordinary telephone lines (the local loops) into the home or office. DSL speeds are tied to the distance between the customer and the telephone company's central office.

**EDI:** Electronic Data Interchange (computer-to-computer transactions).

**Encryption:** The process of transforming information into unintelligible form in such a way that the original information cannot be obtained without using the inverse decryption processes.

**Health plans:** Individual or group plans (or programs) that provide health benefits directly, through insurance, or otherwise. For example, Medicaid, State Children's Health Insurance Program (SCHIP), state employee benefit programs, Temporary Assistance for Needy Families (TANF), and others.

**Healthcare providers:** Providers (or suppliers) of medical or other health services or any other person furnishing healthcare services or supplies, and who also conduct certain health-related administrative or financial transactions electronically. For example, local health departments; community and migrant health centers; rural health clinics; school-based health centers; homeless clinics and shelters; public hospitals; maternal and child health programs (Title V); family planning programs (Title X); HIV/AIDS programs; and others.

**Health information clearinghouses:** Any public or private entities that process or facilitate processing nonstandard health information into standard data elements. For example, third-party administrators; pharmacy benefits managers; billing services; information management and technology vendors; and others.

**HHS or DHHS:** U.S. Department of Health and Human Services.

**IOM:** Institute of Medicine. Prestigious group of physicians that studies issues and advises Congress. The IOM developed a report on computer-based patient records that led to the creation of CPRI. Its most recent popular work is its report on medical errors, *To Err Is Human: Building a Safer Health System* (Washington, D.C., National Academy Press, 1999).

**Incident:** An unusual occurrence or breach in the security of a computer system.

**ISO 17799:** ISO 17799 gives general recommendations for information security management. It is intended to provide a common international basis for developing organizational security standards and effective

424

security management practice and to provide confidence in inter-organizational dealings.

**NIST:** National Institute of Standards and Technology

**Nonrepudiation:** Strong and substantial evidence of the identity of the signer of a message and the message integrity, sufficient to prevent a party from successfully denying the origin, submission, or delivery of the message and the integrity of its contents.

**NPRM:** Notice of Proposed Rulemaking. The publication, in the Federal Register, of proposed regulations for public comment.

**NRC:** National Research Council. Quasi-governmental body that conducted a study on the state of security in healthcare, *For the Record: Protecting Electronic Health Information* (Washington, D.C., National Academy Press, 1997).

**PDA:** Personal Digital Assistant. A handheld computer that serves as an organizer for personal information.

**PGP:** Pretty Good Privacy. Public key cryptography software based on the RSA cryptographic method.

**PKI:** Public Key Infrastructure.

**SNIP:** Strategic National Implementation Process. Sponsored by WEDI.

**SSO:** Single Sign-On or Standards-Setting Organization.

**UPIN:** Universal Provider Identification Number. To be replaced by National Provider Identifier under HIPAA.

**URAC:** The American Accreditation Healthcare Commission (formerly Utilization Review Accreditation Commission).

**Use:** With respect to individually identifiable health information, the sharing, employment, application, utilization, examination, or analysis of such information within an entity that maintains such information. (See Disclosure, in contrast.)

**VPN:** Virtual Private Network. A private network that is configured within a public network.

**WEDI:** Workgroup on Electronic Data Interchange.

**Workforce:** Under HIPAA, employees, volunteers, trainees, and other persons whose conduct, in the performance of work for a covered entity, is under the direct control of such entity, whether or not they are paid by the covered entity. (See Business Associate, in contrast.)

APPENDICES

**From the Regulatory Text**

*§ 162.103*

**Code set:**   Any set of codes used to encode data elements, such as tables of terms, medical concepts, medical diagnostic codes, or medical procedure codes. A code set includes the codes and the descriptors of the codes.

**Code set maintaining organization:**   An organization that creates and maintains the code sets adopted by the Secretary for use in the transactions for which standards are adopted in this part.

**Data condition:**   The rule that describes the circumstances under which a covered entity must use a particular data element or segment.

**Data content:**   All the data elements and code sets inherent to a transaction, and not related to the format of the transaction. Data elements that are related to the format are not data content.

**Data element:**   The smallest named unit of information in a transaction.

**Data set:**   A semantically meaningful unit of information exchanged between two parties to a transaction.

**Descriptor:**   The text defining a code.

**Designated Standard Maintenance Organization (DSMO):**   An organization designated by the Secretary under § 162.910(a).

**Direct data entry:**   The direct entry of data (for example, using dumb terminals or Web browsers) that is immediately transmitted into a health plan's computer.

**Electronic media:**   The mode of electronic transmission. It includes the Internet (wide-open), extranet (using Internet technology to link a business with information only accessible to collaborating parties), leased lines, dial-up lines, private networks, and those transmissions that are physically moved from one location to another using magnetic tape, disk, or compact disk media.

**Format:**   Refers to those data elements that provide or control the enveloping or hierarchical structure, or assist in identifying data content of, a transaction.

**HCPCS:**   Stands for the Health (Care Financing Administration) Common Procedure Coding System.

**Maintain or maintenance:**   Refers to activities necessary to support the use of a standard adopted by the Secretary, including technical corrections to an implementation specification, and enhancements or expansion of a code set. This term excludes the activities related to the adoption of a

426

new standard or implementation specification, or modification to an adopted standard or implementation specification.

**Maximum defined data set:**   All of the required data elements for a particular standard based on a specific implementation specification.

**Segment:**   A group of related data elements in a transaction.

**Standard transaction:**   A transaction that complies with the applicable standard adopted under this part.

### § 160.103

**Act:**   The Social Security Act.

**ANSI:**   Stands for the American National Standards Institute.

**Business associate:**

1. Except as provided in paragraph (2) of this definition, business associate means, with respect to a covered entity, a person who:
    i. On behalf of such covered entity or of an organized healthcare arrangement (as defined in § 164.501 of this subchapter) in which the covered entity participates, but other than in the capacity of a member of the workforce of such covered entity or arrangement, performs, or assists in the performance of:
        A. A function or activity involving the use or disclosure of individually identifiable health information, including claims processing or administration, data analysis, processing or administration, utilization review, quality assurance, billing, benefit management, practice management, and repricing; or
        B. Any other function or activity regulated by this subchapter; or
    ii. Provides, other than in the capacity of a member of the workforce of such covered entity, legal, actuarial, accounting, consulting, data aggregation (as defined in § 164.501 of this subchapter), management, administrative, accreditation, or financial services to or for such covered entity, or to or for an organized healthcare arrangement in which the covered entity participates, where the provision of the service involves the disclosure of individually identifiable health information from such covered entity or arrangement, or from another business associate of such covered entity or arrangement, to the person.
2. A covered entity participating in an organized healthcare arrangement that performs a function or activity as described by paragraph (1)(i) of this definition for or on behalf of such organized healthcare arrangement, or that provides a service as described in paragraph (1)(ii) of this definition to or for such organized healthcare arrangement, does not, simply through the performance of such function

or activity or the provision of such service, become a business associate of other covered entities participating in such organized healthcare arrangement.

3. A covered entity may be a business associate of another covered entity.

**Compliance date:**   The date by which a covered entity must comply with a standard, implementation specification, requirement, or modification adopted under this subchapter.

**Covered entity:**

1. A health plan.
2. A healthcare clearinghouse.
3. A healthcare provider who transmits any health information in electronic form in connection with a transaction covered by this subchapter.

**Group health plan:**   (Also see definition of health plan in this section.) An employee welfare benefit plan (as defined in section 3(1) of the Employee Retirement Income and Security Act of 1974 (ERISA), 29 U.S.C. 1002(1)), including insured and self-insured plans, to the extent that the plan provides medical care (as defined in section 2791(a)(2) of the Public Health Service Act (PHS Act), 42 U.S.C. 300gg-91(a)(2)), including items and services paid for as medical care, to employees or their dependents directly or through insurance, reimbursement, or otherwise, that:

1. Has 50 or more participants (as defined in section 3(7) of ERISA, 29 U.S.C. 1002(7)); or
2. Is administered by an entity other than the employer that established and maintains the plan.

**HCFA:**   Healthcare Financing Administration within the Department of Health and Human Services.

**HHS:**   Department of Health and Human Services.

**Healthcare:**   Care, services, or supplies related to the health of an individual. Healthcare includes, but is not limited to, the following:

1. Preventive, diagnostic, therapeutic, rehabilitative, maintenance, or palliative care, and counseling, service, assessment, or procedure with respect to the physical or mental condition, or functional status, of an individual or that affects the structure or function of the body; and
2. Sale or dispensing of a drug, device, equipment, or other item in accordance with a prescription.

**Healthcare clearinghouse:**   A public or private entity, including a billing service, repricing company, community health management information

428

system or community health information system, and "value-added" networks and switches, that does either of the following functions:

1. Processes or facilitates the processing of health information received from another entity in a nonstandard format or containing nonstandard data content into standard data elements or a standard transaction.
2. Receives a standard transaction from another entity and processes or facilitates the processing of health information into nonstandard format or nonstandard data content for the receiving entity.

**Healthcare provider:** A provider of services (as defined in section 1861(u) of the Act, 42 U.S.C. 1395x(u)), a provider of medical or health services (as defined in section 1861(s) of the Act, 42 U.S.C. 1395x(s)), and any other person or organization who furnishes, bills, or is paid for healthcare in the normal course of business.

**Health information:** Any information, whether oral or recorded in any form or medium, that:

1. Is created or received by a healthcare provider, health plan, public health authority, employer, life insurer, school or university, or healthcare clearinghouse; and
2. Relates to the past, present, or future physical or mental health or condition of an individual; the provision of healthcare to an individual; or the past, present, or future payment for the provision of healthcare to an individual.

**Health insurance issuer:** (As defined in section 2791(b)(2) of the PHS Act, 42 U.S.C. 300gg-91(b)(2) and used in the definition of health plan in this section) An insurance company, insurance service, or insurance organization (including an HMO) that is licensed to engage in the business of insurance in a State and is subject to State law that regulates insurance. Such term does not include a group health plan.

**Health maintenance organization (HMO):** (As defined in section 2791(b)(3) of the PHS Act, 42 U.S.C. 300gg-91(b)(3) and used in the definition of health plan in this section) A federally qualified HMO, an organization recognized as an HMO under State law, or a similar organization regulated for solvency under State law in the same manner and to the same extent as such an HMO.

**Health plan:** An individual or group plan that provides, or pays the cost of, medical care (as defined in section 2791(a)(2) of the PHS Act, 42 U.S.C. 300gg-91(a)(2)).

1. Health plan includes the following, singly or in combination:
    i. A group health plan, as defined in this section.
    ii. A health insurance issuer, as defined in this section.

429

      iii. An HMO, as defined in this section.

      iv. Part A or Part B of the Medicare program under title XVIII of the Act.

      v. The Medicaid program under title XIX of the Act, 42 U.S.C. 1396, et seq.

      vi. An issuer of a Medicare supplemental policy (as defined in section 1882(g)(1) of the Act, 42 U.S.C. 1395ss(g)(1)).

      vii. An issuer of a long-term care policy, excluding a nursing home fixed-indemnity policy.

      viii. An employee welfare benefit plan or any other arrangement that is established or maintained for the purpose of offering or providing health benefits to the employees of two or more employers.

      ix. The healthcare program for active military personnel under title 10 of the United States Code.

      x. The veterans' healthcare program under 38 U.S.C. chapter 17.

      xi. The Civilian Health and Medical Program of the Uniformed Services (CHAMPUS)(as defined in 10 U.S.C. 1072(4)).

      xii. The Indian Health Service program under the Indian Healthcare Improvement Act, 25 U.S.C. 1601, et seq.

      xiii. The Federal Employees Health Benefits Program under 5 U.S.C. 8902, et seq.

      xiv. An approved State child health plan under title XXI of the Act, providing benefits for child health assistance that meet the requirements of section 2103 of the Act, 42 U.S.C. 1397, et seq.

      xv. The Medicare + Choice program under Part C of Title XVIII of the Act, 42 U.S.C. 1395w-21 through 1395w-28.

      xvi. A high risk pool that is a mechanism established under State law to provide health insurance coverage or comparable coverage to eligible individuals.

      xvii. Any other individual or group plan, or combination of individual or group plans, that provides or pays for the cost of medical care (as defined in section 2791(a)(2) of the PHS Act, 42 U.S.C. 300gg-91(a)(2)).

2. Health plan excludes:

      i. Any policy, plan, or program to the extent that it provides, or pays for the cost of, excepted benefits that are listed in section 2791(c)(1) of the PHS Act, 42 U.S.C. 300gg-91(c)(1); and

      ii. A government-funded program (other than one listed in paragraph (1)(i)-(xvi)of this definition):

        A. Whose principal purpose is other than providing, or paying the cost of, healthcare; or

        B. Whose principal activity is:

          a. The direct provision of healthcare to persons; or

          b. The making of grants to fund the direct provision of healthcare to persons.

**Implementation specification:**   Specific requirements or instructions for implementing a standard.

**Individually identifiable health information:**   Information that is a subset of health information, including demographic information collected from an individual, and:

1. Is created or received by a healthcare provider, health plan, employer, or healthcare clearinghouse; and
2. Relates to the past, present, or future physical or mental health or condition of an individual; the provision of healthcare to an individual; or the past, present, or future payment for the provision of healthcare to an individual; and
   i. That identifies the individual; or
   ii. With respect to which there is a reasonable basis to believe the information can be used to identify the individual.

**Modify or modification:**   Refers to a change adopted by the Secretary, through regulation, to a standard or an implementation specification.

**Secretary:**   The Secretary of Health and Human Services or any other officer or employee of HHS to whom the authority involved has been delegated.

**Small health plan:**   A health plan with annual receipts of $5 million or less.

**Standard:**   A rule, condition, or requirement:

1. Describing the following information for products, systems, services or practices:
   i. Classification of components.
   ii. Specification of materials, performance, or operations; or
   iii. Delineation of procedures; or
2. With respect to the privacy of individually identifiable health information.

**Standard-setting organization (SSO):**   An organization accredited by the American National Standards Institute that develops and maintains standards for information transactions or data elements, or any other standard that is necessary for, or will facilitate the implementation of, this part.

**State:**   Refers to one of the following:

1. For a health plan established or regulated by Federal law, State has the meaning set forth in the applicable section of the United States Code for such health plan.
2. For all other purposes, State means any of the several States, the District of Columbia, the Commonwealth of Puerto Rico, the Virgin Islands, and Guam.

**Trading partner agreement:** An agreement related to the exchange of information in electronic transactions, whether the agreement is distinct or part of a larger agreement, between each party to the agreement. (For example, a trading partner agreement may specify, among other things, the duties and responsibilities of each party to the agreement in conducting a standard transaction.)

**Transaction:** The transmission of information between two parties to carry out financial or administrative activities related to healthcare. It includes the following types of information transmissions:

1. Healthcare claims or equivalent encounter information.
2. Healthcare payment and remittance advice.
3. Coordination of benefits.
4. Healthcare claim status.
5. Enrollment and disenrollment in a health plan.
6. Eligibility for a health plan.
7. Health plan premium payments.
8. Referral certification and authorization.
9. First report of injury.
10. Health claims attachments.
11. Other transactions that the Secretary may prescribe by regulation.

**Workforce:** Employees, volunteers, trainees, and other persons whose conduct, in the performance of work for a covered entity, is under the direct control of such entity, whether or not they are paid by the covered entity.

### *§ 160.202*

**Contrary:** When used to compare a provision of State law to a standard, requirement, or implementation specification adopted under this subchapter, means:

1. A covered entity would find it impossible to comply with both the State and federal requirements; or
2. The provision of State law stands as an obstacle to the accomplishment and execution of the full purposes and objectives of part C of title XI of the Act or section 264 of Pub. L. 104-191, as applicable.

**More stringent:** In the context of a comparison of a provision of State law and a standard, requirement, or implementation specification adopted under sub-part E of part 164 of this subchapter, a State law that meets one or more of the following criteria:

1. With respect to a use or disclosure, the law prohibits or restricts a use or disclosure in circumstances under which such use or

disclosure otherwise would be permitted under this subchapter, except if the disclosure is:
   i. Required by the Secretary in connection with determining whether a covered entity is in compliance with this subchapter; or
   ii. To the individual who is the subject of the individually identifiable health information.
2. With respect to the rights of an individual, who is the subject of the individually identifiable health information, regarding access to or amendment of individually identifiable health information, permits greater rights of access or amendment, as applicable.
3. With respect to information to be provided to an individual who is the subject of the individually identifiable health information about a use, a disclosure, rights, and remedies, provides the greater amount of information.
4. With respect to the form, substance, or the need for express legal permission from an individual, who is the subject of the individually identifiable health information, for use or disclosure of individually identifiable health information, provides requirements that narrow the scope or duration, increase the privacy protections afforded (such as by expanding the criteria for), or reduce the coercive effect of the circumstances surrounding the express legal permission, as applicable.
5. With respect to recordkeeping or requirements relating to accounting of disclosures, provides for the retention or reporting of more detailed information or for a longer duration.
6. With respect to any other matter, provides greater privacy protection for the individual who is the subject of the individually identifiable health information.

**Relates to the privacy of individually identifiable health information:** With respect to a State law, that the State law has the specific purpose of protecting the privacy of health information or affects the privacy of health information in a direct, clear, and substantial way.

**State law:** A constitution, statute, regulation, rule, common law, or other State action having the force and effect of law.

### § 142.103

**Code set:** Any set of codes used for encoding data elements, such as tables of terms, medical concepts, medical diagnostic codes, or medical procedure codes.

**Healthcare clearinghouse:** A public or private entity that processes or facilitates the processing of nonstandard data elements of health information into standard data elements. The entity receives healthcare transactions from healthcare providers or other entities, translates the data from a given format into one acceptable to the intended payer or payers, and forwards the processed transaction to appropriate payers and clearinghouses. Billing services, repricing companies, community health management information systems, community health information systems, and "value-added" networks and switches are considered to be healthcare clearinghouses for purposes of this part.

**Healthcare provider:**   A provider of services as defined in section 1861(u) of the Social Security Act, 42 U.S.C. 1395x, a provider of medical or other health services as defined in section 1861(s) of the Social Security Act, and any other person who furnishes or bills and is paid for healthcare services or supplies in the normal course of business.

**Health information:**   Any information, whether oral or recorded in any form or medium, that —

1. Is created or received by a healthcare provider, health plan, public health authority, employer, life insurer, school or university, or healthcare clearinghouse; and
2. Relates to the past, present, or future physical or mental health or condition of an individual, the provision of healthcare to an individual, or the past, present, or future payment for the provision of healthcare to an individual.

**Health plan:**   An individual or group plan that provides, or pays the cost of, medical care. Health plan includes the following, singly or in combination:

1. Group health plan. A group health plan is an employee welfare benefit plan (as currently defined in section 3(1) of the Employee Retirement Income and Security Act of 1974, 29 U.S.C. 1002(1)), including insured and self-insured plans, to the extent that the plan provides medical care, including items and services paid for as medical care, to employees or their dependents directly or through insurance, or otherwise, and —
   i.  Has 50 or more participants; or
   ii. Is administered by an entity other than the employer that established and maintains the plan.
2. Health insurance issuer. A health insurance issuer is an insurance company, insurance service, or insurance organization that is licensed to engage in the business of insurance in a State and is subject to State law that regulates insurance.
3. Health maintenance organization. A health maintenance organization is a Federally qualified health maintenance organization, an organization recognized as a health maintenance organization under State law, or a similar organization regulated for solvency under State

law in the same manner and to the same extent as such a health maintenance organization.

4. Part A or Part B of the Medicare program under title XVIII of the Social Security Act.
5. The Medicaid program under title XIX of the Social Security Act.
6. A Medicare supplemental policy (as defined in section 1882(g)(1) of the Social Security Act, 42 U.S.C. 1395ss).
7. A long-term care policy, including a nursing home fixed-indemnity policy.
8. An employee welfare benefit plan or any other arrangement that is established or maintained for the purpose of offering or providing health benefits to the employees of two or more employers.
9. The healthcare program for active military personnel under title 10 of the United States Code.
10. The veterans' healthcare program under 38 U.S.C. chapter 17.
11. The Civilian Health and Medical Program of the Uniformed Services (CHAMPUS), as defined in 10 U.S.C. 1072(4).
12. The Indian Health Service program under the Indian Healthcare Improvement Act (25 U.S.C. 1601 et seq.).
13. The Federal Employees Health Benefits Program under 5 U.S.C. chapter 89.
14. Any other individual or group health plan, or combination thereof, that provides or pays for the cost of medical care.

**Medical care:** The diagnosis, cure, mitigation, treatment, or prevention of disease, or amounts paid for the purpose of affecting any body structure or function of the body; amounts paid for transportation primarily for and essential to these items; and amounts paid for insurance covering the items and the transportation specified in this definition.

**Participant:** Any employee or former employee of an employer, or any member or former member of an employee organization, who is or may become eligible to receive a benefit of any type from an employee benefit plan that covers employees of that employer or members of such an organization, or whose beneficiaries may be eligible to receive any of these benefits. "Employee" includes an individual who is treated as an employee under section 401(c)(1) of the Internal Revenue Code of 1986 (26 U.S.C. 401(c)(1)).

**Small health plan:** A group health plan or individual health plan with fewer than 50 participants.

**Standard:** A set of rules for a set of codes, data elements, transactions, or identifiers promulgated either by an organization accredited by the American National Standards Institute or HHS for the electronic transmission of health information.

**Transaction:** The exchange of information between two parties to carry out financial and administrative activities related to healthcare. It includes the following:

1. Health claims or equivalent encounter information.
2. Healthcare payment and remittance advice.
3. Coordination of benefits.
4. Health claims status.
5. Enrollment and disenrollment in a health plan.
6. Eligibility for a health plan.
7. Health plan premium payments.
8. Referral certification and authorization.
9. First report of injury.
10. Health claims attachments.
11. Other transactions as the Secretary may prescribe by regulation.

### § 164.501

**Correctional institution:** Any penal or correctional facility, jail, reformatory, detention center, work farm, halfway house, or residential community program center operated by, or under contract to, the United States, a State, a territory, a political subdivision of a State or territory, or an Indian tribe, for the confinement or rehabilitation of persons charged with or convicted of a criminal offense or other persons held in lawful custody. Other persons held in lawful custody includes juvenile offenders adjudicated delinquent, aliens detained awaiting deportation, persons committed to mental institutions through the criminal justice system, witnesses, or others awaiting charges or trial.

**Covered functions:** Those functions of a covered entity the performance of which makes the entity a health plan, healthcare provider, or healthcare clearinghouse.

**Data aggregation:** With respect to protected health information created or received by a business associate in its capacity as the business associate of a covered entity, the combining of such protected health information by the business associate with the protected health information received by the business associate in its capacity as a business associate of another covered entity, to permit data analyses that relate to the healthcare operations of the respective covered entities.

**Designated record set:**

1. A group of records maintained by or for a covered entity that is:
   i. The medical records and billing records about individuals maintained by or for a covered healthcare provider;

ii. The enrollment, payment, claims adjudication, and case or medical management record systems maintained by or for a health plan; or

iii. Used, in whole or in part, by or for the covered entity to make decisions about individuals.

2. For purposes of this paragraph, the term record means any item, collection, or grouping of information that includes protected health information and is maintained, collected, used, or disseminated by or for a covered entity.

**Direct treatment relationship:**   A treatment relationship between an individual and a healthcare provider that is not an indirect treatment relationship.

**Disclosure:**   The release, transfer, provision of access to, or divulging in any other manner of information outside the entity holding the information.

**Healthcare operations:**   Any of the following activities of the covered entity to the extent that the activities are related to covered functions:

1. Conducting quality assessment and improvement activities, including outcomes evaluation and development of clinical guidelines, provided that the obtaining of generalizable knowledge is not the primary purpose of any studies resulting from such activities; population-based activities relating to improving health or reducing healthcare costs, protocol development, case management and care coordination, contacting of healthcare providers and patients with information about treatment alternatives; and related functions that do not include treatment;

2. Reviewing the competence or qualifications of healthcare professionals, evaluating practitioner and provider performance, health plan performance, conducting training programs in which students, trainees, or practitioners in areas of healthcare learn under supervision to practice or improve their skills as healthcare providers, training of nonhealthcare professionals, accreditation, certification, licensing, or credentialing activities;

3. Underwriting, premium rating, and other activities relating to the creation, renewal, or replacement of a contract of health insurance or health benefits, and ceding, securing, or placing a contract for reinsurance of risk relating to claims for healthcare (including stop-loss insurance and excess of loss insurance), provided that the requirements of § 164.514(g) are met, if applicable;

4. Conducting or arranging for medical review, legal services, and auditing functions, including fraud and abuse detection and compliance programs;

5. Business planning and development, such as conducting cost-management and planning-related analyses related to managing and

operating the entity, including formulary development and administration, development or improvement of methods of payment, or coverage policies; and

6. Business management and general administrative activities of the entity, including, but not limited to:

   i. Management activities relating to implementation of and compliance with the requirements of this subchapter;

   ii. Customer service, including the provision of data analyses for policy holders, plan sponsors, or other customers, provided that protected health information is not disclosed to such policy holder, plan sponsor, or customer.

   iii. Resolution of internal grievances;

   iv. The sale, transfer, merger, or consolidation of all or part of the covered entity with another covered entity, or an entity that following such activity will become a covered entity and due diligence related to such activity; and

   v. Consistent with the applicable requirements of Sec. 164.514, creating de-identified health information or a limited data set, and fundraising for the benefit of the covered entity.

**Health oversight agency:**   An agency or authority of the United States, a State, a territory, a political subdivision of a State or territory, or an Indian tribe, or a person or entity acting under a grant of authority from or contract with such public agency, including the employees or agents of such public agency or its contractors or persons or entities to whom it has granted authority, that is authorized by law to oversee the healthcare system (whether public or private) or government programs in which health information is necessary to determine eligibility or compliance, or to enforce civil rights laws for which health information is relevant.

**Indirect treatment relationship:**   A relationship between an individual and a healthcare provider in which:

1. The healthcare provider delivers healthcare to the individual based on the orders of another healthcare provider; and

2. The healthcare provider typically provides services or products, or reports the diagnosis or results associated with the healthcare, directly to another healthcare provider, who provides the services or products or reports to the individual.

**Individual:**   The person who is the subject of protected health information.

**Inmate:**   A person incarcerated in or otherwise confined to a correctional institution.

**Law enforcement official:**   An officer or employee of any agency or authority of the United States, a State, a territory, a political subdivision of a State or territory, or an Indian tribe, who is empowered by law to:

1. Investigate or conduct an official inquiry into a potential violation of law; or
2. Prosecute or otherwise conduct a criminal, civil, or administrative proceeding arising from an alleged violation of law.

**Marketing:**

1. To make a communication about a product or service that encourages recipients of the communication to purchase or use the product or service, unless the communication is made:
   i.   To describe a health-related product or service (or payment for such product or service) that is provided by, or included in a plan of benefits of, the covered entity making the communication, including communications about the entities participating in a healthcare provider network or health plan network; replacement of, or enhancements to, a health plan; and health-related products or services available only to a health plan enrollee that add value to, but are not part of, a plan of benefits.
   ii.  For treatment of the individual; or
   iii. For case management or care coordination for the individual, or to direct or recommend alternative treatments, therapies, healthcare providers, or settings of care to the individual.
2. An arrangement between a covered entity and any other entity whereby the covered entity discloses protected health information to the other entity, in exchange for direct or indirect remuneration, for the other entity or its affiliate to make a communication about its own product or service that encourages recipients of the communication to purchase or use that product or service.

**Organized healthcare arrangement:**

1. A clinically integrated care setting in which individuals typically receive healthcare from more than one healthcare provider;
2. An organized system of healthcare in which more than one covered entity participates, and in which the participating covered entities:
   i.  Hold themselves out to the public as participating in a joint arrangement; and
   ii. Participate in joint activities that include at least one of the following:
       A. Utilization review, in which healthcare decisions by participating covered entities are reviewed by other participating covered entities or by a third party on their behalf;

    B. Quality assessment and improvement activities, in which treatment provided by participating covered entities is assessed by other participating covered entities or by a third party on their behalf; or

    C. Payment activities, if the financial risk for delivering healthcare is shared, in part or in whole, by participating covered entities through the joint arrangement and if protected health information created or received by a covered entity is reviewed by other participating covered entities or by a third party on their behalf for the purpose of administering the sharing of financial risk.

3. A group health plan and a health insurance issuer or HMO with respect to such group health plan, but only with respect to protected health information created or received by such health insurance issuer or HMO that relates to individuals who are or who have been participants or beneficiaries in such group health plan;

4. A group health plan and one or more other group health plans each of which are maintained by the same plan sponsor; or

5. The group health plans described in paragraph (4) of this definition and health insurance issuers or HMOs with respect to such group health plans, but only with respect to protected health information created or received by such health insurance issuers or HMOs that relates to individuals who are or have been participants or beneficiaries in any of such group health plans.

**Payment:**

1. The activities undertaken by:

    i. A health plan to obtain premiums or to determine or fulfill its responsibility for coverage and provision of benefits under the health plan; or

    ii. A healthcare provider or health plan to obtain or provide reimbursement for the provision of healthcare; and

2. The activities in paragraph (1) of this definition relate to the individual to whom healthcare is provided and include, but are not limited to:

    i. Determinations of eligibility or coverage (including coordination of benefits or the determination of cost sharing amounts), and adjudication or subrogation of health benefit claims;

    ii. Risk adjusting amounts due based on enrollee health status and demographic characteristics;

    iii. Billing, claims management, collection activities, obtaining payment under a contract for reinsurance (including stop-loss insurance and excess of loss insurance), and related healthcare data processing;

    iv.  Review of healthcare services with respect to medical necessity, coverage under a health plan, appropriateness of care, or justification of charges;

    v.  Utilization review activities, including precertification and preauthorization of services, concurrent and retrospective review of services; and

    vi.  Disclosure to consumer reporting agencies of any of the following protected health information relating to collection of premiums or reimbursement:

        A.  Name and address;

        B.  Date of birth;

        C.  Social security number;

        D.  Payment history;

        E.  Account number; and

        F.  Name and address of the healthcare provider and health plan.

**Plan sponsor:**  As defined at section 3(16)(B) of ERISA, 29 U.S.C. 1002(16)(B).

**Protected health information:**  Individually identifiable health information:

1. Except as provided in paragraph (2) of this definition, that is:
   i. Transmitted by electronic media;
   ii. Maintained in any medium described in the definition of electronic media at § 162.103 of this subchapter; or
   iii. Transmitted or maintained in any other form or medium.
2. Protected health information excludes individually identifiable health information in:
   i. Education records covered by the Family Educational Right and Privacy Act, as amended, 20 U.S.C. 1232g; and
   ii. Records described at 20 U.S.C. 1232g(a)(4)(B)(iv); and
   iii. Employment records held by a covered entity in its role as employer.

**Psychotherapy notes:**  Notes recorded (in any medium) by a healthcare provider who is a mental health professional documenting or analyzing the contents of conversation during a private counseling session or a group, joint, or family counseling session and that are separated from the rest of the individual's medical record. Psychotherapy notes excludes medication prescription and monitoring, counseling session start and stop times, the modalities and frequencies of treatment furnished, results of clinical tests, and any summary of the following items: diagnosis, functional status, the treatment plan, symptoms, prognosis, and progress to date.

**Public health authority:**  An agency or authority of the United States, a State, a territory, a political subdivision of a State or territory, or an Indian tribe, or a person or entity acting under a grant of authority from or contract with such public agency, including the employees or agents of such public agency or its contractors or persons or entities to whom it has granted authority, that is responsible for public health matters as part of its official mandate.

**Required by law:**  A mandate contained in law that compels an entity to make a use or disclosure of protected health information and that is enforceable in a court of law. Required by law includes, but is not limited to, court orders and court-ordered warrants; subpoenas or summons issued by a court, grand jury, a governmental or tribal inspector general, or an administrative body authorized to require the production of information; a civil or an authorized investigative demand; Medicare conditions of participation with respect to healthcare providers participating in the program; and statutes or regulations that require the production of information, including statutes or regulations that require such information if payment is sought under a government program providing public benefits.

**Research:**  A systematic investigation, including research development, testing, and evaluation, designed to develop or contribute to generalizable knowledge.

**Treatment:**  The provision, coordination, or management of healthcare and related services by one or more healthcare providers, including the coordination or management of healthcare by a healthcare provider with a third party; consultation between healthcare providers relating to a patient; or the referral of a patient for healthcare from one healthcare provider to another.

**Use:**  With respect to individually identifiable health information, the sharing, employment, application, utilization, examination, or analysis of such information within an entity that maintains such information.

### § 164.504

**Common control:**  Exists if an entity has the power, directly or indirectly, significantly to influence or direct the actions or policies of another entity.

**Common ownership:**  Exists if an entity or entities possess an ownership or equity interest of 5 percent or more in another entity.

**Healthcare component:**  A component or combination of components of a hybrid entity designated by the hybrid entity in accordance with paragraph (c)(3)(iii) of this section.

**Hybrid entity:**  A single legal entity:

1. That is a covered entity;

2. Whose business activities include both covered and noncovered functions; and

3. That designates healthcare components in accordance with paragraph (c)(3)(iii) of this section.

**Plan administration functions:**   Administration functions performed by the plan sponsor of a group health plan on behalf of the group health plan and excluding functions performed by the plan sponsor in connection with any other benefit or benefit plan of the plan sponsor.

**Summary health information:**   Information that may be individually identifiable health information and:

1. That summarizes the claims history, claims expenses, or type of claims experienced by individuals for whom a plan sponsor has provided health benefits under a group health plan; and

2. From which the information described at § 164.514(b)(2)(i) has been deleted, except that the geographic information described in § 164.514(b)(2)(i)(B) need only be aggregated to the level of a five-digit zip code.

## § 142.304

**Access:**   Refers to the ability or the means necessary to read, write, modify, or communicate data/information or otherwise make use of any system resource.

**Access control:**   Refers to a method of restricting access to resources, allowing only privileged entities access. Types of access control include, among others, mandatory access control, discretionary access control, time-of-day, and classification.

**Authentication:**   Refers to the corroboration that an entity is the one claimed.

**Contingency plan:**   Refers to a plan for responding to a system emergency. The plan includes performing backups, preparing critical facilities that can be used to facilitate continuity of operations in the event of an emergency, and recovering from a disaster.

**Encryption (or encipherment):**   Refers to transforming confidential plaintext into ciphertext to protect it. An encryption algorithm combines plaintext with other values called keys, or ciphers, so the data becomes unintelligible. Once encrypted, data can be stored or transmitted over unsecured lines. Decrypting data reverses the encryption algorithm process and makes the plaintext available for further processing.

**Password:**   Refers to confidential authentication information composed of a string of characters.

**Role-based access control (RBAC):** An alternative to traditional access control models (e.g., discretionary or nondiscretionary access control policies) that permits the specification and enforcement of enterprise-specific security policies in a way that maps more naturally to an organization's structure and business activities. With RBAC, rather than attempting to map an organization's security policy to a relatively low-level set of technical controls (typically, access control lists), each user is assigned to one or more predefined roles, each of which has been assigned the various privileges needed to perform that role.

**Token:** Refers to a physical item necessary for user identification when used in the context of authentication. For example, an electronic device that can be inserted in a door or a computer system to obtain access.

**User-based access:** Refers to a security mechanism used to grant users of a system access based upon the identity of the user.

# About the Authors

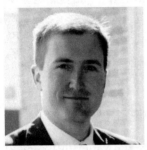

As founder and principal consultant of Principle Logic, LLC, Kevin Beaver has over 15 years of experience in IT and specializes in information security. Before starting his own information security services business, Kevin served in various information technology and security roles for several healthcare, e-commerce, financial, and educational institutions. In his most recent position, he was the Information Security Manager responsible for securing the information assets of a $50B global B2B marketplace for the tire and rubber industry. His areas of information security expertise include network and messaging security, security assessments, and incident response.

Kevin is author of the upcoming book *Ethical Hacking for Dummies*, Wiley Publishing. He is also author of the new book *The Definitive Guide to Email Management and Security* by Realtimepublishers.com, and is a contributing author and editor of the book, *Healthcare Information Systems, Second Edition,* Auerbach Publications. In addition, he is technical editor of the book *Network Security for Dummies*, Wiley Publishing.

Kevin is a regular columnist and information security and HIPAA expert advisor for SearchSecurity.com and SearchMobileComputing.com. Kevin also serves as an advisory board member and contributing author for "HCPro's Briefings on HIPAA" newsletter and is a Security Clinic Expert for ITsecurity.com. In addition, his information security work has been published on SecurityFocus.com, Computerworld.com, as well as in the *HIMSS Journal of Healthcare Information Management* and *ADVANCE for Health Information Executives.* He is an information security instructor for the Southeast Cybercrime Institute and frequently speaks on information security at various workshops and conferences around the United States.

Kevin is the founder and president of the Technology Association of Georgia's Information Security Society and serves as secretary of InfraGard Atlanta. In addition, he is an active member in the SHARP Workgroup and serves as an IT advisory board member for several universities and corporations around the southeast. Kevin earned his bachelor's degree in Computer Engineering Technology from Southern Polytechnic State University and master's degree in Management of Technology from Georgia Tech. He also holds CISSP, MCSE, Master CNE, and IT Project+ certifications.

Kevin can be reached at kbeaver@principlelogic.com.

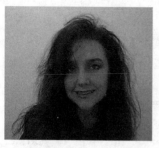

Rebecca Herold is Vice President, Privacy Services and Chief Privacy Officer at DelCreo, Inc. and has provided security and privacy services to organizations from a wide range of industries. Rebecca was the editor and a contributing author for *The Privacy Papers,* an executive-level book about privacy that was released in December 2001. Rebecca has also authored chapters for several books, including:

- *Law, Investigations and Ethics Domain: The Total CISSP Exam Prep Book,* Auerbach Publishers, July 2002
- *Information Protection: Organization, Roles and Separation of Duties; Information Security Management Handbook,* 4th Edition, Volume IV, Auerbach Publishers, Dec. 2002
- *HIPAA Privacy in the Healthcare Industry; Healthcare Information Systems Handbook,* Auerbach Publishers, Dec. 2002

Rebecca authored and developed all the content for the NetIQ HIPAA and 21 CFR Part 11 VPC software modules, and also authored and developed the PrivaPlan HIPAA privacy and security rule risk assessment PrivaGuide. Rebecca also created and delivers a HIPAA Privacy and Security Workshop. Additionally, Rebecca authors a monthly privacy column in the CSI Alert newsletter. Rebecca has written numerous articles for magazines and newsletters on information security and privacy topics, and is a frequent presenter on a wide range of security and privacy topics at conferences and seminars.

During her years as a consultant, Rebecca has led a large number of projects for Fortune 500 organizations, private organizations, and government agencies. Prior to consulting, Rebecca was instrumental in developing the corporate information protection department at Principal Financial Group (PFG), where she worked for 12 years. Prior to working for PFG, Rebecca taught secondary school math and computer education in Missouri. She has a B.S. in Math and Computer Science and an M.A. in Computer Science and Education. Rebecca is a Certified Information Systems Security Professional (CISSP), a Certified Information Systems Auditor (CISA), and a Fellow of the Life Management Institute (FLMI). Rebecca has been a member of the Information Systems Audit and Control Association (ISACA) since 1990 and has held all board positions throughout her membership in the Iowa chapter. Rebecca is a charter member of the Iowa InfraGard chapter that was formed in 2000, and a member of the International Association of Privacy Practitioners (IAPP).

Rebecca can be reached at rebeccaherold@rebeccaherold.com, rebecca@delcreo.com, or 515.491.1564.

# Index

# Index

# Index

ARO (annual rate of occurrence), 182
Attorneys, 253
Audio instruction, 323
Audit controls, *190*, 204
Audit trail, 423
Auditors, 253
Authentication, *190*
  controls, 267
  definition of, 423, 443
  in technical safeguard requirements
    (Security Rule), *175*, 204
Authorizations, 91
  definition of, 423
  healthcare providers, 218–219
  mandatory contents of, 135
  in organizational privacy policies, *115*
  for uses and disclosures, 53–55
Automatic log-off
  in applications and data bases, 269
  in operating systems, 277
  in technical safeguard requirements
    (Security Rule), *174–175*, 204
Availability of data, 160
Awareness programs, 319–320
  awareness and training groups, 321
  documenting, 328
  getting support for, 328–329
  measuring effectiveness of, 329–330
  options in, 326–328
  practical checklist, 331
  in privacy policies, 376
  training, 321–323
  training design and development,
    324–326

## B

Background checks, 377
Backup generators, *170, 174*
Banking laws, 229
Banks, 253
Baylor University Medical, 24
Billing and printing services, 253
Biometric identifiers, 68, 249
Biometrics, *172*, 268
Birth dates, 68
Brochures, *169*, 327
Bulk eraser, *173*
Business associate contracts, 41
  compliance in, 147
  in contingency plans, 202

definition of, *171*
  mandatory documentation of, 146
  safeguard standards, *38*
  sample document, 365–373
Business associates, 11, 69
  compliance deadlines, *255*
  and covered entities (CEs), 255–257
  definition of, 253–254, 427–428
  of healthcare providers, 217–218
  inventory of, *195*
  limited data set, 59–60
  in organizational privacy policies, *115*
  practical checklist, 257
  in privacy policies, 375
  requirements, 254–255
  security and privacy practices of, 89

## C

California, *122*
Case laws, 117
Case studies, 345–359
  metropolitan area healthcare system,
    348–351
  multi-state health insurance plan, 354–359
  small physician's office, 351–354
CD-ROMs, *170, 174*, 270
CERT (Computer Emergency Response
    Team), *293*
Certificate numbers, 249
Certification, 423
Change management, 17–20
Chief Information Officer (CIO), *293*
Chief Privacy Officer (CPO), 87, 362–364
CHS (Certified in Healthcare Security), 308
CIA (confidentiality, integrity, and
    availability), 423
CISA® (Certified Information Systems
    Auditor), 307
CISM (Certified Information Security
    Manager), 308
CISSP® (Certified Information Systems
    Security Professional), 307, 423
Civil penalties, 12–13
Classroom training, 323
Code sets, 13–14
  in Administrative Simplification, 5
  definition of, 425, 433
  maintaining organizations, 426
Cold sites, 300
Collection agencies, 253